The Golden Treasury of Natural Health Knowledge

JOHN H. TOBE

LC: 73-83219
ISBN: 0-8397-3015-2

Provoker Press
St. Catharines, Ontario

Paul S. Eriksson
New York
Printed In Canada

TABLE OF CONTENTS

CHAPTER

1

MY PHILOSOPHY

It's often good to get things off your chest or you might say, to bare one's soul. I am not a crusader, I am not a fighter, I am not a do-gooder and I have no desire or intent to lay down my life for my fellow man. I am best described as a crap-disturber. There may be kinder terms for this kind of an individual but this is the bluntest and probably the most direct. If you sought to be kind to me you might say I was an iconoclast.

It so happens that by nature I am simple, frank and candid. I do not seek fame or renown. I don't even seek wealth. I don't buy sweepstake tickets because I'm afraid I might win and I wouldn't know what to do with the damnable money.

You think I'm kidding, but friend, you never made a bigger mistake in your life . . . I'm serious. All that a million dollars could

1

do for me would be to bring me trouble. I have a family and if I were to suddenly strike it rich, then I would have to give them a large share of it and that would destroy their instincts, their ambitions and becloud their horizons. I don't want to do that to my family. I want them to struggle a bit and I want them to reach the top by their own efforts. While occasionally there are people who can handle money and do not allow it to go to their heads, in most cases money — especially quick money — does much more harm than good. Therefore, I don't want to be rich.

Oh, I wouldn't mind owning a couple of hundred thousand dollars which would give me a good income and permit me to travel and write and do the things I want to do. When I say I don't want to be famous or renowned, I mean that from the bottom of my heart, because from what I have seen and learned most people who gain fame and renown also gain a lot of troubles. Their lives are no longer their own and I don't want that to happen to me. I want to live my own life in my own way and I don't want reporters or newsmen or other nosy people continually barging into my private affairs.

Yes, I've done a fair share of television appearances, radio broadcasts and lecturing but its work that I don't particularly enjoy and I do it only because I think perhaps some people can be helped by that appearance. But I would prefer not to do any of them.

I used to do a fair amount of public speaking but I practically refuse to accept appointments and I only do so under pressure or in certain circumstances . . . because I don't feel I can do enough good by making speeches. I claim I am not an entertainer and at speeches most people want to be entertained with funny stories interjected into the speech. I say if you want entertainment . . . go hire Georgie Jessel.

It is my belief that I do my best work by means of my writing and I want to disseminate it as far and as wide as possible. That, ladies and gentlemen, is the full and complete extent of my ambitions.

Through the years I have been laughed at and ridiculed, I have been debased and insulted, and although I usually can defend myself quite capably, I still don't like to become involved in these encounters. It leaves me with an indescribable pain in my heart and I'd rather not be subjected to it. Therefore, I prefer to stick to my writings.

However, I do feel that I owe a duty to my fellow man. Let me cite the case of one of my brothers whom I saw dying ten years before he died. One day he resented my pointing out the wrong things that he was doing to himself and he turned on me and gave me a vigorous tongue-lashing. When he was finished, I said to him, "You are blind or you refuse to see. I am not blind and I see you walking towards certain disaster. You are my brother . . . what am I supposed to do? Stand by and watch you destroy yourself when I have a voice and the knowledge that can save your life?"

He didn't have very much to say after that and I didn't have too much to say, either.

They told him he was a healthy man . . . at least, his doctors told him that . . . but he died about three or four years later of cancer combined with tuberculosis and probably a dozen other things.

Now I knew exactly where he was heading. And the same thing applies to many of my friends and acquaintances and generally speaking, my fellow man. I see where some of them are heading and I feel it my duty to warn them or at least try to tell them. When they don't follow after I tell them well, I have no more responsibility. I have fulfilled my duties.

I have an employee — a woman — who has been with me now for 27 years. She is a dedicated, loyal employee and a woman with a high character, good intelligence, attractive and personable . . . a woman whom I admire and respect as much as any woman I have ever known. Well, she smokes and for at least 17 or 18 of these 27 years I have tried to get her to give up smoking. I get somewhere but

3

I don't get far enough. In any event, as of today she still hasn't given up smoking.

Because of the continued mentioning of her bad habit, I sort of felt that I was getting on her nerves or perhaps doing her a disservice so I stopped mentioning anything about smoking and said little to her about it for perhaps two years. Then one day I came to her and I said to her, "Pearl, I've had a nasty dream and I want to tell you about it. I dreamt you called me from the hospital and told me that you had cancer of the lungs. I went to visit you and at this visit I said to you, 'I am responsible for your condition!' Then you said, 'Oh, that's nonsense. You know you're not!' But I insisted and said, 'Oh, yes, I am!' In this dream I told you I was responsible and I explained it this way, 'When I quit badgering you about smoking, I let you down. Had I tried harder, had I insisted or had I even compelled you by threat of dismissal, I could have saved your life. Now you have contracted lung cancer and I feel that I am to blame.' "

Well, even that story didn't work. However, I'm still trying. By the same token I am still trying to help my friends. I feel that it is a cardinal sin to remain silent where one can be of help. I feel that you fail your duty as a decent human being if you do not fulfill your purpose. It is my belief that for a man to remain silent in the presence of outrage and criminal action or genocide is to degrade the reason for living and human dignity.

I admit that it is hard to be present and see before me the tragedy of my brothers, my sisters, my kinfolk and fellow man being slowly but most assuredly done to death. However, it would be much harder for me to stand idly by and watch these goings-on and do nothing about it with my voice or my pen. And I guess that is the way it will ever be. I don't think I'll win but I'll go down trying . . . with my pen poised!

Frequently I'm asked about my status, "Are you a vegetarian? Are you a raw fooder? Are you a vegan? Are you a lacto-ovo vegetarian? Are you a hygienist? Are you a naturopath? Are you a fruitarian?

In truth I am none of these and yet some of all of them. My philosophy about eating is somewhat similar to that of the Chinese. I'll eat anything that is fit to eat. If it grows, if it walks, if it runs, if it flies, if it moves, if it lives on the earth, below the earth or above the earth I will eat it.

I have for years believed in the hygienic way of life, but I cannot stomach a philosophy that is narrow and bigoted so I had to break away from the fold. They believe in distilled water, they don't eat anything that is fermented. They will not eat any vegetable that is pungent, like pepper, radish, onion, garlic, leek, chives and many others. They will not use honey, they will not use seeds and grains and they will eat only the good tasting fruits and vegetables. They believe in food combinations. For example, if they eat melons they will eat nothing with them. They say eat them alone or leave them alone. I have repeatedly asked for the basis, the proof, the scientific research that would establish their rhyme and their reason but little or none is forthcoming.

I've investigated the macrobiotic philosophy and I find it borders on the ridiculous. Still it gives good results frequently but this is easy to explain. After the horrors in the conventional diet — tea, coffee, French fries, hamburgers, cakes, cookies and other bakery horrors and Coca Cola, Pepsi Cola and other soft drinks, or beer and alcohol — the change to the macrobiotic way is indeed like coming out into the open air after being stifled in a cellar.

There is no hesitation on my part in stating that the best and finest way of life is that of the strict vegetarian but with one proviso . . . that all vegetables be uncooked and no resorting to any processed or contemptible foods just because they are meatless. That is the big mistake that vegetarians make. They flee from anything that contains animal matter and in their mad rush to get away from it they eat some of the most contemptible processed foods in the world and the British vegetarians are the worst offenders and the sickliest. This is not a knock at the British or British vegetarianism. It

5

is just taking them to task for the food horrors they perpetrate. I'm a firm believer in the raw food system of eating. If you must eat meat, if you must eat fish, if you must drink milk and use dairy products then make sure they are not heated, not treated and not pasteurized then at least you'll be getting the food value contained in the food.

My own diet consists of 100% raw food for all but one meal a day. Whether I eat two meals, three meals or four meals a day only one can consist of some cooked food.

I try to allow 10 to 12 hours to go by every day without eating. That is, from my last meal in the evening until morning . . . 10 to 12 hours fasting every day. I find it suits me and my way of life. This pattern sometimes changes when I have visitors. So I don't know what you would class me as but whatever I am that is what I am.

Under no circumstances should you take tobacco, alcohol, drugs, narcotics, tea or coffee. I also recognize that gluttony is one of man's greatest crimes and one of the most difficult to control. I oppose the use of drugs, medicine, inoculations, vaccines, X-rays, blood transfusions or hypnotism. Vitamin pills and food supplements are not part of my life and do not belong in anyone's life unless they won't or can't eat proper food. However I do grant that they are far better to use than drugs or medicines.

For beverages I use a herb tea, or a cup of hot water with a dash of milk. I rarely eat out and never knowingly eat any food that contains a chemical additive.

CHAPTER

2

HEALTH TODAY IS NO ACCIDENT

Health is generally regarded as something to which every human being is entitled at birth. Basically I am confident that nature intended that every creature born should possess this gift that we know as health.

Health to one person may be something entirely different to what it means to another person.

I recall quite vividly in my youth that everybody was considered healthy unless he was confined to a hospital. Only then it was felt that he was not healthy. But years of experience have taught me that there are varying degrees of health . . . all dependent upon what each individual regards as being health.

I meet people practically every day of my life who consider

themselves healthy. Yet I know they look ghastly ... with sallow skins, poor posture, lack-lustre eyes, coughing and wheezing, with a step that denotes the onslaught of premature age and physical insecurity. Yet they tell me they're healthy. I don't know whether they are trying to kid me or themselves.

Some smoke two packs of cigarettes a day, smell like walking out-houses, with a breath that would make a skunk shy away, yet they say they're healthy. If you think I'm exaggerating, look around about you and see how many people fill this bill.

Most people only recognize sickness or lack of health when they are struck down by a serious disease. Things like a little headache or a cough or a cold or a wheeze or stiffening muscles or pains in the back and shoulders and the legs or griping pains in the stomach, indigestion or poor vision and poor hearing ... these are not regarded as signs of sickness. They just think it is the inevitable — old age — and when you hear people of 40 or 50 saying this, then do you wonder that I wonder?

So as you can see, health means many different things to many different people. While we all regard health as being our inherent right (and it is) yet upon examination it is much more complex than that. By and large, you have a right to expect that your parents give you a good start in life and give you a healthy body and a sound mind. But health doesn't just come by a snap of the fingers ... even if you were born healthy, you must do something to retain or maintain that health.

To begin with, let us postulate. Health is the absence of disease and there is no need to say good health, perfect health or excellent health ... health means the absence of disease and therefore you are in the pink.

Good health, basically, is seldom an accident. Today, most positive, good health is never an accident ... especially if you can claim good health after you are 40, 50 or 60 years of age or better.

For 50 years I made it a practice, whenever I saw an old person, who appeared to be in good health, to ask him what his or her secret or formula for health was. And believe it or not, through the years I have gathered sufficient knowledge from these oldsters to guide me and lead me to the secret that Ponce de Leon sought for all his life ... the secret of perpetual youth. And that, dear friends, is health! No, I didn't get all the answers but I found many of them and then I traipsed around the world even to remote places to get more answers.

It is my profound belief that no man or woman ever reaches the age of 50 to 70 and beyond in good health without having earned it. It is agreed that people reach the age of 60, 70 and 80 in comparatively good health and yet they have violated consistently all of the rules of health ... but please believe me, these are the rare, rare exception and never the rule.

By the same token I have seen men fall 50 feet and land unhurt or with only a few minor bruises. But you know and I know that the chances of anyone falling 50 feet and remaining unhurt are as rare as hen's teeth. And by that token, so is the individual who reaches a ripe old age and has violated all the laws of nature.

Even when I was a young man and did not know about or follow the principles that I know and follow today concerning good health, I was still alerted to the fact that these so-called health nuts, vegetarians or kooks had some of the answers. Strange as it sounds these health kooks didn't drink coffee, didn't smoke, didn't touch liquor, didn't eat meat and did those crazy exercises ... but I did recognize that these so-called peculiar people did appear healthy, did have more stamina, did have more vim, vigor and vitality, yes, and did live longer than the conventional individual. In those days this sort of puzzled me but I still recognized it as being a positive fact. I didn't then know why it should be so, because I felt that by living conventionally I was doing the right thing. Wasn't that what most people were doing? Therefore, it must be right! After all, I was eating and doing things according to what I was taught in school and through the various government agencies.

At that time I had tremendous faith in my government, in government officials, my doctor, the hospitals and all of these organizations. I felt that they were looking after me and guarding me at all times . . . looking after my welfare and seeing to it that I would be healthy and live to a ripe old age.

Boy, oh, boy, let me tell you this . . . that was the biggest blunder I ever made in my life. And if you follow those precepts, let me tell you, fella, it will be the biggest blunder you ever make in your life, too. Yes, and you'll pay for it with your health and life.

There is no doubt about it, if you care, if you try, if you want to be healthy and live long, you will do something about it. And the chances are you will attain the goal that you set for yourself, providing you don't wait until the eleventh hour and fifty-nine seconds before you take action.

Without argument I will also agree that I have known some individuals who waited till the eleventh hour and well on to the last few seconds before they started and they still cheated the angel of death by a few years or more.

Obviously this is some kind of a philosophy because I've met quite a few people in my life who have said to me, "I'll quit smoking when I get lung cancer," or "I'll quit eating all those refined carbohydrates and all the foods that I like when I get diabetes," or "I'm not worried, my doctor will fix me up!"

Well, even in these instances I've seen many of them make the changes and still get many more years of life out of the deal.

The answer to all these strange, fanciful and unusual happenings is that the human body is a tremendous force . . . a force that cannot be comprehended or is incalculable to even the greatest minds who ever lived.

I have seen and known people who were terminal cancer cases and in spite of the fact that they did nothing to help themselves but just kept on violating all the rules and laws, yet they got remissions and lived quite a few years after the chips were down.

Don't ask me how or why it happens but it does happen. But again these are the rare, rare exceptions and I suggest you don't count on them.

I would strongly urge you to do something about it and the wonderful, the glorious and the beautiful thing about doing something about it is the fact that it practically always works . . . there is seldom a failure. I can say to you in all sincerity and without stretching the truth even one degree that seldom have I seen a failure when an individual seeks to embark upon the venture of following nature's practices and principles, no matter how sick he is.

Give nature and your body a chance and they'll respond to a degree that will utterly amaze you just as it has and still continues to amaze me.

Please believe me, and follow this last statement that I will make in this chapter and that is that I feel in my heart and in my soul and with all of the intelligence or intellect that I may or may not possess that 95% of the ills and the ailments that afflict mankind could be stopped, could be driven back, and health earned, if only people would follow a course of proper eating and living . . . which means a balanced diet composed of raw vegetables, grains and fruits, with wholesome uncontaminated drinking water, good air and a sanitary, sensible mode of life.

CHAPTER

3

A MOMENT OF DECISION

The time is either at hand or fast approaching where we as human beings must make a decision ... an important, a vital, earth-shattering decision. We must choose between man and nature or if you prefer, man and God. This actually came about in my mind when I received a letter from a dear friend with whom I have been corresponding for many years. She lives in Utah. She is one of those who think along natural lines like myself but her father does not go along with that idea. He believes in science and in chemistry and in technology.

So one day she said to her father, "Dad, do you believe that man is greater than God?" Here I'll tell it as she described it.

"He looked at me with an expression that said, 'Don't be ridiculous'. But before he could speak I went on, 'Now please listen a minute. I know that you believe in God and that you believe that he created man. Well, if God created us then he knows everything about us. Man has learned a lot about the human body but it is only a drop in the ocean to what God knows. Because God created our bodies he knows absolutely everything about them. Exactly how they work and the type of fuel they need in order to perform with precision. So after he created our bodies he created fruits, vegetables, nuts, grains and seeds to feed our bodies properly. Then here comes puny man and he is so puffed up with his scant knowledge that he thinks he can improve upon what God has made. He takes this perfect food and he cooks it, adds to it, takes away from it, pulverizes it, pasteurizes it, processes it, sprays it and a dozen or so other things and then this nervy man has the audacity to tell you that he has made it better than it was originally, that he has improved upon God's creation! Therefore the question — Is man greater than God?' My Dad was silent for a few seconds and then he said thoughtfully, "Ya know Margaret, I believe you've got a point there."

Actually my young friend has said it as succinctly as possible and the situation is covered but now we have to sort of delve into it. First we must decide whether natural foods are better than processed foods; whether natural healing is better than trying to heal with drugs; whether food should be as nature made it or processed and cooked; whether we lead a synthetic existence or whether we go back to nature.

When I presented my case to a very close friend of mine and asked him to challenge me so that I might defend nature he said, "After all, in many ways man has done better than nature. For example, he took a cow that gave a couple of quarts of milk a day and turned it into a milking machine that gives 20 quarts of milk a day. Can you deny that this is a genuine achievement on the part of man and a triumph of man over nature?"

It so happened that I had argued this point before and was quite prepared. There is no argument whatsoever that man has made "Bossy" produce many, many times more than she did in the good old days when she was on her own. First of all, it has not been

14

proven that milk is proper food for man. Then no one can deny that we have shortened the lifespan of the cow. We must have a veterinarian handy to look after the cow because of her tremendous milk giving capacity and because she gives milk for such a long period of the year her body breaks down and she gets sick frequently. Therefore the milk cannot be up to standard . . . we get more milk but it is milk from a sick cow. I am fully acquainted with the process of running a dairy farm. I visit one or another more than once a week.

I am not denying that man is capable, very capable. His mental potential is much greater than even the most informed of us believe and know but I still do not think that man is greater than nature or God. Now with all of man's knowledge it is clear as clear can be that the lifespan of man on earth has been drastically shortened . . . not increased as some people and certain statistics or statisticians would make us believe. I'm not calling everybody a liar but I have carefully investigated statistics and my interpretation of these statistics clearly indicates that man has definitely not increased his lifespan but man can manipulate statistics to make it appear as though he has. However, that argument is covered elsewhere in this book, so back to my point.

We must make a decision . . . either we follow man or we follow nature. Which is it going to be? If we follow man, in my opinion we are not only courting disaster but we may end life on this planet once and for all or at least for hundreds or maybe thousands of years. We are now near the brink and some scientists even claim that disaster cannot be averted. I have followed mankind's progress as far as literature or history can lead me and frankly I don't think we are getting anywhere.

Let's trace our civilizations. Let's go back as far as we can. Can't you see that it has been one disaster after another or would you call it one triumph after another? Civilizations, which constitute progress, come and go every few hundred years. What was once great is buried and something else springs up instead. Or are we running true to nature like an annual flower that sprouts, grows and thrives,

15

blossoms and sets seed and then dies . . . only to be resurrected another year? A plant does not have the ability to reason, at least so we think, as yet. A man can reason and perhaps because of this his span or cycle lasts more than a year but it's unlike an animal, a perennial or a bi-annual that has a fixed or an established life cycle. With man it appears that his life cycle or the cycle of civilization depends entirely upon how man has learned to handle the situation during that specific civilization.

Granted, in this book we are not concerned with the future of civilization — we are concerned with man's health at this time and it is precisely because man has interferred so boisterously, so unscrupulously, that he is causing havoc with the health of humanity, especially in the western world. His interference through scientific or so-called scientific endeavour is creating a situation never before encountered in the history of mankind. Then too, is mankind to blame when but a mere handful are the cause and the perpetrators of the outrages and problems? Now economics becomes involved, followed by wealth and then things really become complicated. At the present moment man doesn't know where to turn and more and more people are beginning to realize that we are reaching or have reached the end of our tether. I still believe there is a way out — a sane way, a safe way but I know man won't listen. Things are too good. Those signs of decay, those cracks that appear are noticed by the scant few. What can they do?

So there we have it. We have to choose between man and nature and I am afraid that man will choose to follow man. That, in my opinion, means certain disaster.

CHAPTER

4

YOUR HEALTH YOUR RESPONSIBILITY

I refuse to accept the thesis that health, be it that of the individual or the nation, is dependent upon doctors or healing institutions or any government department or authority. The idea that the world needs medicare, hospitals, drugs and various other therapeutic measures, including all of the fields of healing, such as, osteopathy, homeopathy, naturopathy, chiropractic, etc., is nothing but sheer ignorance or mesmerism. To suggest that a man is incapable of protecting his own health is an insult to any decent man and his creator. Any animal, even of the lowest order, knows how to stay healthy . . . except mighty man . . . he needs a whole healing arsenal.

No, I am not thinking or dreaming of a Utopian state where everything is perfect and everyone follows a set of rules and behaves according to a pattern or an ideology. I am thinking only in terms of common sense, humanity, civilization and realism.

17

The first principle that should be taught to a child, even before he learns what to call his mother and his father, is the simple truism that his health and his very life depend entirely upon himself . . . and therefore it is entirely in his own hands. The idea that a child must depend upon a mother or anyone else is dead wrong. Agreed, from birth and during the period of infancy and the tender ages a child has to depend upon a mother or a guardian for sustenance and guidance. So when the first sign of intelligence appears, or the ability of the child to think for himself, we must implant quickly in his mind that his health and his very being depend upon his own actions.

It was indeed a sad day for man when he was led to believe or taught to accept the theory that he must rely upon a healer or a medicine man of some field of healing. I feel that man erroneously believes that someone else can do a better job than he can do in most fields of endeavour. We go to an artist if we want a painting, we go to an architect if we want a design for a house, we go to a play-wright if we want a play, we go to a miller if we want wheat milled, we go to a carpenter if we want a carpenter's job done, we go to a plumber if we want a plumber's job done, and so on down the line. This is mainly due to the age of specialization.

It was but a few short years ago that a friend of mine set out to build a house. All he could manage to do was raise sufficient money to purchase the lot and lay the foundation and then he got a mortgage. Then he set about building the house with his own two hands. Now I'm talking about building a house in a town in this day and age. Yes, he succeeded in building the house. He did his own cement pouring, he did his own roughing in, he did his own carpenter work, he did his own electrical work, he did his own plumbing work and then he did his own painting. The house stands today and it is worth seeing, the work of one man. It is much better than most houses, at much, much higher prices, and it is as attractive as any house on the street.

Perhaps every man is not so gifted but this man was a plain ordinary Joe who had the desire to build his house, the willingness and the temerity, and I do not know of one single quality that he possessed over any other man I've known except he was willing to try and to work. Yet this selfsame individual became a sick man and is now much sicker because he relied upon his doctor to keep him well.

Frankly, I don't think that a man should depend on anyone else to do his job for him . . . even though he can afford to pay to have it done. The excuse that we are too busy with our own occupation permits us to have others do the job for us. Well, that's too much like sound unionism, where no man dares to even touch the work of another man.

Strange, but throughout my lifetime — even in my early youth — I always felt that I could do as good a job at anything as any other man. This came about because I always watched, wherever I could, other men doing their job . . . brick layers, electricians, carpenters, automobile mechanics, machinists . . . and I saw at once that there was no special skill or magic or special know-how involved but it was intelligence and a wee bit of practice. I think these are faculties that one could easily acquire.

No, I am not suggesting that every man become a jack-of-all-trades but I am encouraging the idea of self-reliance. I know people who would call a doctor if they pricked themselves with a pin. I'm not exaggerating . . . this is true! Not too long ago one of my closest employees got a couple of fingers and part of her hand stuck in a machine. Her thumb was squeezed until it was almost as flat as a pancake. I rushed to the scene, upon being notified, and helped her to extract her hand. It was bleeding and a horrible sight. Everybody said we should rush her to the hospital so I said to her, "What do you want to do?"

She asked, "What do you suggest I do?"

I said, "First go over there and wash your hand and then let's take a look at it."

19

She was in agony but she did wash her hand and I said, "I don't see any obvious serious damage, lacerations or macerations. If I take you to a hospital or to a doctor, they'll fill you full of shots, then they'll x-ray you and then they'll probably cut in to see what has been done inside . . . and who knows what else. You'll be laid up for a couple of weeks and probably be sick from the shots, the x-rays, the exploratory affairs and treatments and who knows what will happen? I suggest that you gradually move your fingers and gradually massage all around them, take a little rest and play it by ear from there. If complications arise, then you can decide what to do."

Today she doesn't have a single sign or blemish or mark indicating where the damage was done. Had she gone to a doctor or a hospital, need I tell you what would have happened? I could cite dozens of cases that would illustrate the way the specialists would have handled it . . . and the bigger the specialist the greater would have been the problems, the troubles and the tribulations . . . and as a joke, I would say she would probably have had her fingers amputated and probably her wrist and maybe the elbow or the whole arm due to fear of lockjaw or gangrene setting in.

O.K., laugh and suggest that I am exaggerating and that I am off beam. But you laugh . . . I won't!

Of course, a casual employee would have liked the idea of going to a doctor because no doubt he would have told her to stay home for at least six weeks and probably two months. Again you think I'm exaggerating. But before you say I'm exaggerating, smile . . . because I have been an employer for 45 years and a good number of employees have passed through my hands in that time and I tell you I am not exaggerating.

On rare occasions I have visited doctors. When I was twenty-two I organized a group of young men into a lodge and part and parcel of the deal was that they had to have a physical examination by a doctor. So I wheeled well over a hundred individual boys and young men to the doctor for an examination and I was there every single time one was examined. I saw the examination, I heard the questions asked and I was also there when they had problems. I saw each one of the more than one hundred young men in their nakedness and imperfections. I heard the discussions and the questions asked and the answers given. My opinion then, and it has been cemented now, was that the doctor only knew what his patients told him. That taught me a very positive lesson.

When I have a slight problem that I think requires medical attention I sit down and say to myself, "Now what is the doctor going to ask me? And what am I going to tell him?" So I play doctor and patient with myself. Realizing that the doctor relies upon my answers for his decision and actions, I do the job myself and it has worked so well for me for 45 years that I think I can handle my own problems much better than any doctor could handle them for me and I want you to know that I know many capable, splendid physicians and surgeons.

I do admit that if I were in an accident or even ran into a dental problem or such a thing as a prostate problem, I would have to consult with someone acquainted with such things ... but only because the civilized way of life has led me into this trap. When I tell my friends that I wouldn't be a bit afraid to live on a desert island or in a remote area near the equator or the Arctic Circle, they say, "How would you get along without a doctor?"

I would reply, "More important, how is the doctor going to get along without me?"

They might say, "You might get appendicitis or a gall bladder attack!"

My reply is, "I know enough about how to live to prevent such conditions from arising."

Right here if you're astute, dear reader, you might say to me, "Well, how about that prostate condition you mentioned ... why can't you avoid it?"

21

I would not seek to stall or pass the buck and I would say, "All of my studies have left a blank when it comes to a solution for a prostate condition. I do not know the answer. I think I do but I'm not positive."

As far as diabetes, heart disease, arthritis, kidney infections, kidney stones and asthma are concerned, I am not the least bit worried, because through the years I have learned that a proper pattern of living and diet can make those conditions obsolete. I think the same applies to the prostate but once the damage is done to the prostate gland it does not always respond to natural methods of treatment.

If we were taught that our lives are in our own hands, our whole approach to health and living would be different. For instance, no man would ever light a cigarette because he would know that it was going to do him various degrees of damage and he would be bringing grief and disease upon his own head and body. The same would apply to drinking alcoholic beverages.

Yes, of course I recognize that drinking various forms of these beverages can be pleasant for it allows people to forget their worries, it breaks down barriers, it makes people do things they normally wouldn't do and it makes them talkative, friendly and sociable and also darned unsociable, too. I'm well acquainted with all that part of the deal. But at this time we're talking about benefits and advantages to the human body. And alcohol in any form performs no service or benefit to the human body, even if you do enjoy it.

By the same line of reasoning you could not drink coffee, because it definitely causes harm. Any burnt substance is a carcinogen and coffee is positively a burnt substance.

You would quickly learn that you must only take into your body such substances as will benefit your body or at least not do it any harm. This would, of course, mean that you would have to read the labels of any purchased or processed food that you might eat. And the moment you saw chemicals that are not foods you'd have to pass it by. In fact, this would eliminate most processed foods.

If you would be your own guardian of health, you would not permit recognized, known and established harmful agents to enter your body. But as long as you feel that a doctor is responsible for your health, because you have life insurance, health insurance, drug insurance or other medical or such participation, you say to yourself, "Who in heck cares? I can do all these things and let the doctor worry about it! He's got to fix me up. I'm covered".

Now you may think that this attitude is a bit ridiculous yet it is the precise attitude of the largest segment of our population. I wouldn't want to say 90% but I think I'd be closer to right if I did say 90%. Some people have the ridiculous idea that it's the doctor's business to keep people healthy. But, my dear folks, I want to assure you that this is not the doctor's business or his aim in life. He studies medicine with the avowed intention of learning a profession that will provide him and his wife and family with sustenance in comfort and in luxury for ever and ever.

Then he has many other ambitions and considerations . . . probably to be the highest earner of his group, to be the most skillful in his profession and to achieve prominence in his profession. And somewhere down the line it was written or prescribed or avowed that he would help the sick. But from what I have learned from doctors, they are more apt to think, "Why these stupid dolts, if they haven't got any more sense than to eat the things they do, to drink the things they do, to smoke the things they do and put these things into their system as they do, hell's bells, they don't deserve any consideration!"

My statement of this attitude on the part of the doctors is not an insult to the medical profession . . . it is precisely what the people who do these things deserve. Relatives, dearly loved ones, friends and associates have been dying all around me for years — men whom I loved, men whom I liked and men whom I respected — and of most of them I say, "He didn't deserve to live longer. He was asking for it and he got it. He would do nothing to help himself. He violated every biological principle. He flaunted nature, he derided nature and scoffed at her, and dared her to do her worst." Yes, and nature struck back . . . nature seldom forgives.

Then there were those who took calculated risks and said so. There were others who hoped and prayed they'd get away with it and tried to kid themselves and everybody else. Then there is another school who say, "Don't tell me — don't tell me — I don't want to know. I like what I'm doing and I want to keep on doing it and I don't want anybody to tell me it's wrong or point out the dangers. Just leave me alone and mind your own business!"

There are others who just go blithely along their way of life asking no questions, seeking no answers, evading anything resembling an issue concerning health and laughing and giggling and doing as they want to do and enjoying life to the utmost . . . until . . .

At my mother's knee I learned that he lives who wants to live.

At times friends have challenged me on this statement and we have discussed its pros and cons. Admitted, a man who has a fractured skull in an accident may want to live but the fates decree otherwise. It is admitted that a person born with a congenital disease would like to live but the fates have dealt him a rather foul blow. Well, these situations could be multiplied but I have known people — terminal cases — who wanted to live and who were told and taught how to live and who followed the rules and who gave themselves many days, weeks, months and years of added life because they wanted to live.

Please understand, wanting to live implies that you will do something about it, even if it means effort, even if it means sacrifice, and even if it means turning away from the conventional and going down the long narrow winding road alone.

Do not ignore the tremendous unyielding force of the words "I want to live!" Faith moves mountains. Will can move chains of

24

mountains or even mountain systems. There is not one person alive who hasn't seen demonstrations of man's indomitable will. One man's indomitable will brought forth the world's greatest religion. One man's indomitable will conquered the world. One man's indomitable will helped turn the tide of the greatest military machine that ever existed. And I'm sure if you looked around you, you could find innumerable other instances of what a man's will can accomplish.

Well, you can accomplish health, long life and freedom from disease. You can conquer sickness — any sickness, including the dreaded cancer — if you have the will, the sheer will to do so. I don't know of anything on earth that a man could not accomplish if he had the will to do so!

I ask myself, "Where do I stand about helping my fellow man to health?" Please listen. My one aim in life is to pass along information on natural health or the ways and means of achieving natural health, freedom from disease and long life. I will not counsel or advise anyone who refuses or hedges about accepting full personal responsibility for his own health and welfare. I cannot cure anyone. I would not cure anyone. I do not believe or accept the thesis of a cure. I positively refuse to help those who will not help themselves. I do not believe in miracle foods, I do not believe in drugs in any form, I do not believe in health foods. I maintain that you must accept nature and follow her laws and her rules. It simply means that you must follow biological rules and laws in order to remain healthy and live your full life.

I maintain that the world could readily be helped back to health and long life if all the healers in the world told their patients, "I am by choice and location a healer. I can help you heal your body and achieve good health. But when you come to me, remember, I will assist, I will help and I will guide and instruct you, but you must never lose sight of the fact that it is you who is sick, it is you who has the disease and not me, and therefore while I am willing to assist you, it is not my responsibility nor my disease. You must never forget this for one minute. You can be well if you want to be well, if you want to follow the practices and principles that will make you well. You must be willing to do all things that are required to return your body to good health but you must never lose sight of the fact that the problem and the responsibility is entirely yours and you are the one who will pay the piper. You must have a strong enough desire to be well to do everything that is required to be well."

CHAPTER

5

PERFECT HEALTH TODAY — CRIPPLING DISEASE TOMORROW

Ever so often I hear or actually come face to face with a case where a man in apparent perfect health is stricken and hospitalized . . . or worse, the attack results in immediate death. Common sense indicates that a body in perfect health will not be suddenly stricken. It just doesn't happen that way. It is like a nut that looks perfectly sound on the outside but when cracked it is found either empty or rotten. As with the nut, this condition just didn't happen while you were cracking the shell.

I would judge that 90-99% of the adult population of the United States either drinks alcohol in one form or another, uses tobacco in one form or another or drinks tea or coffee. I categorically state that no human being who drinks alcoholic beverages, uses any form of tobacco or drinks tea or coffee can be in perfect health. It is utterly impossible. However, the human body is a wonderful machine and it does its best to fight off its enemies even if the enemies are self-inflicted. But the damage that these habits or products inflict upon the body eventually takes its toll.

No, I'm not going into the intricacies of how this happens and in all probability no one really knows exactly how but we certainly have ideas on the subject. But the true fact is that you cannot keep poisoning the body with these substances without causing damage. Usually there are indications of things going wrong. For example, if you have a cold or a headache or are indisposed or not feeling so good or occasionally you are tired . . . there are literally hundreds of signs. But, unfortunately most of us do not recognize these signs for what they really are or we take any one of a hundred different medications to drive off these warning signals the moment we feel them. Taking analgesic or pain killing drugs is like shutting off an alarm system. What good is the world's best system if you prevent it from working so that you won't be alarmed?

I recall that when I was in my 30's and early 40's I used to go to a doctor or clinic for a physical check-up and when the doctor eventually announced that everything was fine, that I was in good health and there was no apparent sign of an immediate breakdown I left the doctor's office with a buoyant feeling that all was well. Actually, what I was doing was paying the physician's fee just to give me some buoyancy and sort of make me click my tongue and say "Well, in spite of all the abuses that I'm doing to my body I'm still doing all right".

Now it is hard for me to imagine that any man who drinks or smokes can really think that he is not endangering his health or at least chipping away at it. Truthfully, I can't visualize a human being being so utterly stupid as not to realize that he is doing damage of varying degrees.

To illustrate this entire concept I'd like to quote from a letter that appeared in the magazine, "Lancet".

"Doctor Warns Against Over-Confidence In 'Checkups' — One

of the most irrational and comfortable delusions held by the layman is the notion that his body is really a kind of a motor-car. 'I feel much better now you've given me a thorough overhaul' is a remark I have heard on many occasions.

"Some doctors foster this delusion when they make remarks such as, 'You'd better come in for a complete check-up.'

"Behind all this lies the delusion that the physician is likely to remedy defects as he finds them — applying a little oil here, fitting a replacement there, and possibly clearing out a blocked pipe. Businessmen and high-up executives like to have 'complete check-ups' at regular intervals, when they can go into a clinic for a lot of expensive investigations.

"This emphasizes their importance and also it gives them a feeling of security, as they come out of the clinic rejuvenated by a comforting illusion of physical decarbonization. But the analogy with motor-car engines is false, and the only point where it applies is that when the trouble is very serious the patient is likely to be returned to his Maker."

I recall in my youth that over the week-end, starting Friday night, we had parties that would continue off and on until late Sunday night and Monday morning. Understandably I would not be in very fine fettle or at my best on Monday. But probably by Tuesday or so I'd be all right again and it never occurred to me for many years that what I was doing was really burning the candle at both ends and that this situation could definitely not continue very long without some breakdown or that the damage I was doing could be irreparable. But such is youth that these things don't even enter their heads. It never occurred to me that headaches, pains in the back of the head, stomach upsets, lack of energy and finding it very hard to get up in the morning was nature's way of illustrating that I was doing much that was wrong and should change my ways.

Looking back I often wonder how I could have kept telling myself that I was in perfect health on Tuesday, Wednesday, Thursday and Friday and then run the gauntlet over the week-end. Today, I know that any departure from normal or perfection like being overtired, lacking full pep, excessive yawning, a slight pain somewhere in my anatomy or heartburn or even burping indicates something is amiss. Mind you, I haven't had anything of this nature for many years because I just don't do the things that will bring this about. Yet, on looking back, all of these things happened almost daily and I did not recognize that they were warnings and that it was a cause and effect or symbiotic arrangement. I was doing this and my system was doing that as a direct result.

Furthermore, nowhere are we taught by health authorities or by the government or by the medical profession that health is a cause and effect arrangement. Well, this only illustrates how blind, how stupid and how ignorant we really are in matters pertaining to the most important thing in our lives . . . . our health.

No, you cannot possibly be in perfect health today and be stricken tomorrow by a crippling or killing disease. It just does not happen that way . . . you must earn the disease that afflicts, cripples or kills you.

CHAPTER

6

WHERE CAN WE LEARN ABOUT HEALTH?

It was in 1939, more than 34 years ago, that I suddenly became alerted to the serious dangers to my health, that surrounded me. It was a series of events that brought this about. I was the father of four children and it dawned upon me that it was encumbent upon me that I stay healthy and alive if I were to do justice to my children. It also happened that I temporarily lost my sexual drive. And frankly, this frightened me out of my wits. While searching for a means of bringing back my virility or my sexual prowess, I started on the trail of the long search for health.

There you have it...I have been ardently, avariciously, searching for the truth about health for more than 34 years. Now the climb has not been easy. The first dregs of information that I gleaned came hard. I didn't know where to turn...I didn't know where to seek health. At the start I sought it from qualified medical doctors, from food technologists and from government agencies, but I quickly learned that if I were going to gain any knowledge about health it would not be from any of those sources. If the truth must be told, I would say that it appears that they are allied and joined together to prevent mankind from acquiring true knowledge about food.

Please believe me, what I say is absolutely true. It was in the early stages of my quest for health knowledge that I learned that those three sources were definitely not the answer. Yet they appeared to me to be the logical places to go for health knowledge. Even today I am telling you that those three sources are not the place to search for knowledge about health.

If you went to the public library tomorrow and you asked for books on health, they would direct you to one or all of the three sources that I have mentioned.

Now most of the food processors publish literature on health and some go to great lengths to pass on not only the merits of the foods that they process, but the advantages of refined, chemicalized foods. For example, The Bakery Foundation publishes regular booklets and pamphlets on health. Heinz publishes a book on health, apart from other health pamphlets and such. The processing industry in general, I would say, spends millions every year sending out literature about health. But the health that they teach you is the kind of health that brings them heavy returns by millions and millions of dollars.

It's understandable that the food processors will not tell you to follow John Tobe's system of health through raw foods. And of course the doctors won't tell you to read John Tobe's "Guideposts To Health and Vigorous Long Life". You see, none of this knowledge would put any money in their pockets . . . in fact, it might cause them to become empty.

In any event, as soon as I learned positively that I could not find the knowledge I was seeking from those sources, I turned to other sources. And believe me, there are a lot of sources, too darned

32

many . . . but very few of them give you the true knowledge.

I was pleased and greatly enlightened with the knowledge contained in the books written by the pioneers . . . Benedict Lust, Henry Lindlahr, Russel T. Trall, J. H. Tilden, Otto Carque, John H. Kellog, Horace Fletcher, Wm. H. Hay, Bernarr MacFadden, John Richter, Alfred McCann, James C. Thompson, Herbert M. Shelton, Doris Grant, Ellis Barker, Gaylord Hauser and later Adele Davis, Cathryn Elwood, Linda Clark and many others . . . all of which gave me an insight into new knowledge which was a tremendous improvement on the ridiculous nonsense promulgated by the three sources mentioned at the start of this chapter.

I kept striving, I kept trying and I kept sending for literature and reading books and pamphlets . . . and then eventually the picture began to take shape. I found that no one author and no one book told anything near the whole true story of health. It seemed that each individual author had his own individual system. Some were much closer to the truth than others but practically all of them were slanted.

One author, who is among those that I consider the truly greats, Herbert M. Shelton, spoiled his approach and his writing by devoting phrase after phrase, interjected throughout his work, with tirades about the medical profession . . . calling them nasty, horrible names. I have long felt that, in spite of the fact that this writer gave the best information of all writers on health to his readers, he could have done much, much better or could have made a much greater contribution had he not shown his hate for the medical profession.

Mind you, he no doubt was fully justified in his tirades but if it dims the value of his writing, he is doing himself a disservice as well as his readers.

Nevertheless my quest continued, as it still continues today, but I can now see the trees in the forest . . . I can now understand many things that I didn't understand before.

I recall that about five years ago I thought I had the answer — the whole answer. It suddenly all became clear . . . the way to a long healthy life. I was so enthused that I almost broke through my skin, I swelled up so much.

I don't know why I kept on reading because I was sure I knew all the answers but I kept plugging away and lo and behold, the real truth dawned upon me . . . and that was that neither I nor all the rest had all the answers. I had some of them and I had many of them and maybe more than most men ever get, but I still didn't have all the answers. And I knew then, as I know now, that I never ever will have all the answers.

But if you read what I have to say, you will see that I am trying earnestly to pass on to you the gist and the benefits of what I have learned and I feel that it can be of great and tremendous benefit to those of you who take the time and the trouble to investigate.

CHAPTER

7

WHO DO WE BELIEVE AND WHAT TO BELIEVE?

One of the most frequent questions that is thrown at me is . . . "There is so much conflicting literature on health, who am I to believe and what am I to believe?"

Somehow I've always felt that if I were presented this two sided story I could judge which was wrong and which was right. Perhaps this is just ego on my part but through my lifetime when I've had a chance to hear both sides of the argument I don't recall of ever having made a mistake. I maintain that you have that ability to as great or a greater degree than I have. I maintain that you are just as capable of choosing right from wrong as I am, probably even more capable.

I recall about 25 or so years ago when the fluoride question was just rearing its ugly head I was presented with the fluoride side,

35

that is the advantages and the benefits of fluorides. I was completely sold on the value and merit of fluoridation and for a short time I shouted from the housetops how wonderful it was and how stupid everyone was who didn't embrace and follow this wonderful new idea.

Then I got into an argument with someone and I remember telling this party that he was impeding progress and preventing needy children from getting the benefits of fluorides. I also recall that at that time I couldn't conceive of ever being presented with evidence that could shake my faith in the benefits of fluorides. Then this party said to me, "Would you be willing to listen to the other side of the story?".

This touched my Achilles heel since I've always prided myself on having an open mind and I said of course I would and then this party placed some literature in my hand and said, "Do I have your promise to read this material?"

I promised and that night when I poured over the literature that gave the other side of the fluoride story I was shocked, I was troubled, I was amazed and most of all I was ashamed. Since then I've been a foremost believer in the strongest possible opposition to the fluoridation of water or the use of fluorides, both sodium fluoride and calcium fluoride in any manner, shape or form as food or drink for human beings. I contend that no human being with normal intelligence could examine the evidence of both sides and still believe that added chemical fluorides have a place in the health of human beings.

I also recall when the theory of raw food was first presented to me. It was totally untenable to my way of life and to my way of thinking and when the challenge was thown at me and I was told to investigate before I closed my mind I accepted the challenge and again I was shocked from the top of my head to the bottom of my feet.

From that day on I've never turned back from raw food and

natural living ... but I'll listen to any argument, I'll stand by and hear any presentation and I'll never close my mind to anything or to any knowledge again as long as I live. I feel that every human being is capable of knowing right from wrong and good from bad. So therefore when people come to me and say, "I'm troubled, I don't know who to believe, I don't know what to accept" I quickly say, "Read both sides and there will be no problem. You'll know who to believe and you'll know what to accept".

Right at the moment for example, I'm involved with two serious contentive questions. One is concerning the use of distilled water and the other is concerning the use of grains in the human diet. I have examined every bit of literature I can find on both subjects from any angle. I beg information, I beg knowledge, I beg data and I contend it is simple to make a decision when the evidence is presented clearly before you. I believe that grains or seeds that are palatable are good food, in fact among the best food on earth. I contend that distilled water has no place in the human anatomy. Although I feel that the evidence is overwhelming, still if anyone wants to present me with new evidence I'll take the time and listen.

In the field of nutrition we have on the one side the government, the medical profession, the food processors and industry in general ... all together. Then we have the side of thinking individuals who do not accept as gospel everything the Department of Health and Welfare, the A.M.A., the food industry and other profit organizations have to say and put into print. Yes, there are many of us with enquiring minds who desire to learn for themselves what is proper food and take the trouble to investigate and do honest research to learn the truth, and who are not afraid to admit that mother nature still knows something. There are many other supporters as well. I contend that raw food is the only food fit for human beings or animals. All other food is either lacking in nutrients or positively toxic.

So again, who do you believe? The evidence is there if you want to see it. Try feeding any group of creatures on the face of the earth with cooked food or processed food and another similar group on uncooked or raw food. See which one will remain healthier, see which one will live longer. You'll know in a matter of weeks, or months. Well, such research, such experiments, such records are available. It has been done and is being done. There is no question as to who is right and who is wrong.

Then the challenge is thrown at me, "If it is wrong to eat processed and cooked food why do the government, the AMA and others recommend it?" That's an easy question to answer. It is simply a matter of dollars . . . the economy, you know. And when dollars count the value of human life is ignored.

Anyway, if you want knowledge, if you want truth . . . investigate and the truth will be yours, clear and unmistakable. I say throw off the shackles that bind you and then remove the rose colored glasses that you have been wearing too long.

CHAPTER

WHERE IS RESEARCH LEADING US?

There is no doubt in my mind that every boy, at least at one time, has stood in awe of science. Science was the greatest of studies and a scientist was the greatest of men, and I somehow feel that most boys in their early days at school dream of being a great and renowned scientist.

In my case it took quite a lot of prodding, shocking, amazing and misadventures to uproot my awe and respect for science and scientists. It was only when error upon error, lie upon lie and folly upon folly became so evident that I had to sit down one day and re-evaluate my thinking about science and scientists. And don't you ever think that the very root of my existence wasn't shaken!

To begin with, I believed that science was always right and never in error. Secondly, I believed that a scientist was invariably a dedicated man who placed science and truth, which should be synonymous, above anything else on earth. Third, I believed that a scientist had to study deeply and intently and ferret out every truth for himself. Fourth, I believed that a scientist would choose to die rather than disgrace the name of science.

Well, poor, innocent, stupid dolt that I was, I believed all the above until I learned they were false. Oh, yes, there are still a few scientists in the world who might fit this description but they are so few that you would need Diogenes and a much bigger light than he had to find them. But I definitely admit that they do somewhere exist.

Now I don't know who is more guilty, the assassin or the man who hired the assassin, but that's not for me to decide. Somehow, by some stupid logic, I reasoned that every scientist was a researcher and that he spent his life in the interests of his fellow man and that he sacrificed sleep and food and his health and his love life for science. Boy, what a dreamer I was!

To me, to even think of questioning the findings of a scientist was the highest heresy. I would have fought to the death any man who impunged the reputation or the name of a scientist.

Now I ask myself, "Was I wrong about science originally or has something happened to make scientists different to what they were?"

That's a burning question! When I think of scientists like Newton, Magendie, Einstein, Semmelweis, Galvan, Faraday, Kelvin and Watt, I somehow feel certain that I was right in my first analysis of a scientist but that something has happened to him or his image in the past 50 years. And a bit of investigation will quickly reveal what has happened to him.

Back in the old days a scientist worked in a wee laboratory or a hole in the ground or a cellar, he worked for himself usually and by himself, or a few scientists worked in a university or some institute of learning, and there were no offending or tempting third parties involved. Today scientists in the main are hirelings of the chemical and generally speaking, industrial and business world. Today a scientist doesn't do what he wants to do or what his inherent mental make-up tells him to do . . . he does what he is told to do by the people who pay his salary.

I suggest that with few rare exceptions every scientist in the world today is shackled and bound. He either works for the government, a university or an industrial corporation. Well, the industrialists who hire the scientists for their own business also give most of the money to the universities for research and therefore they control the research projects and the scientists who perform them. And those who work for the government do what the government tells them to do. But big business tells the government what to tell the scientists to do. After all, without the revenue from big business neither the universities nor the government would be able to exist.

So today there is no such thing as an honest and courageous scientist. At least, he is a very rare breed. In fact, I don't know how he would make a living if he didn't belong to one of the three groups I mentioned. So it becomes strictly a matter of economics.

You can readily understand why scientists do not undertake research unless there is the likely possibility that it will make money for someone.

I am suggesting that today science is busily engaged in doing everything humanly possible to destroy the human race. Actually, the suggestion of this is even absurd because no one really wants to destroy himself . . . yet that's what I'm telling you that scientists are doing. I need only point to the atom bomb and the use of pesticides to prove that I am absolutely correct in my summation or supposition.

Of course their defenders will say that science has made a better world. But I would say quickly, "Where is that better world?"

41

I suggest they have corrupted every principle, every conviction and everything that we hold dear. Today in the progress of science absolutely nothing is sacred. Before long they'll be up there kicking God off his throne and putting a robot that will take orders there in his place. And they'll quickly tell you that God has done a lousy job . . . he's permitted wars, he permitted it to rain for 40 days and 40 nights, he kills millions with earthquakes, he brings hurricanes and other sheer madness to the people of the world. The scientists no doubt feel that they can control the weather and elements, they can get to the moon and they can also blow up all these planets if they so desire . . . and they probably will. So obviously science is greater than God. Who can deny it? Who will deny it, except a few religious fanatics?

I'm sure I can't tell you whether or not other people in this world are as disenchanted with science as I am but today I see science as the most potent factor on earth for evil. I am sorry to say that I see very little if anything good that science produces. Oh, yes, I recognize that they have given us electricity and they have given us leisure and comforts. Why, right at this present time there are places in Chicago, for example, where a man can be born, live and die without putting his foot outside the one building . . . and he can lead an interesting, comparatively healthful and fascinating existence, yes, from infancy to the grave at 70 or more!

No, no, I'm not fooling . . . this is an absolute truth. In fact, they'll probably bury him right below there in the cellar, too. They can put him in a tomb or if he wants his ashes scattered over the Seven Seas, well, they have a quay right there of their own . . . I saw it with my own eyes. And the buses drive into the terminals there and so do the trains. Then I understand they have a helicopter that will pick you up off the top of the building and then land at the airport and you can go anywhere on earth.

So who needs God? God made all this in seven days and science can destroy it in seven seconds.

One thing you must recognize, whether you go along with my

tale or not, is that no one in the world — no government on earth — has the power to curb the scientists. Scientists are gods unto themselves.

Any man can set up a laboratory and do what he wants to do. He can cross a gorilla with an elephant, he can create storms, he can breed a human being in a glass tube and he can replace the heart of a man or any other organ for that matter with that of a monkey. They will no doubt soon be taking the brains of men like Einstein, when they are old and decrepit, and putting them into fresh new young bodies. This could go on endlessly. There is just no stopping the scientists.

Now I'm asking you . . . is this good or bad? Have we pulled the cork and allowed the genii to get out? I sometimes think that we have gone too far already.

Now while part of this dissertation was a bit of whimsy and I allowed my imagination to run riot, I think we should give a sober thought as to whither or whence science is leading us.

CHAPTER

9

MEDICAL MEN ARE NOT MIRACLE MEN

Through the years I have been privileged to read the writings of a great number of doctors. Doctors do write books. Some are good, some are bad, some are fair and a few are excellent. But most books by doctors are, in my humble opinion, mediocre.

Any man who has not read the writings of Oliver Wendell Holmes and Sir William Osler has missed some mighty good reading and some mighty good philosophy and general counsel. Now there are lots of other medical writings that perhaps come close to this caliber but generally I have found that books by doctors aren't worth reading.

Some of the best medical writings that I have ever come across dealt with doctors who were sick ... that is, books dealing with doctors as patients. Here I read some of the finest literature that it has ever been my privilege to read. It was written by doctors themselves who, when they became afflicted with a disease, wrote and described the situation and condition and I shall be forever grateful to these doctors who documented their experiences for the world to know and understand.

In my opinion it takes a great deal of courage, strength and love of one's fellow man for a doctor to write about his own personal sickness . . . that is, how he got sick and how he behaved and reacted when he was sick. It must be tragic when he has to admit that neither he nor his colleagues, nor the whole world of medicine can make him well. I could have wept through some of these tales and through it all I got the impression that the doctors as a group were mighty, mighty fine human beings. In fact, I felt a kinship or closeness to them that I had never felt before.

I read such articles closely and digested and sought to experience the feelings that they described. Nevertheless, through it all there were certain truths that appeared in their stark nakedness and these truths are worthy of enumeration.

The first tremendous denouement came when I realized that when it came to disease and sickness the doctors were just as helpless as you and I or the man on the street or the average housewife. Believe it or not, this came as quite a shock to me because they made it crystal clear that with all their skills, with all their fame, with all their knowledge, with all their conveniences and mechanics, and with all the thousands upon thousands upon thousands of volumes of scientific data and proofs and experiments, when disease struck they were as helpless as a new-born babe.

Truthfully, most of the doctors who wrote these articles were quite honest and courageous about it. They did not weep or seek mercy, nor did they pretend to any great bravery. They admitted they were struck, they were sick and they were dying, and they were prepared to meet their Maker.

In practically every instance they used their skills to the

highest degree. They did not stop short ... using every weapon at their command, which included every drug they ever heard of or knew of or was recommended and the surgeon's scalpel, x-rays and radiation. They used everything that was usable according to the principles, practices and useages of the medical profession.

Let me here enumerate some of the diseases from which these doctors suffered: alcoholism, drug addiction, heart disease, arthritis, cataract, multiple sclerosis, schizophrenia, etc.

Practically all of them died ... and in my estimation they died much sooner than they would have died had they not been treated in their own way and if they hadn't been doctors. I feel certain that with few exceptions they died quicker because they were given the best treatment in the world. It is my sincere belief that they would not have died so soon had they been neglected or just given ordinary treatment. I am suggesting that this over-indulgence in one way or another contributed to or caused their earlier death.

As you well know I am not a healer of any field. I do not hold any degrees from any universtiy in the world. I would not and will not accept any degrees. I know nothing about disease, sickness or pathology. But I will suggest that I do know something about health.

Well, it is my feeling that if they had followed the advice given in my writing, practically every single one of them could have brought himself back to good health or at least added months or years to his life.

Remember, I could have done nothing for any of them but I could have shown them how they could have helped themselves and thus added months or years and perhaps many years to their lives ... to the benefit of all mankind.

Egad! This should make you wonder and perhaps you are smarting to ask me a question like, "Do you mean to suggest that you, a lousy layman without any degrees or without any accreditation from any university or school of learning, know more about health than the whole medical profession?"

By all that's holy, if you were to put that theoretical question to me boldly, I would look you square in the eye and just as boldly snap back at you "Yes, that is exactly what I mean!"

Then if you gave me a few more minutes, I would continue by saying, "I have watched many — I repeat, many — medical students start off on their careers and they bury themselves in their work. Most medical students study hard and work hard to attain their degrees. Very few take risks of being flunked out and I contend that very few are flunked out, especially after the second year. Most of these boys or young men eat, sleep and breathe medicine. They study anatomy, physiology, pathology, histology and whatever subjects are pertinent to their studies. During their heavy study years I doubt if they read very much, if anything, apart from that which pertains to the subjects that I have outlined. They become steeped in their studies and as most of them want to get good grades they toil relentlessly to absorb the knowledge that is taught them or to which they are directed. The result is a sort of computer that spouts materia medica through the oral opening without any thinking process."

From those medical men whom I have known intimately, plus the thousands about which and whose works I have read, my impression is that they are the most neglected, the most naive, the most uninformed men of any profession in America. They have even drowned their normal natural instincts, many of which are protective, in their search for knowledge of drugs and medicine and surgery. To the minds of nine doctors out of ten it is unthinkable that anything could affect the health of an individual other than drugs, medicines, surgery and radiation. That is what they have been taught, that is what they believe and that is what they practise. That is what they have permitted to be instilled into them.

Please understand that I am not condemning them nor am I apologizing for them, nor am I seeking to draw sympathy for them or from them. I am relating facts plus my own understanding and

48

feelings of the situation.

So, the end result of all this is that we have a group of men who had brains — a higher incidence than normal — who had the ability to gain knowledge and who have spent hard years at toil of studying, with the end result that they have neglected anything and everything that did not appear in the prescribed texts.

It is only after taking all of these matters into consideration that I can understand why doctors are the shortest lived of all the professions or businesses. Most people believe or are told that the doctors die young because they are so devoted to their fellow man and they work so hard and struggle so valiantly for others that they neglect themselves and, so to speak, kill themselves. But my understanding is entirely different. I maintain that that is absolutely not true. I grant, without fear or favor, that most medical men do work hard and do work long hours . . . because unlike a business or some of the other professions, if a doctor should become ill or incapacitated, his income usually stops dead. That is the reason why so many doctors work so hard for at least the first ten or fifteen years of their practice . . . until they have made themselves a little nest egg upon which their families can rely for the future, especially in the event of their demise.

So while I do not deny that doctors work hard, I do maintain, however, that they don't work a darn bit harder than I work or that most men who own private individual businesses work. What I am saying is that most business men, especially independent business men, work as hard as the average doctor . . . and it doesn't kill the business man. So why should it kill the doctor?

Of course, some doctors say that it does kill business men, but I dispute that just as vigorously, too.

In any event, the reason that the doctors die at a younger age than business men do is because a business man might have an open mind about some other form of living or treatment which would be to his benefit. The medical doctor would not be amenable to ideas or treatments that are not medically oriented because it's contrary to what he has been taught, to what he believes and what he accepts.

So they pay with their lives for what they believe in. I guess that's just retribution or poetic justice, eh?

CHAPTER

10

A DISCUSSION ON MEDICAL RESEARCH

I don't know how many millions, or perhaps I should say billions, of dollars are being spent this year on medical research. The government of course is the biggest contributor to medical research. The contribution that the various disease funds make is also no small matter. These funds, remember, collect hundreds of millions of dollars from the public and they do allow a trickle to seep out which goes into research. Then, of course, there are many universities who have a lot of foundation and other moneys left to them as endowment which they give out for research purposes as well. Besides this, there are independent donations from people who leave money in their wills and of course the various industrial organizations in America also donate millions of dollars towards medical research.

All in all, I would suggest that the whole affair runs into a billion or a couple of billion dollars a year.

51

Just tonight over the radio I heard an announcement saying that medical science has eliminated death from our young folks... they exhorted motor car drivers not to kill the young people. So obviously we are told or led to believe that nobody dies now until they reach 70 or 80 because the medical profession takes credit for extending the life span of the average man to beyond 70 years.

I am sure that the average individual walking around the streets today — every Joe Blow and his uncle — is confident and knows for a certainty that he is going to live to be 70 and beyond and collect the old age pension and social security. This is the actual concept and the feeling that many people have because this is what they have been taught and this is what they are led to believe and it is absolutely true that most of the general public do believe that the life span has definitely been extended by twenty or thirty years or more.

Four of my brothers and sisters have passed on. One of them reached the three score and ten but the others died at 57, 63 and 64 years of age. They'll probably come back and haunt the perpetrators of the outrage that told them they were going to live to be 70 and beyond.

From the obituaries that I read in the newspapers it would appear that not very many of them make the coveted three score and ten and beyond. So I begin to ask myself, who is kidding whom? Among my friends, Bert Sheppard 61, Jack McMillan 47, Don Lauder 66, Alex Williamson 60, Tommy Phipps 68, Linc Quinn 64 ... not one single one of them made the grade to 70.

I am suggesting that the reason these stories are spread is so that the medical profession can get more and more grants, so they can keep us living not only to 70 but to 80 and 90.

Well, let's stop here for a moment and really examine the records. It is an established scientific fact that we haven't had an outbreak of small-pox in a good number of years yet each and every year a goodly number of people die from vaccination for small-pox. It seems a little crazy, doesn't it? Nobody dies from small-pox but a goodly number die from vaccination against small-pox.

With the billions of dollars that are being spent annually on research let's ask ourselves how many specifics we have against diseases. That is, how many diseases can the medical profession positively cure. Of course the first one that comes up quickly is that they have a specific for pneumonia. Yet a friend of mine recently died from pneumonia. So obviously they don't have a specific for pneumonia. Do they have a specific for cancer? No. Do they have a specific for heart disease? No. Do they have a specific for arthritis? No. Do they have a specific for asthma? No. Do they have a specific for prostate disease? No.

Well come now, just what do they have a specific cure for? We are told they have these many, glorious, fearful and wonderful cures . . . well, just what in blazes are they curing? Rheumatism, Emphysema, Multiple Sclerosis, Muscular Dystrophy, Kidney Disease, Ulcers, Colitis, Varicose Veins and Hemorrhoids?

I'm deeply wrapped in thought now and perhaps I'm going to show my ignorance but I don't know one single specific cure that they have for any disease.

I can hear someone saying, "Malaria!"

In the first place, cinchona, which is used for malaria, was not a medical discovery. And secondly, it doesn't cure it . . . it only relieves it. It keeps coming back.

Do they have a specific for leprosy? For Hodgkin's disease? For Parkinson's? Of course, the answer comes back, "NO!"

Well, what's all the research for?

Ah, that's a good question and one that deserves an answer . . . but I don't think the answer will be forthcoming.

53

There's the cancer fund, the heart fund, the muscular dystrophy fund and the arthritis fund and oh so many more funds. All of these funds collect a total of hundreds of millions of dollars every year and of course the idea is that you give your money, they'll do the research, they'll find a cure and then you won't have to suffer from the disease and you won't have to die or give any more money. It's supposed to be a sort of self-liquidating program. Every year these medical funds need more money, put on bigger drives, collect more money, spend more money and the diseases and the number of afflicted continue to increase.

Now there is an exception here. Evidently T.B. was supposedly conquered. I don't know who conquered it or who konked it but for quite a few years the number of T.B. patients decreased and dropped to practically nothing. Of course the Christmas Seal Fund and perhaps others took the credit for it. But the stories I get now say that it is coming back. So who got rid of the T.B. or tuberculosis? The medical profession or the tuberculosis fund? No one can answer that question because nobody knows but it certainly isn't because the people with tuberculosis are cured . . . it is just that people don't get tuberculosis any more than they get small-pox or diphtheria or cholera or bubonic plague any more.

What I am trying to point out to you as clearly as I can and as emphatically as I can is that giving this money, whether it's for these funds or to the research foundations, doesn't eliminate the disease or cure anything . . . it just gives folks a lot of money to play with in a laboratory. With this money I guess they buy test-tubes, scientific equipment, dogs and other animals to work on, and the researchers earn their Bachelors, Masters and Ph.D. degrees doing it. So it works out very nicely for everybody concerned . . . but the disease goes merrily on and on and on.

No doubt that's the way it should be, I guess, because if by giving money you eliminated the disease, then you wouldn't have to give any more money . . . and that would never do.

Obviously it is in the best interests of all of these funds and

54

researchers not to come up with any cure because a cure means the end of their prosperity. Anyway, don't worry about it, there is no danger of any cures being found and there is no danger in the researchers being eliminated or the funds being eliminated because it's big business and billions of dollars are involved and just nobody in their right mind will do anything to interfere with this golden egg laying goose. Besides, nobody is going to cure anything. The curing and the healing of the sick is something that lies in the hands of Mother Nature and the human body itself . . . one or the other or both.

So I prophesy that these health or disease funds and these research projects will go on forever and a day. And the cure will be just around the corner. The cure is imminent and it may break any day. There will be a great breakthrough . . . soon.

Well, if I recall correctly the breakthrough has been coming since Hippocrates first made his first diagnosis and we're just as close now as we were then. The healers of any of the healing professions can't cure a carbuncle or a cuticle because there is no such thing as a cure. The return to health is strictly the prerogative of nature. And that is why the heads of these funds can sit smugly, snuggly and securely and thumb their noses at guys like Tobe because the money will keep rolling in, more and more with each succeeding year, with never a danger of a cure being found.

One thing for certain that I know is this. Tobe, you're in the wrong business!

I wonder what fund I can start. Why can't you start a fund? After all, there are still a lot of diseases in the medical books for which a fund has not been set up. What are you waiting for? Get cracking . . . it's a business that's a natural and a perennial and it will go on forever and a day!

CHAPTER

11

WHO LIES?

In the course of a year I receive thousands of letters — I should say, tens of thousands. Not all of them are flattering or complimentary.

One letter that recently reached me — my staff didn't spare me by removing it or throwing it in the waste paper basket — was from a woman who said, "What makes you think that we have to come to the likes of you to be given information on health and proper food? You are not qualified, you are untaught, you are unlearned, you are unscientific and a nobody. If we want information about food and health, we can get it from the National Research Council, the National Council on Foods, The National Academy of Sciences and from the various government agencies, from our universities, from our libraries, from our clinics and from our doctors. They are competent, they are properly trained and they have the facilities and the records to give us the information that we require."

Well, that put John H. Tobe right in his place where he belongs . . . squat on his donkey (ass).

I didn't bother answering the lassie but I am answering her now, if she ever gets to read this.

Dear Lassie,

The places you mention are precisely where I went to get information on health when I first started my search for the truth on health matters about 20 years ago. When I went to school — even from kindergarten upwards — I was indoctrined with health knowledge from these same sources through the medium of my teachers. They taught me to brush my teeth with toothpaste, to gargle my throat with Listerine, they taught me to drink pasteurized milk, they taught me to get my tonsils out, they taught me to eat white enriched bread, they taught me to eat white sugar, they taught me to get eye-glasses, they taught me to sleep eight or ten hours a day, they taught me to cook my food, they taught me to use chlorine and fluorine in my drinking water, they taught me to use iodine and hydrogen peroxide to kill germs in wounds and cuts, they taught me to use aspirin for a headache, they taught me to use milk of magnesia for a laxative, yes, and they taught me hundreds of other bad habits — sickness-creating habits — for each and every one of the things that I have just mentioned are positively harmful to the human anatomy. Yes, even the brushing of the teeth with abrasive, caustic chemical substances. And I can conclusively prove to any sane, open-minded individual that all of the above practices are harmful!

Let me also tell you this, the government, the universities, the libraries, the medical profession and the health organizations you mention are teaching you many more harmful, disease-creating habits than those I have mentioned. They have taught us to become drug addicts. They have taught us to smoke and to drink liquor, beer, wine, coffee and tea. They have taught us to use sleeping pills, tranquilizers and anti-pregnancy pills. Yes, they have taught us all the bad habits that we know today and which are bringing our nation to the depths of degradation.

Unfortunately, those who realize and recognize that something is wrong and that the agencies mentioned are misleading us, have no other recourse than to come to crack-pots like Tobe and others in order to learn how to stay alive and healthy in a poisoned world.

For your further enlightenment, dear lassie, there is nowhere else you can go to get truly honest and factual information about food and drugs and health but to these selfsame sources that you despise.

Who else would warn you about the evil and harmful effects of cyclamates, monosodium glutamate, the deadly red dye as well as hundreds of other chemical food additives and drugs that have been positively known to cause diseases of various kinds, including cancer?

I would be most naive if I did not recognize the fact that I and a few others like myself are not the only people who know the truth as we see it.

I am fully aware that the government, the politicians, the libraries, the universities, the doctors, the clinics, the mass advertising media and the scientific bodies mentioned earlier know the truth, too. Of course they know the truth. I have never suggested at any time that they didn't know the truth. Sure they know it . . . but they don't tell it to you and the world at large. Does this all come as a shock to you?

Now you are more enraged than ever and I can hear you saying, "Why you villain! You scoundrel! How dare you insinuate that these great men — these humanitarians, these public servants — are withholding the truth from the people?"

I quite unabashedly say, "Of course they are scoundrels, villains and worse! They know the truth but they speak otherwise because their incomes depend upon keeping people like you in ignorance."

I know, as sure as the sun rises and sets, that the chemical laboratories that make the cyclamates knew for years that the cyclamates were harmful. How do I know they knew? Because I have read the evidence that they have presented for years. The same applies to the manufacturers of the "pill" and of monosodium glutamate and a thousand and one other chemicals, drugs and food additives. They too, know and have known that they are harmful but they play innocent. And why not, when it means profits of millions and hundreds of millions and perhaps billions of dollars?

No, I am not begrudging anyone the right to make money. And I am not an anarchist, a monarchist, a fascist or a communist. I like to make money myself, too, and maybe that's why I'm doing the fighting . . . because they refuse to pay me off. But the fact still remains that I have nothing against anyone who makes money but I am against those who do serious harm to their fellow man in their quest for money.

I would be so bold as to suggest that the doctors who perform those millions of tonsilectomies and millions of appendectomies and hysterectomies and hundreds of other "ectomies" on organs, know for certain that they are removing most of them needlessly. I am suggesting that most doctors who give or prescribe drugs know that most of those drugs do more harm than good. And the same goes for veterinarians and the cattle they treat. You can go down the line further to include government officials, university professors, researchers, scientists and others . . . they all know of the evil that they do, but it's a living . . . often a darned good living. Most of them would prefer not to think about it. They are just doing their duty and they would rather not talk about it.

So if you want information — true information, factual information and scientific information — about these and such things, then you've got to go to crack-pots like Tobe.

CHAPTER

12

LIFE EXPECTANCY FIGURES

Just what do they mean when they specify "life expectancy"? They tell us that a child born today can expect to live to be about 71 years of age. What this really means is a comparative guarantee. In other words, say your baby is born this day it will be alive 71 years from now without much doubt. Well, who am I to argue with science? But I frequently do and I have good cause. However, statistics and figures and scientists tell us that this is so . . . an infant born of this day can expect to live to be 71.5 years of age.

You know I think somebody ought to tell all those corpses in all the cemeteries that they were supposed to have lived to be 71 and not have died at 6, 7, 45, 56 and 68. Now really and truly just what is wrong with these life expectancy figures? I lost a sister and two brothers and they didn't get to 70. I have a number of nieces and nephews and three of them already have gone and they didn't get to

70 and let me tell you that none of these was shot by a burglar or a criminal and none of them was killed in the war. They weren't even killed in automobile accidents. They just up and died.

Practically every day I come across reports from the various newspapers, magazines, radio and television telling me that at the University College in London they've learned how to mix certain food preservatives to make mice live a lot longer. At the University of Notre Dame they have another experiment and the research makes mice live longer, too. Then they have a system of lowering the human body temperature at the University of Southern California which would add a few more years to a man's life.

A report in the Medical Journal of Australia of June 27, 1970 says, "A child born today can expect to live about 70 years . . . a little less if he is a man and a little more if she is a woman."

Here are some of the flaws in the life expectancy figures. To begin with, in order for a man to be 70 years of age he would have had to be born around 1902. Now at the turn of the century there were few if any reliable records kept. As a matter of fact, in many countries throughout the world, even the advanced countries, vital statistics, where there was compulsory registration of births and deaths and such did not commence until well into the century — that is, around 1910 and 1920. Therefore, any figures that go back beyond this date are sort of taken out of the air and are not reliable or factual.

To give credit to the medical profession or to science for the increase in man's life span is utterly preposterous and ridiculous when you consider that most of the medical techniques in use today were not known 50 years ago. Most of the drugs in use today were unknown 25 years ago. Science as we know it today fits in about the same predicament as the medical profession. Fifty years ago science was dragging along like a cow's tail. To claim that science and medicine have given us an increased life span borders on the absurd.

If I were asked what have been or are the main contributors

to the high life expectancy figures I would have to admit my ignorance and say I do not know. It so happens that both my parents and my grandparents lived beyond the three score and ten and that's more than can be said for most of our family, that is their children and their grandchildren. So the increase in the life span is most definitely not apparent in our family and I'm not so sure that it is apparent or existent even in your family or most of the families in America. It is agreed that today 80% of all deaths are due to heart disease and to cancer, (55% to heart disease and about 25% to cancer). Medical science agrees that heart disease as it is known today was unknown 60 years ago. In those days cancer was a disease of the aged. That is, people beyond 50 or 60 got cancer. Today, it afflicts people of all ages, starting in infancy. Does that tend to indicate that our life expectancy has been increased?

From my viewpoint the only channel where life expectancy has definitely made progress is in the decrease of infant mortality. The figures on the infant mortality rates dating back to the turn of the century are rather wild. Judging by these statistics it appears that 25% of all children who were born then did not live to see five years of age. Today, less than 2% die before the age of five. So that's a saving of about 250 people out of a 1,000 who are alive today who were not alive at a comparable age before the turn of the century. As far as I can see, that is the only case where we have made gains in an increase in the life span. I have asked, I've inquired, I've searched for facts and figures that would truly indicate that we are living longer but I have not come up with any indication or proof of any kind. Yet we are told over and over and over again that our life expectancy is increasing and that soon just everybody will live to be 100 and beyond.

It is claimed that there are today in the United States 13,000 people who are more than 100 years old and we are also told that this sub-group of the population is increasing faster than any other group. They would have us believe that soon everyone will live to be 100 and beyond. The increase in the number of doctors, the increase in the number of hospital beds, the increase in the nursing profession and the healing arts in general would certainly emphasize the lie or the fallacy in that statement. Remember, every individual who has reached the grand and glorious three score and ten had to be born prior to the turn of the century and I can't see how the medical profession or science can take one fragment of credit for that.

If any credit is due anywhere it would be due to the fact that these individuals practically in every instance lived on natural food and did not have the processing or the chemical additives in their food that we have today. I recall clearly that in my youth or childhood, that is 60 years ago, the only canned food that you could buy was a tin of tomatoes and everything we ate at our table was prepared in our home. The ingredients were purchased perhaps at the marketplace but the preparation was done entirely in the kitchen, that is the home kitchen and not a food processor's kitchen.

I contend that the prime reasons for the poor health of the people of America today are the food processors and the chemicalized, fragmented so-called foods that they produce.

I don't know whether or not we have more accidents today or less. In the olden days there were a goodly number of farm accidents. Today the highest incidence of deaths is caused by automobiles but I doubt if automobile deaths have any great influence upon our life expectancy rates. In any event, I'm convinced that life expectancy figures have little relevance or meaning. In the simplest language at my disposal I say figures don't lie but liars sure know how to juggle figures.

CHAPTER

13

PROPER FOOD FOR MAN

The most perplexing question facing any nutritionist or individual who is interested in food is, "What is man's proper food?"

At the outset let me make myself crystal clear. Any man or woman, sage or seer, wise man or fool, who attempts to set himself up as an authority and is willing to attest to what is rightfully man's proper food is either a liar, an ignoramous or an egotistical jackass.

It is my sincere belief that I have searched as widely and as deeply as any man living or dead concerning man's proper food and I haven't found any conclusive proof as to what is or what might be the proper food for man. I must reluctantly admit that from my extensive travels and searching I found no proof whatsoever that would in the slightest degree indicate what man's proper food is. The only thing about proper food for man or beast or insect that I know of is that honey is the proper food for a bee and that milk from the mother's breast is the proper food for an infant. Beyond that, I challenge any man to state that he can say or prove for certain what is proper food for man.

I wish, with all my heart and soul, that I could stand before you and say that this or that or the other is the proper food as ordained by God or nature and that is what you should eat to give you health and long life. However, none — I repeat, none — of the literature of the world offers the slightest clue. I have, with great deliberation, searched everywhere where a clue might be found and not a sliver of a positive nature emerged.

Oh, yes, friends . . . please believe me . . . I have searched through the Bible but regarding proper food the Bible is most contradictory or elusive. I can show you where they tell you to eat pulses but I can also show you where they tell you to eat locusts and the clean beasts and not to eat the unclean ones.

However, from this mass of data no one knows or can decide which is right. Then too, one very important factor is omitted . . . the Bible does not tell you whether to eat your food cooked or raw. In fact, most of the instructions deal with cooked, burnt, heated or fired foods.

So be ye theologian, scientist, sage or seer, I challenge you to prove that any one food is proper food for man.

Now about an opinion . . . ah, that is different! I claim to be some sort of a judge (I definitely and deliberately avoid the word "authority") because I have, in the course of my life, eaten practically every blamed kind of food that exists . . . running the gauntlet of the normal foods eaten by anyone on the North American continent or Europe or Asia or Africa or Australia or South America, plus rattlesnake, frogs' legs, baby bees, octopus, quail's eggs, rabbit, beetles, grasshoppers and many other insects . . . I had better stop there, but I could go on.

No, I did not necessarily enjoy all of those or any of them but I did positively eat them at one time or another. If need be, to prove a point, I would eat living worms (in fact, I'm sure I have frequently in apples), humming bird's tongue, dog meat or candied mice. And for those of you whose stomachs I turn when you read this, don't put on any airs, because none of those things that I have mentioned are as filthy or dirty as your ham, bacon, pork or even chicken. A chicken and a pig eat anything and are most unclean. So don't put on any airs with me. Any of you who eat pig meat or chicken meat have sunk to the lowest depths of eating. You see, I've lived long enough to see and know what a pig eats and what a chicken eats and no creature on earth eats anything as vile or filthy.

When a writer or an expert on food and nutrition starts out by telling you what to eat, I know right off the bat that he is an ignoramous or a fool or should I say, a novice, to treat him kindly.

A dear Chinese friend of mine told me that in China if it walks, crawls, flies, swims, moves or grows, it is potential food. And as far as mankind and his food is concerned, I believe that Chinese adage is the most apt description of man's food that I have ever heard.

As you well know some people learn from experience and others don't learn through experience or any other way. We all have our dislikes and likes concerning food. Also food habits run in families. I would say that about 90% of all the people on earth eat like either their father or their mother or a mixture of both. But seldom do we go beyond the limits or food habits and preferences of our parents. If you have any doubts as to the truth of what I am saying, check it out for yourself and you will see that the type of food that is served on your table was served on the table of your parents or your wife's parents ... and you can go back as many decades as you like.

Admitted that new foods — like those of the present age — come and go, some stick and some fade but still we eat the foods that were eaten by our parents and our grandparents and you can go back as far as you like. It is claimed that less than 300 species of plants comprise 90% of the food of man. When you learn that there are more than 300,000 different plants on earth, you can grasp how little we know about what is proper food.

Haggis was probably eaten by the Scots when they first moved into Scotland from Scythia; and roast beef was eaten in England when the first ancient Briton konked a bull on the bean; and the Irish ate pigs when the Emerald Isle first emerged from the sea and the Jews ate Gefilte fish when they reached out from the Ark and hooked a fish . . . and they all continue to eat these foods even today!

Man has been eating the wrong foods as long as literature and records exist. What he ate prior to the time that history was recorded I do not know but I am absolutely certain that he has been eating the wrong kind of foods since any records have been kept. Nowhere — not in one bit of literature — is there any evidence that man knew what to eat.

The closest that anyone ever came to proper food was when Daniel refused to eat from the king's table and he asked for pulses. The only question that arises there is whether or not those pulses were eaten raw or cooked. I'm betting, in fact I'm sure, they were eaten raw, otherwise he would not have been so "fair of flesh".

Everywhere and every time I open my mouth I am dubbed a vegetarian and I have to apologize and tell people that I am not a vegetarian, even though I would like to be one and although my diet consists of more vegetables than any vegetarian ever ate. The fact is that I do eat fish and occasionally meat. Meat I do not eat by preference; fish, I select and choose.

From my actual experiences and from sifting through the knowledge and from what I have learned from conversation and investigation, the finest, the best, the most natural and the most desirable food for man is grass. Yes, I can hear the derision, the weeping, the moaning, the shock, the surprise, the amazement and the utter desperation of those of you who will read this. But I'll repeat it . . . grass is man's best food . . . and that is why nature has made it the most abundant food on earth. There is more grass on the earth than all the other types of plants and animals together.

I say that nature knew what she was doing. The fact that we don't eat grass or eat very little of it just proves our stupidity and our ignorance and the proof that we are eating the wrong food is evidenced by the number of people who go to doctors and fill up our hospitals and our mental and other institutions.

If man overnight became a grass-eating creature, then doctors, hospitals, nurses and most of our health and penal institutions would be rendered totally and completely unnecessary. O.K., so you think I'm kidding. Well, you can laugh, you can bellow till your sides burst, but I'm telling you the truth and I mean every single word of it.

Oh, I know you won't start eating grass . . . but if you did so you'd see the results so fast that you'd be liable to shock yourself to death. That's right, friends, ten days on a strict diet of green vegetables would make such a drastic change in your well-being that you would be liable to drop dead of the shock. But if you sustained the shock and continued on the vegetable diet you'd probably live to be one hundred.

Now if you think I am so utterly stupid as to make a statement like the above that I know will be sneered at and scoffed at, without proper proof, then you're crazy. There is ample true, scientific evidence available to conclusively and without a shadow of doubt prove that grass is the earth's best food. And anyone who bothered to make a survey or to do a research project on the subject would quickly prove to the whole world that every word I say is true. But it won't be done because it would bankrupt too many people . . . and who would be so stupid as to subsidize a project of this nature? Certainly not Heinz or Gerbers, or Del Monte or the packing houses or the chemical companies or the drug houses or the American Medical Association or the government, for that matter. If the government ever dared try such a stunt, well, they'd be turned out at the next election . . . not because they wouldn't be able to prove what they're saying but because they would be able to prove it and ruin 90% of the business establishments in America.

O.K., so grass could be or is your best food. That's established, even though I said before that no one knows what is proper food for man.

Now I want to warn you about eating grass. Here you can see what a louse I am — I've got you to the stage where I have convinced you at last that grass is the best food in the world and now I warn you about it.

No, I'm not contradicting myself. The fact is that grass is the most sprayed, the most dusted and the most chemically treated food on the face of the earth. They spray the grass along the waysides and roadways, in the fields and in the forests, and they dust it from the heavens with planes and they douse the leaves on the trees with powerful spray apparatus. So, with all those poisons on the world's best food, then it becomes the world's worst food . . . the most dangerous food.

O.K., I can see you writhing in agony . . . but don't feel too badly because I've been writhing in agony about this for a long time.

I consider one of the best foods that we have to be leaf lettuce — not the head lettuce — and the leaf lettuce or the grasses in general contain more surface, as you can understand, than any other type of plant or food, so when you eat a big leaf of lettuce that might contain a fraction of a calorie and some chlorophyll and some minerals and a wee bit of fat and a smidgin of carbohydrate, you get a whole tankful of spray. By comparison, when you eat a one inch cube of meat, you've probably got enough food there to last you a day, if need be, and it can't be sprayed. But it might contain some antibiotics and maybe some diethylstilbestrol . . . but only a bit considering the amount of nourishment you've got there.

In order to get the same amount of nourishment as is found

70

in that one inch cube of beef, you'd have to eat about two huge bunches of lettuce with enough spray and poison on them to destroy a regiment. So where do we go from here?

Yes, there is an answer and there is a way out . . . grow your own and be sure to eat your share of grass seeds, wheat, rye, barley, oats, corn, rice and others. Grass is like eating sunlight . . . what better can you eat? But don't ever lose sight of the fact that greens or grass are the world's best food items. And if you don't believe me, try it for a week or ten days or a month and that good health that was once yours many long years ago may come back like a spring freshet.

CHAPTER 14

VEGETARIANISM — THE RIGHT WAY OF LIFE

When I was a youth I knew some people here or there, but very few, who were vegetarians and they were thin and they didn't look very robust and I used to kid them or tease them sometimes unmercifully. But they were good natured, strange to relate, and they took my kidding and we remained friends or at least, we remained on speaking terms.

It took about 25 years from that point in my life to learn that vegetarianism wasn't just a way of life that nuts or lunatics or kooks accept but it had a sound scientific basis, apart from the moral viewpoint. So I began to look around, I began to dig and investigate, and vegetarianism began to appear sensible and logical. I continued my digging and my searching and lo and behold, it dawned upon me that there was something really worthwhile in vegetarianism . . . that it was the best way of life.

First and foremost, let me admit that the appeal of vegetarianism was strictly on the basis of logic and health. It had nothing whatsoever to do with the moral or the ethical viewpoints. These can be dealt with separately. I assure you that on moral or ethical grounds they have the whole affair tied up in a knot and no one can dispute it. But here I'm dealing with it primarily from the point of view of health.

From my many years of study of nutrition I gleaned that a human being could not remain healthy and live long on a strict vegetarian diet. Of course many vegetarians have attested to the fact that they could. But my studies did not reveal this to be a fact.

Also my reading tells me that many scientists today still boldly assert that a man cannot be healthy on a strict vegetarian diet. They claim there are certain amino acids and certain vitamins that he cannot derive from a vegetarian diet.

As I began to dig deeper and glean a bit of knowledge, I learned that these great scientific boys didn't know everything. I began to ask, for example, if a man can't live on vegetables alone, then how does a horse get along or a cow or an elephant? The answer always came back to the tune that these other animals had special digestive processes that allowed them to derive nutrients from the vegetables that man could not derive because of the difference in his anatomy or his digestive system.

At first I accepted this argument. But I continued to seek knowledge and more information appeared and then I found and proved that this was not true . . . that man's digestive system was capable of assimilating most if not all of the nutrients found in vegetable foods.

You may ask how come I found this out when all these great and wonderful scientists throughout the ages didn't find this out?

There is a simple answer to this and it's like the story of the bumble bee. "According to the aerodynamic engineering scientists a

74

bumble bee, because of its peculiar anatomical structure, because its wings are much too weak for its body, because of many other factors that nature did not take into account when creating the bumble bee, the bumble bee cannot fly . . . so the scientists tell us". But strange to relate, the bumble bee, not knowing anything about science or aerodynamics, flies anyway and he makes a darn good job of flying, too.

The same thing is true with vegetarians. The scientists tell you that a vegetarian can't live and be healthy but, shucks, man, there are millions of vegetarians all over the world and they live to be 60, 70, 80 and 90 years old. You see, they don't know anything about the story that science says they can't live and be healthy on only vegetable foods, and that's why they go on living anyway. Yet, strange to relate, they as a rule are much healthier and have a longer life span than meat eaters.

The secret of the situation, folks, is that back about 1928 a scientist by the name of Sumner of Cornell University isolated the first enzyme and we learned there and then that there was a substance in raw food that sort of took the food apart when you put it into your body and made its nutrients available to your whole body. But this substance or enzyme was destroyed by heat.

So the story is this . . . meat suffers less than vegetables from cooking. If you cook vegetables, they suffer, in most cases catastrophically, from heat. Therefore, the meat-eater, eating cooked meat, still gets most of whatever nutrients were in the meat. However, the vegetable-eater, when he eats cooked vegetables, gets very little of the nutrients, because of the destruction by heat.

There we have the big secret. Most scientists haven't yet got around to understanding the function of the enzyme in nutrition and that is why they haven't learned that one can live and be healthy or healthier on a vegetarian diet than he can on a meat diet that is cooked.

The raw food vegetarians are healthy and strong, with

75

tremendous powers of endurance, whereas a cooked food eating vegetarian is, comparatively speaking, the sorry sight that you know as a vegetarian.

Please, Mr. Vegetarian, don't be annoyed with me when I call you a sorry sight because most of your are sorry sights . . . that is, the processed food eating vegetarians.

I recall when I took some members of my staff to their first vegetarian meeting. They listened to a good lecture and at the end of the meeting they said, "Everything they say makes sense. We like the people, we like their way of life, but why do they all look so weak, so sickly and so puny?"

Believe me, this hasn't been asked of me once or twice but it's been asked of me so many times that I am tired of answering. My usual reply is that most people adopted vegetarianism and their way of life because they were sick to begin with on a meat diet, they were ailing or slowly dying. So you see this was the only way that they could save themselves from going to an early grave. They were sick, ailing and emaciated before they started on a vegetarian diet. So don't blame the good wholesome vegetables and the finest way of life for that.

I have said on many occasions, and I say it again, the vegetarian way of life is the finest, the healthiest and the most ethical way of life that exists on earth. Most of the vegetarians that I know – in fact, all of them that I know – are of a higher mental caliber, of a higher moral caliber and they are usually much healthier than their counterparts who are not vegetarians.

But please, vegetarians, don't rely upon cooked and highly processed vegetable foods to give you health, strength and long life because they won't. Learn to eat your vegetables raw and if possible, eat organically grown vegetables. Then you vegetarians, while you may be lighter of flesh than the others, will be much healthier, have much more stamina and be much better looking, too.

I had a great deal of respect for Mohandas K. Gandhi. He was one of the truly great men of his century and probably one of the truly great men of all time. But I'll let history in the future evaluate his qualifications. I just want to state here that I respected the man very, very much and hold his name in high esteem.

Of course you know that Gandhi was killed by an assassin, supposedly a mad assassin, and that cut short the life of a man who could have helped lead his country to a higher degree of greatness than it so far has achieved. The millions in India would have followed Gandhi or adopted his teachings much quicker than they would have those of any other man, of any generation in India.

Now whether or not you know this, Gandhi became a food nut just like Tobe and he sought to live the proper way without the use of animal products and he did it nobly. He tried and tried hard. But unfortunately he was just a wee bit ahead of his time. The nutritional knowledge that could have enabled him to succeed in his endeavour was not yet available . . . or should I say, had not yet reached his ears or his eyes. He tried to live entirely on vegetable food without the use of animal or milk products of any kind.

In any event, he got sick. His experiment didn't work and he was forced most reluctantly to admit, "On account of this and several similar experiences, I have been forced to admit the necessity of adding milk to the strict vegetarian diet. But I am convinced that in the vast vegetable kingdom there must be some kind, which, while supplying those necessary substances which we derive from milk and meat, is free from their drawbacks, ethical and other.

"In my opinion there are definite drawbacks in taking milk or meat. In order to get meat we have to kill. And we are certainly not entitled to any other milk except the mother's milk in our infancy."

Then he went on to say, "Now let us consider mixed diet. Man requires food which can supply tissue building substances to provide for the growth and daily wear and tear of the body. It should also contain something which can supply energy, fat, certain

77

salts and roughage to help the excretion of waste matter. Tissue building substances are known as proteins. They are obtained from milk, meat, eggs, pulses and nuts. The proteins contained in milk and meat, in other words, the animal proteins being more easily digestible and assimilable, are much more valuable than vegetable proteins. Milk is superior to meat. The medicos tell us that in cases where meat cannot be digested, milk is digested quite easily. For vegetarians milk, being the only source of animal proteins, is a very important article of diet. The proteins in raw eggs are considered to be the most easily digestible of all proteins."

To illustrate that Gandhi was not well informed on food and nutrition, it is a known fact today that no one is forced to admit the necessity of adding milk to a strict vegetarian diet. There are ample products for food in the vegetable kingdom which are more nutritious than milk and supply all of the required nutrients in the form of amino acids, to nourish and keep the human body in perfect health.

Now when Gandhi said, " . . . the animal proteins being more easily digestible and assimilable, are much more valuable than vegetable proteins," he made a terrific, terrible, horrible blunder. In the first place, the proteins in milk and meat or animal proteins are definitely not more easily digestible and most emphatically and positively they are not more assimilable. And even in stronger terms I would say that they are definitely not "much more valuable than vegetable proteins."

You see, today there is ample positive scientific proof, based on research projects, that vegetable proteins are not inferior but are definitely superior. They are not less assimilable but more assimilable. They are not less digestible but more digestible.

Now I did not write this article to discredit Gandhi. I am just pointing out that while Gandhi was a great man, he did not know the truth at that time. And I regret this on many counts. Few people at that time, if any, knew the whole story. But Gandhi was a brave man and he made the experiment in spite of the fact that he did not have the knowledge. He made it possible for us to have the knowledge. He at least tried and risked his life in so doing because he did become very, very ill.

Today any person who wishes to follow a strict vegetarian diet, for moral, aesthetic or health reasons, can do so with full confidence that he is not depriving his body of anything but is in fact giving his body the finest, the most nourishing, the most valuable and the very best food on earth.

I wish to emphasize boldly and unmistakably that one of Gandhi's greatest errors was the fact that he did not eat all of his food raw. However, very few people realized in those days that it was in the heating that most of the valuable nutrients were harmed, lost or destroyed. No one knew then that raw leafy vegetables and grains were the perfect diet and good, tasty and succulent fruits would provide dessert or candy.

So let it be remembered — it is scientifically proven — that neither meat, fish, milk nor dairy products of any kind are essential to maintain the body in good health and fitness. In fact, it is positively true that the body can be kept in the best possible condition only on a diet that omits meat, fish, milk and all other dairy products.

CHAPTER

15

GUIDEPOSTS FROM THE BIBLE

Today we are going to have a bible lesson. Get out your bible and turn to Daniel. Now please understand I'm not a bible student and I'm not religious and I don't intend to force the bible down your throat but I want to just bring home a very clear point to you and this happens to be my way of doing it. Assuming you are not a believer in the bible and that you think it's all bosh and hooey, let me first state that practically all of the incidents and facts mentioned in the chapter of Daniel which took place approximately 2600 years ago have been verified by archaeologists. Now if the archaeologists verify all of the things mentioned in the book of Daniel referring to that period of history and conclusively prove them to be true then you must be broad enough to admit that the facts that I am going to bring to your attention from this chapter of the bible can also be true and this deals with the eating of proper food.

So we read chapter 1, vs. 5. "And the King appointed them a daily provision of the King's meat and of the wine which he drank so nourishing them three years that at the end thereof they might stand before the King". Then in vs. 8 we read, "But Daniel purposed in his heart that he would not defile himself with a portion of the King's meat nor with the wine which he drank; therefore he requested of the prince of the eunuchs that he might not defile himself". In vs. 10, "And the prince of the eunuchs said unto Daniel, I fear my lord the king, who hath appointed your meat and your drink: for why should he see your faces worse liking than the children which are of your sort then shall ye make me endanger my head to the king". Vs. 11-17, "Then said Daniel to Melzar whom the prince of the eunuchs had set over Daniel, Hananiah, Mishael, and Azariah, Prove thy servants, I beseech thee, ten days; and let them give us pulse to eat, and water to drink. Then let our countenances be looked upon before thee, and the countenance of the children that eat of the portion of the king's meat: and as thou seest, deal with they servants. So he consented to them in this matter, and proved them ten days.

"And at the end of ten days their countenances appeared fairer and fatter in flesh than all the children which did eat the portion of the king's meat. Thus Melzar took away the portion of their meat, and the wine that they should drink; and gave them pulse. As for these four children, God gave them knowledge and skill in all learning and wisdom: and Daniel had understanding in all visions and dreams."

The point I am making here is that here Daniel ate only pulses which means beans and peas and greens of all kinds and they grew healthy and looked good and were strong and above all things they were mentally brilliant on this diet because they were the greatest, wisest, most handsome and most brilliant in the land. If you would read further as to what Daniel achieved then you might get a glimpse of what you can do for yourself by eating pulses or as I say a raw vegetable, grain and fruit diet. Now I don't care whether or not you believe in the bible. It would be better if you did but it is not necessary. You can be the biggest heathen or the biggest agnostic or free thinker on earth and that is your right and your privilege and I

DANIEL

1 In the third year of the kingship of Je·hoi′a·kim the king of Judah, Neb·u·chad·nez′zar the king of Babylon came to Jerusalem and proceeded to lay siege to it. 2 In time Jehovah gave into his hand Je·hoi′a·kim the king of Judah and a part of the utensils of the house of the [true] God, so that he brought them to the land of Shi′nar to the house of his god; and the utensils he brought to the treasure house of his god. 3 Then the king said to Ash′pe·naz his chief court-official to bring some of the sons of Israel and of the royal offspring and of the nobles, 4 children in whom there was no defect at all, but good in appearance and having insight into all wisdom and being acquainted with knowledge, and having discernment of what is known, in whom also there was ability to stand in the palace of the king; and to teach them the writing and the tongue of the Chal·de′ans. 5 Furthermore, to them the king appointed a daily allowance from the delicacies of the king and from his drinking wine, even to nourish them for three years, that at the end of these they might stand before the king. 6 Now there happened to be among them some of the sons of Judah, Daniel, Han·a·ni′ah, Mish′a·el and Az·a·ri′ah. 7 And to them the principal court-official went assigning names. So he assigned to Daniel [the name of] Bel·te·shaz′zar; and to Han·a·ni′ah, Sha′drach; and to Mish′a·el, Me′shach; and to Az·a·ri′ah, A·bed′ne·go. 8 But Daniel determined in his heart that he would not pollute himself with the delicacies of the king and with his drinking wine. And he kept requesting of the principal court-official that he might not pollute himself. 9 Accordingly the [true] God gave Daniel over to loving-kindness and to mercy before the principal court-official. 10 So the principal court-official said to Daniel: "I am in fear of my lord the king, who has appointed YOUR food and YOUR drink. Why, then, should he see YOUR faces dejected-looking in comparison with the children who are of the same age as YOURS, and [why] should YOU have to make my head guilty to the king?" 11 But Daniel said to the guardian whom the principal court-official had appointed over Daniel, Han·a·ni′ah, Mish′a·el and Az·a·ri′ah: 12 "Please, put your servants to the test for ten days, and let them give us some vegetables that we may eat and water that we may drink; 13 and let our countenances and the countenance of the children who are eating the delicacies of the king appear before you, and according to what you see do with your servants."

14 Finally he listened to them as regards this matter and to put them to the test for ten days. 15 And at the end of ten days their countenances appeared better and fatter in flesh than all the children who were eating the delicacies of the king. 16 So the guardian kept on taking away their delicacies and their drinking wine and giving them vegetables. 17 And as for these children, the four of them, to them the [true] God gave knowledge and insight in all writing and wisdom; and Daniel himself had understanding in all sorts of visions and dreams.

18 And at the end of the days

won't take it away from you but facts are facts and truth is truth and there you have it. Pulses . . . vegetables are the best food for man and it was known 2600 years ago.

But still assuming a few of you might by accident believe in the bible I want you to turn to Leviticus, chapter 3, vs. 17 and read, "It shall be a perpetual statute for your generations throughout all your dwellings, that ye eat neither fat nor blood." Please also now take a look at Leviticus 7, vs 23: "Ye shall eat no manner of fat, of ox, or of sheep, or of goat."

Please bear in mind that Leviticus was written almost 3500 years ago, 1490 years before Christ. Within the last decade or two science and medical men have discovered that fats, animal fats specifically, are one of the main causes of heart disease. I believe it is fairly clearly established that if human beings did not consume any animal fats whatsoever there would be no heart disease. No one would die of a heart attack and if you will refer to your statistics you will learn that right at this time 54% of all deaths in America are caused by heart attacks. Now catch the significance here . . . if we had any common sense and followed the laws taught us in Leviticus and what Daniel taught us, between 54% of all the deaths, premature deaths, deaths before their time could be avoided.

Hold now — before you call me a madman or say I'm off my rocker I'm asking you to examine the proof that I've offered you. Here we have Leviticus in the bible telling us not to eat any kind of animal fat whatsoever. In fact, prohibiting its use in any Jewish household and they don't care whether it's from a goat or a sheep or an ox. Animal fat is prohibited. I would humbly suggest that this is the greatest health knowledge ever presented to man and he has chosen to ignore it, to mock it, to ridicule it. So the price we pay is untimely death. If you want to live long the first step is to follow the proven principles laid down here from the bible.

CHAPTER 16

I DARE TO QUESTION

I dare to criticize the Bible. First let me clarify. I am a believer, a firm believer of Jehovah and His great universe. I accept and I read and study the Bible. However, I complain bitterly that the Bible has let mankind down. There is insufficient information on food and diet in the Bible and as a result mankind suffers untold miseries. I realize that too few of us follow the admonitions in the Bible and we would no better follow any other counsel that the Bible might have given . . . still I feel something is wrong when the world's greatest work, the Bible, does not tell us to eat raw vegetables, grains and fruit.

Leviticus 3:17 — "It shall be a perpetual statute for your generations throughout all your dwellings, that ye eat neither fat nor blood." Nothing could be more explicit, but these positive taboos are almost totally ignored. I have never known a vegetarian Rabbi. How can any person who believes in the Bible justify the eating of fat?

There is no mention anywhere in the Bible concerning the evils of cooked food and the benefits of uncooked natural food. The Bible does lay down dietary laws governing the kinds of animals and fish . . . also, dairy products and flesh foods. It also specifies how meat is to be treated before eating. There are certain religious groups today who do stress the merit of food in their way of life — the Mormons, the Seventh Day Adventists, Jehovah Witnesses, Buddhists and Moslems.

The immunity that the Jews have acquired through almost 6,000 years of following the dietary laws in Leviticus are now being violated because the Rabbis are either asleep on the job or have sold out to the chemical and food processing interests. I make this charge clearly that the Jewish people have been betrayed by their leaders and they are suffering the consequences. I believe the Jews have today the highest rate of cancer of any people, besides an abnormally high incidence of diabetes and heart disease. This would not be so if their leaders directed them according to the laws of Moses.

Leviticus 7:23 — "Ye shall eat no manner of fat, of ox, or of sheep, or of goat."

The Hebraic law furthermore was iron-clad in its strictness, in its prohibition of cruelty to animals. Therefore, no animal that is treated the way animals are treated today could ever become food for the Jewish people if the laws laid down by Moses were enforced. According to the law even the beasts of burden were to be free on the hallowed Sabbath, not incarcerated and manicled any day let alone seven days and nights of the week.

Let me quote from Corinthians 9: 9. "Doth God take care for oxen" and Timothy 1: 5, 18. "And the laborer is worthy of his reward". Deuteronomy 25: 4 "Thou shalt not muzzle the ox when he treadeth out the corn. 22: 10 — "Thou shalt not plow with an ox and an ass together". 22: 4 — "Thou shalt not see thy brother's ass or his ox fall down by the way".

The way our food animals are treated today is an adomination in the eyes and the sight of the Lord. Therefore, the animals cannot be fit food for man.

When Adam lived in the Garden of Eden he ate raw food. Methusalah lived to be 969 years, Jared 962 years, Noah 950 years, Adam 930 years, Seth 912 years, Cainan 910 years, Enos 905 years, Mahalaleel 895 years, Lamech 777 years. Man was kicked out of the Garden of Eden for disobedience and after the flood he began to cook his food and then his lifespan dropped to 120. Well, he wasn't happy with his cooked food or vegetables so he wanted meat and when he added meat to his diet his lifespan dropped to 70 and according to statistics today his lifespan is now dropping below 70, even though the statisticians in America tell us life expectancy is somewhere around 71. But the figures in the obituary columns and the years on the stones in the cemetery tell me that the average man does not live to be 70 and beyond.

I advise man to go back to eating the way he did in the Garden of Eden. Life will be pleasanter and longer.

CHAPTER 17

THE BENEFITS OF A RAW FOOD DIET

Does this sound most unappetizing and perhaps uncivilized?

Frankly, I am bold and honest enough, even if unwise, to admit that the idea of eating only raw food as my means of sustenance does not strongly appeal to my gastronomical tastes. I am a cooked food eater from 'way back.

The only raw food ever eaten in my home when I was a lad was an apple and rarely a banana or an orange. Oh, yes, I must admit that come the festive season we did get a few nuts. And I must also admit that we did eat raw onions fairly regularly. I'm trying hard to think of any other raw foods that we ate at home but I'm afraid that was the sum and substance and the extent of our raw food diet in my early childhood.

Then a little later, when my sister became old enough to go out and earn a living, she used to add radishes, lettuce, cucumbers, celery and some tomatoes to our raw food regimen. By then I was about 10 or 11 years old. So you can gather from what I am telling you that raw food eating was certainly not part of my way of life.

The first man who gave me a talking-to about raw food caused me great dismay and frankly I thought that he was completely out of his mind. When he said he ate only raw food, I felt that I had heard the heighth of some or other stupidity. And when he left, I thought to myself, "Man, oh, man, how crazy can a man get?"

However, he had flicked a switch in my brain and the darn thing bothered me and it kept coming back and it kept coming back and I kept saying to myself, "But he is a fairly intelligent man. But raw food only! Nothing cooked, nothing baked, nothing fried and nothing steamed! Aw, the guy must be nuts!"

It hounded me, it annoyed me and it worried me. I guess it had struck a vibrant chord somewhere and I couldn't rest and I had to dig and dig and dig and investigate.

When the truth began to dawn upon me, it brought graver dismay than ever to me . . . because I was an epicurean hog. I knew only the delight of cooked foods. Sure, an apple or a pear or some other nice fruit was very delicious, but only as an adjunct to a good cooked meal.

Well, it tortured me then as it's torturing me today. I was appalled to think that I must give up all those cooked delicacies that I knew . . . Italian cookery, Jewish cookery, Greek, Hungarian, yes, Polish, Japanese and Chinese cookery, too. Man, those are marvelous foods . . . that's living! And I'm supposed to live on raw salads, raw fish, raw carrots, raw parsnips, raw turnips and the like. What are you saying?

That's the way it happened, friends. I could hardly believe my ears. I didn't want to accept it. I hated to accept it. But there was the conclusive, undeniable proof in my hands, from the best scientific sources on earth. Aw, man, I'm ruined!

So today I still eat some cooked foods but as much as I enjoy them, I look upon them as my deadly enemies . . . and so they are my deadly enemies and yours too. By raw food I mean vegetables, grains, fruits without treatment or processing of any kind or sort. You can also eat raw meat, fish, eggs and dairy products. A little experimenting will prove these can be made not only palatable but delicious.

Unfortunately I have to challenge the world. I maintain in clear-cut, terse language that no food for a human being or an animal was ever improved nutritionally by cooking or heating.

Most scientists do and will continue to attempt to disprove what I have said. In fact, I can show you a great deal of proof that claims that I am wrong . . . that is, scientists who maintain that certain foods are made more nutritional by cooking or treating. But even if they have proof, I maintain that their proof is wrong, in error or a deliberate lie. I will stand and fight to the death the statement by anyone that any food is improved nutritionally by heating or treating. Remember, I am fighting the most renowned nutritionists in America and the world with degrees from America and the world's greatest Universities, like Harvard no less.

Now in most cases I can prove conclusively to anyone's satisfaction that most foods lose nutritional value in the heating or cooking and my proof would be the United States Government's Handbook No. 8 and anyone can buy it for a couple of dollars. They give the nutrient values of cooked and raw foods. I am giving you the above reference in case you need proof. I have long recognized the merit of the raw food diet . . . I don't need statistical proof.

So even though a few claim that certain foods are nutritionally enhanced by cooking, I say I don't care who says it or who doesn't say it, I stand four-square and will live or die by the statement, "No food is improved nutritionally by cooking, heating or processing!"

I realize that some of the things I say here are repetitious but I don't think I can be too repetitious in this instance because the health and the very lives of humanity rise and fall on the basis of this thesis.

No scientist has ever attempted to bring enzymes into the raw food picture but I use the enzyme factor as my trump card and I couch it in the simplest language at my command, to illustrate scientific proof. When you eat cooked food the nutrients or the components in that food are rendered inactive. Therefore, if your body wants the calcium or the phosphorous or the magnesium or the iron or any one of the other elements, it must go to work and remove it from the food and assimilate it so that it can become cells or tissue.

On the other hand, when you eat raw food, the whole structure of the food has been unimpaired. It is left in its original state and when you put it into your mouth and then let it pass down into your stomach, the structure is of no concern to the body and the body doesn't have to do the breaking down. From the stomach it passes into the intestines and then into the blood stream and all of the elements are automatically picked up by means of the blood stream and allotted to the various tissues and organs for cellular structure and regeneration.

A simple analogy would be an automobile assembly line. The parts come down the line and a team of men stand by to pick up each component part as it comes along and fit it into its proper place to eventually build the finished automobile. This is the cooked food way.

In the raw food way, the parts come down the assembly line and there is no team of men to put each part in its proper place . . . it is all done automatically, for it is done inherently by nature.

By cooking you impede the progress and the functions of nature. With raw food you allow nature to perform the function that it was intended to perform.

To more positively implant in your mind the tremendous superiority of raw food over cooked food and at the same time clinch the argument with undisputable scientific proof, I offer you the Kouchakoff experiment. I'll give you this experiment in complete detail so that when some Doubting Thomas tells you that you are nuts, just as they have told me for years, then you can throw this at them and let them argue with Kouchakoff.

THE INFLUENCE OF FOOD COOKING ON THE
BLOOD FORMULA OF MAN
by
Paul Kouchakoff (Suisse), M.D.
of the
Institute of Clinical Chemistry, Lausanne, Switzerland
PROCEEDINGS: FIRST INTERNATIONAL CONGRESS
OF MICROBIOLOGY, PARIS, 1930
Translation by Lee Foundation for Nutritional Research,
Milwaukee 1, Wisconsin

The living organism is very sensitive to all harmful influences and reacts against them immediately.

We see this when we make an analysis of our blood during simple and infectious illnesses, when extraneous substances are introduced into our system, etc.

In such cases the number of white corpuscles changes and the correlation of percentage between them is disturbed. This is one of the indications of a pathological process going on in our system.

After every dose of food, we also observe a general augmentation of white corpuscles, and a change in the correlation of their percentage. This phenomenon has been considered, until now, a physiological one, and is called a digestive leukocytosis.

93

We use, for our food, raw foodstuffs, foodstuffs which have been altered by means of high temperature, and manufactured foodstuffs. How then does each one of these foodstuffs separately act on our blood formula?

We find that, after taking raw foodstuffs, neither the number of white corpuscles nor the correlation of their percentage has changed. Ordinary unboiled drinking water, mineral water, salt, different green foodstuffs, cereals, nuts, honey, raw eggs, raw meat, raw fish, fresh milk, sour milk, butter — in other words, foodstuffs in the state in which they exist in nature, belong to the group of those which do not call forth any infringement in our blood formula.

After the consumption of the same natural foodstuffs, altered by means of high temperature, we find that the general number of white corpuscles has changed, but the correlation of their percentage has remained the same.

After consumption of manufactured foodstuffs not only has the number of white corpuscles changed but also the correlation of percentage between them.

To this group belong sugar, wine, chocolate in tablet form, etc.

All our experiments have shown that it is not the quantity, but the quality of food which plays an important role in the alteration of our blood formula, and that 200 milligrams or even 50 milligrams of foodstuffs produce the same reaction as large doses of them. The experiments also show that the reaction in our blood takes place at the moment the food enters the stomach, while the preliminary mastication of food in the mouth softens the reaction.

We have already said that raw foodstuffs, altered by means of high temperature only call forth an augmentation of the general number of white corpuscles.

Does this occur only when such foodstuffs are heated to

boiling point, or is the same phenomenon called forth by lower temperatures?

It appears that every raw foodstuff has its own temperature which must not be surpassed in heating, otherwise it loses its original virtues and calls forth a reaction in the system.

Ordinary drinking water, heated for half an hour to a temperature of 87 degrees (C.) does not change our blood, but this same water heated to 88 degrees (C.) changes it.

We have given the name "critical temperature" to the highest degree of temperature at which a particular foodstuff can be cooked for half an hour in bain marie, and eaten, without changing our blood formula.

This critical temperature is not the same for all raw foodstuffs. It varies within a range of ten degrees. The lowest critical temperature for water is 87 degrees; for milk it is 88 degrees; for cereals, tomatoes, cabbage, bananas, 89 degrees; for pears, meat, 90 degrees; for butter, 91 degrees; for apples and oranges, 92 degrees; for potatoes, 93 degrees; for carrots, strawberries and figs, 97 degrees. (See conclusion for conversion to Fahrenheit)

Our experiments show that it is possible to paralyze the action of a foodstuff, once its critical temperature is surpassed. There exist strictly definite laws for this, and the critical temperature plays the first role here.

If a cooked foodstuff is eaten along with the same product in a raw state there is no reaction.

The raw product has neutralized the action which this same product, with its critical temperature surpassed, would have called forth. In other words, the raw product has, so to say, re-established the virtues of the product altered by high temperature. Such a re-establishment is also possible when two different products have been absorbed, but with one condition; their critical temperature must either be the same, or else the critical temperature of the raw product must be higher than the critical temperature of the overheated one.

If the critical temperature of a raw product is lower than that of the overheated one, the reaction is sure to take place; in this case, even the augmentation of the quantity of the raw products does not help.

This law remains the same when the raw product is mixed with several overheated ones of the same critical temperature.

If several cooked foodstuffs are taken, each with a different critical temperature, along with raw food, reaction takes place, even if the raw product has a higher critical temperature than that of any of the cooked foodstuffs.

Now we pass on to the 3rd group of foodstuffs, such as sugar, wine, etc. obtained by complicated manufacturing processes, and producing double reaction in our organism. These products may also be consumed without calling forth any reaction, but only when they are introduced into our organism conjointly with no less than two raw foodstuffs of a different critical temperature. Even one raw product has a beneficial influence on this 3rd group, and deprives them of one of their properties, namely the power of altering the correlation of percentage of the white corpuscles.

As regards the proportions in which raw products must be added to cooked foods, there is an irreducible minimum. For water, for example, it is 50%.

CONCLUSIONS

After over 300 experiments on ten individuals of different age and sex, we have come to the following conclusions:

1. The augmentation of the number of white corpuscles and the alteration of the correlation of the percentage between them

which takes place after every consumption of food, and which was considered until now as a physiological phenomenon, is, in reality, a pathological one. It is called forth by the introduction into the system of foodstuffs altered by means of high temperature, and by complicated treatments of ordinary products produced by nature.

2. *After the consumption of fresh raw foodstuffs, produced by nature, our blood formula does not change in any lapse of time, nor in consequence of any combinations.*

3. *After the consumption of foodstuffs produced by nature, but altered by means of high temperature, an augmentation of the general number of white corpuscles takes place, but the correlation of percentage between them remains the same.*

4. *After the consumption of foodstuffs produced by nature, but altered by manufacturing processes, an augmentation of the general number of white corpuscles as well as a change in the correlation of their percentage takes place.*

5. *It has been proved possible to take, without changing the blood formula, every kind of foodstuff which is habitually eaten now, but only by following this rule, viz: — that it must be taken along with raw products, according to a definite formula.*

6. *In a healthy organism, it is not possible, by the consumption of any food to alter the correlation of percentage between the white corpuscles, without augmenting their general number.*

7. *Foodstuffs do not seem to have any influence on the transitional and the Polymorphonuclear Eosinophiles and the correlation of percentage between them is not altered.*

8. *We can change our blood formula in the direction we desire by dieting accordingly.*

9. Blood examination can only have significance as a diagnosis if it is made on an empty stomach.

FOOD	CRITICAL TEMPERATURE
Drinking water	191 degrees F.
Milk	191 degrees F.
Cereals	192 degrees F.
Tomatoes	192 degrees F.
Cabbage	192 degrees F.
Bananas	192 degrees F.
Butter	196 degrees F.
Apples	197 degrees F.
Oranges	197 degrees F.
Potatoes	200 degrees F.
Carrots	206 degrees F.
Strawberries	206 degrees F.
Figs	206 degrees F.

I don't know how many experiments — that is, scientific experiments — are conducted annually but they run into the tens of thousands. Through the years the only positive experiments on the merits of raw food, to the best of my knowledge, are the Kouchakoff experiments and the one by Dr. Francis C. Pottenger, Jr. with his cats. ("The Effect of Heat — Processed Foods and Metabolized Vitamin D Milk On The Dentofacial Structures of Experimental Animals, Francis M. Pottenger Jr., M.D., F.A.C.P. Reprinted from American Journal of Orthodontics and Oral Surgery, St. Louis, Vol 32, No. 8, Oral Surgery, Pages 467-485, August, 1946).

The reason these experiments are so scarce or practically non-existent is simple. The greatest contributors to research in America are the food processors, the chemical corporations, the drug companies and industry. None of these groups can profit from raw food experiments or establishing that raw food is superior to cooked food. In fact, to the contrary, they benefit only if they can keep this truth well buried or hidden.

I do not know of one experiment ever conducted at the universities that sought to establish the pros and cons or the merits of cooked food as compared to raw food. And of course the reason again is quite clear. Any researcher would understand that the chances are he would come up with the same conclusions as Pottenger and Kouchakoff.

Where there is no one to benefit then obviously the work will not be done. It takes money today — real money — to conduct a scientific experiment of any duration and to make the experiment valid and acceptable it would have to be conducted over a period of at least a couple of years. And this, as I said before, costs real money and unless someone has an angle or a profit factor in mind he would not invest in this experiment. And as no one except the general public stands to benefit from such an experiment, it won't be done . . . unless the general public pays for it.

In truth, the government should sponsor such an experiment, but who is our government? The people? Of course not! The government is the moneyed interests, I'm ashamed to admit, and they will permit no such experiments at the expense of the public treasury.

Understandably, that would explain why there are no experiments to prove the superiority of raw foods over cooked or processed foods.

CHAPTER 18

THE ENZYME STORY

The Bible says the days of a man shall be three score and ten. But elsewhere it says that the days were 120 years. Methuselah lived to be 969 years and Adam, Noah, Seth and others lived to ripe old ages.

Well, I'm not satisfied with the three score and ten (I'll be lucky if I make it!). I want four score and maybe five score. At least I'm going to try to make it.

Now I feel absolutely confident that I could have made 100 had I known about the proper way of life years ago. I curse — yes, I mean curse — the people, the organizations and the governments that deprived me of the knowledge that would have made it possible for me to reach 100 years or more in good health and well-being. I have been denied that opportunity by a government that let me down, as it is letting down the millions of people today. Corruption, bribery and lobbying are cutting down the life span of the people of America.

Oh, yes, I know that they have shown statistics that our life span has been increased but that's another story. If you want to argue that point, I'm willing to argue or debate it with you any place in the world. Our life span has not been increased but it has been decreased.

I will admit that up until 30 years ago or so it was only by luck that a man reached three score and ten and beyond, but with the knowledge that we have today everyone should live to be more than three score and ten. Now this may sound like the blandishments of a blithering idiot, which is me, but I'm telling you that what I say is true. Any Tom, Dick and Harry can live to be 70, 80 and 90 years of age if they are taught the principles of life and living.

I can hear you saying, "Well, Tobe, if you're so smart, how come the whole wide world through all these eons of time didn't learn the secret? Who are you that this secret was given to you? How come you alone know how to get men to live to be 80, 90 and 100 years of age and you can guarantee this to the whole population?"

I agree, those are good questions, chum. But the fact is that until a man by the name of James B. Sumner isolated the enzyme in 1926 it was never known or understood that a man could live indefinitely. He isolated the enzyme, Urease, in microscopic crystalline form. He was a true pioneer in the field of enzymes. I am trying to convey to you the message that when we first learned about the enzyme — that is, it was isolated and that enzymes were destroyed at 120 degrees and higher — it was then that the secret of long life and health was out and every school child had an opportunity to hear about it and learn about it.

I only heard about this less than 15 years ago and I wrote the first book about enzymes by a layman. Many others have been written since but I demonstrated in my book about enzymes, just exactly what enzymes meant in the health and longevity of man. In the simplest terms that I can master the knowledge of enzymes told me that the only proper food for mankind was food that was not heated or treated, because if you kill, harm or destroy the enzymes you are destroying your chance at health and long life. This meant giving up boiling, stewing, baking, frying, roasting, and going back to eating the fruits and vegetables as nature provided them.

Please understand me and please listen to me . . . I don't hate cooked foods, I don't hate processed foods, but it's just that there is positive, absolute and undeniable proof that all food is harmed by cooking and processing. So you can understand what I am trying to tell you. Your very life depends on enzymes.

I have nothing to sell you. I am not trying to sell you packages of enzymes and make money on you. I am only selling knowledge to you. I am trying to get it through your thick skull.

O.K., you've heard my story so let's for a moment go back to the Garden of Eden where it all started. Now I don't care whether you're a believer or a non-believer . . . we're going back to the Garden of Eden anyway, even if it is only an imaginary trip.

There in the Garden man had his choice of all the finest vegetables, fruits, grains and nuts on earth . . . all there for the picking. But man wasn't satisfied with that, he started to cook his food, for reasons that have never been established, and when he cooked it of course he ruined not only his food but his health. Man didn't have to be kicked out of the Garden of Eden . . . he loused it up so badly there was no use staying there any longer.

You know, that old Bible is quite a document. I maintain that somewhere along the line there was someone who knew the truth about that allegorical incident and they said that Adam and Eve ate of the forbidden apple. Well, it wasn't the forbidden apple . . . it was the forbidden cooking. Man lost everything when he learned to cook his food. The apple and fig leaf story sounds much more romantic and acceptable.

103

So thousands of years elapsed before the error was discovered and it was only with the advent of the isolation of the enzyme that the reason became apparent. Up until then we had been taught, we had been led to believe that cooking was the proper thing and that food was improved nutritionally and culinarily by all the various heating processes, whereas the truth is that we destroy most of its value and we pay for it in the ill health that follows.

I maintain it was when man started to cook his food he discovered it was inadequate and then he sought meat. But while meat was satisfying it caused many diseases and that's when his life span dropped down to 70.

It is my belief that man on the average never lived to be 70. Most died before then. It was only the one of many who got to 70 . . . that was the goal to hope for.

Nevertheless, my story is that you cannot have good health and long life on anything else but raw food. Oh, yes, there are many who limp along, with aches and pains and suffering, to reach their three score and ten but anyone can reach it and well beyond easily on a raw food diet.

How long will it take mankind to wake up?

CHAPTER 19

AMINO ACIDS

As soon as anyone begins to get interested in nutrition, he begins to use words like proteins, carbohydrates, fats, calories, essential amino acids, non-essential amino acids, enzymes and so on. I used to be greatly impressed when individuals, nutritionists and medical men started throwing these 25c words at me. But after close to twenty years of intensive studies on health, I have reached the conclusion that these words are not only meaningless but actually lead you off the track.

Seldom does a day go by that I do not gorge myself on scientific literature concerning health and nutrition, chemistry, biochemistry, physiology, pathology and other scientific and pseudo-scientific literature. And my conclusion is that all these big-wigs and experts and big-shots, scientists, nutritionists and biochemists, when they start talking about nutrition, are plainly talking mumbo-jumbo and they are showing their deep profound ignorance. Now this goes for men who have their B.A.'s, B.Sc.'s, M.Sc's, D.Sc.'s or Ph.D's. I know men who have all of these qualifications, from accredited universities from various parts of the world, and I've never yet met one of them who actually talked sense or should I say, knew what he was talking about.

O.K., wise guy, now ask me if I know what I am talking about and I'll answer, "When it comes to nutrition and health, no living man knows what he is talking about. It's just that some know less than others and others think they know more than they know."

I have heard nutritionists on the radio, on the television and I have heard them lecture in many places and I have also frequently engaged them in conversation . . . and every statement that I have made above is absolutely true. Yes, this goes for all those vaunted authorities whose books are widely circulated throughout the English-speaking world. I would also state that I am personally acquainted with most of them and they're all good, decent people. They are knowledgable people, they are mostly intelligent people, but when they talk about nutrition and health, they don't know what they are talking about.

Now I know what you're thinking and that is, "If Tobe claims nobody knows what he is talking about, why is *he* doing so much talking?"

So listen to me and I'll try to explain myself as clearly and as quickly as possible.

The modern knowledge of nutrition in America was started in the 1880's by a researcher known as W. O. Atwater. It was followed by such authorities as Thos. B. Osborn and L. B. Mendel, Carl Voigt, G. Bunge, I. P. Pavlov, Casimir Funk, Wm C. Rose, R. H. Chittenden, E. V. McCollum, H. C. Sherman, Max Rubner, C. A. Pekelharing, Emil Abderhalden, C. Eijkman, J. C. Drummond and many others . . . but these are the ones whose experiments and writings I have studied. All of these men were good scientists and as far as I

106

know, but I am not sure, none of them did their work for any of the chemical companies or for feed and food corporations . . . they did it for science. Only on rare occasions did one scientist re-do the experiments of the other. That is, most of them accepted without question or investigation the work done by their predecessors.

I did notice that some of the researchers struggled to establish the merits of certain foods and this work I recognize as being supported by some food processor or dollar interested party. So you see even back at the turn of the century research was "rigged".

Here I want to make a few shocking or revealing statements . . .

Did you know that practically all of the knowledge that we have gained about nutrition is based upon studies with rats and dogs? The whole story of nutrition is based on the rate of growth of rats fed on special foods. The experimenters fed them amino acids derived or crystallized from casein. When the rats grew normally, they considered that optimum. So they removed certain items and added others and when the rats didn't grow normally, they assumed these amino acids were essential. And the ones that didn't affect their growth were considered non-essential.

Pavlov did his work with dogs and our knowledge of the gastro-intestinal system of man is based mainly upon Pavlov and the controlled reflexes of the dogs that he worked with.

However, there was one experiment that dealt with a human being and it was an accidental one. A trapper by the name of Alexis St. Martin was accidentally shot in the stomach and evidently they couldn't perform surgery that was required to close up the wound so a Dr. Wm. Beaumont who was called to the scene worked out a deal with Alexis whereby he would sort of put a window in the man's stomach so he could watch what went on. He also took fragments of meat and other foods and put them on the end of a string and dipped them into his stomach through the hole and extracted them . . . and oh, he did a lot of things.

107

From the studies of Atwater and Mendel and Osborn and from Pavlov on the dogs and with Beaumont on Alexis St. Martin and a few others, we have the complete foundation of the whole study of nutrition as it is accepted and believed throughout the scientific world. There are so many inaccuracies, and there are so many stupidities and blunders, that one could write ten volumes describing them . . . yet everything they said and did is accepted as sacred by all of the nutritionists throughout the world.

Now I want to emphasize that the rats, on which everything is based, never ever were fed proper food for a rat, whatever that may be . . . cheese, meat or grains. They were fed fractions of casein which isn't even milk . . . it's a substance made from milk.

I'm probably the only man in the world interested in health and nutrition who refuses to abide by and accept the work of these researchers on rats, dogs and a hole in a man's stomach as the bedrock of my nutritional knowledge.

Here while we're being anti-establishment, let me cite another instance . . .

First let me tell you that I am a nurseryman by profession and have been actively engaged in this pursuit for over 40 years. I'm telling you this so you will understand that I do know a little bit about plants and trees and agriculture.

Early in my career I learned most emphatically and definitely that the scientists regarded corn as a much superior grain to oats and that oats were considered superior to wheat. Well, I'd had a very wide association with these three vital grains of mankind and I couldn't readily accept the fact that corn was the king-pin. I did hear that corn would fatten hogs quicker than oats or wheat but I was somewhat reluctant to buy the bill of goods that it was so far superior to both of these other grains.

When I questioned the superiority of one over the other, I was quickly put in place by this authority who said, "McCollum positively proved the superiority of corn in an experiment with cattle." Then he went on to tell me the story that one group of cattle was fed corn and another was fed oats and another was fed wheat. The ones on the wheat didn't do very well at all. They were sickly, they were ill-kempt and they couldn't give birth to their young alive. The ones on the oats did much better but they didn't look as good as the ones on the corn. They gave birth to their young alive but they were not as sleek and as fat and as active as the ones on the corn.

This practically drove me up a wall because it was contrary to what my lifetime with nature had taught me and I just couldn't buy that bill of goods. So after it had been shoved down my throat about fifty times I became annoyed and I resolved to get a copy of the research experiment conducted by McCollum and read every detail for myself . . . and that's precisely what I did.

What did I find? That the animals on the wheat were fed the wheat from the field, along with the wheat straw. The cattle on oats were fed the oats from the field, along with the oat straw. The cattle on the corn were fed the corn from the field, along with the corn stalks. Now I don't know whether or not you have caught the point but if you have ever been on a farm or know anything about a farm, you'd quickly recognize that wheat straw is inedible, oat straw is barely edible and animals will eat it if they don't have other things to eat but corn stalks — man, oh, man — that's food! Yes, green corn stalks are real food! So the combination of the corn stalks and the corn really hit the gong.

So you see, it wasn't the fact that the corn was superior to the oats and the wheat . . . it was the fact that those wonderful, big, husky, green and delicious corn leaves and stalks went along with the corn.

Isn't it strange that nobody but Tobe ever bothered to investigate and learn this?

So of course I know today and so should you and so should

anybody who investigated that corn is not better than oats and oats are not better than wheat.

Now that you've heard all this I feel that I had better give you a list and tell you a little bit about the amino acids. Obviously amino acids have some significance and do have some tangible part to play in nutrition. What it is we don't exactly know. Furthermore, the story is told to us that there are 20 amino acids, of which 8 are essential and the other 12 are non-essential. This is pure bunk or hypothesis. If you tried to feed me a diet of only essential amino acids, I'd tell you what you could do with them. I want food containing all the amino acids if I can get them, whatever that may be and also the full complement and not just the essential ones. I don't think nature is playing games with anyone. Nature made food containing all of the amino acids and that's what you should eat.

Again, we're told that there are about 20 amino acids but some more or better informed writers will tell you that there are 21 or 22. But the truth is that I have a record of 25 amino acids and I understand there are 40 that have been isolated. I'm still going to try to dig up the others but in the meantime I'm giving you the list of the 25 so that when somebody asks you about amino acids you'll be able to jam them down his throat. At the same time you'll also know that he has swallowed the usual nonsensical nutritional bait or has been thoroughly brainwashed.

AMINO ACIDS

Alanine	Leucine
Arginine	Lysine
Aspartic acid	Methionine
Cysteine	Norleucine
Cystine	Phenylalanine
Glutamic acid	Proline
Glycine	Serine
Histidine	Threonine
Hydroxyglutamic acid	Thyroxin
Hydroxyproline	Tryptophan

110

AMINO ACIDS

Iodogorgoic acid

Isoleucine

Citrulline

Tyrosine

Valine

CHAPTER

20

MIRACLE FOODS AND NUTRITION EXPERTS

I am fully aware that most of the nutritionists and most of the health writers do have their favorite foods or supplements or vitamins and some of them boldly call them "miracle" foods. Some of these nutritionists and writers are among the most famous and best established names in the health field. One raves about blackstrap molasses, yogurt and brewer's yeast. Another about high protein or vitamin E. Some stress the merits of magnesium or potassium and another claims you can't be healthy without distilled water. One attacks wheat, some claim all grains are no good. One in the group tells you that synthetic vitamins are as good as natural vitamins. Then a few stress the superiority of certain manufactured and processed products. Probably they are paid to plug them or they are part owners of the company that makes these products.

Well, they have every right to express their opinion and tell you about these foods that they think are so wonderful. I also admit that I do not have any of the degrees that some of these people have. They have been to college and they have earned or bought and paid for their degrees. I have earned no degrees and I apologize for this . . . not because I feel that I am cheated but because you expect me to have degrees, and for that I apologize.

Frankly, I wouldn't take a degree if all the colleges in the country offered one to me. I would consider it a serious handicap. To me a degree means only one thing and that is that you have permitted yourself to be brainwashed in order to get the degree, because if you didn't acquiesce and accept what you were taught you could never get a degree. You had to learn what they wanted you to learn, you had to study what they wanted you to study and you had to commit to memory, for now and evermore, what they wanted you to commit to memory . . . otherwise, again, you would not have graduated.

I read what I wanted to read. I read what I needed to read. I learned what I needed to know. I am still searching and I am still studying and I am still groping . . . all because I do not have a degree. I, unlike the others, cannot point to my degree and say, "There, that proves that I am intelligent, that proves that I am knowledgable and that proves that I am learned." So, not having that glorious decorative instrument, I have to work day and night so that I might perchance know what I am talking about. So blessed be they who have degrees and can sit on their fannies . . . and cursed am I who has no degrees and has to keep boning, boning, boning.

Besides all of this, I am basically a professional horticulturist and I am stupid enough to believe that agriculture is the highest culture. I have found that my agricultural training has stood me in good stead. For example, I don't think that corn is a better food for animals than oats or wheat, I don't think that sunflower seeds are better than pumpkin seeds or squash seeds or even cucumber seeds, I don't think that yogurt is one darn bit better than clabbered milk, and I don't think that brewer's yeast is one iota better or even as good as a handful of sesame seeds.

114

I admit my ignorance but I have never been able to read or learn that any food contains any miraculous qualities that cannot be found in other foods. I don't think, for example, that carrot juice is any better than turnip juice or parsnip juice or beet juice. It may be that carrot juice is more palatable but nutritionally you won't make me believe it is any better.

Basically, I believe that no one food or no group of foods is the whole answer. I believe that nature intended man to take part of many foods in his diet. That's why nature provided about half a million different plants for the use of man and beast. I believe, for example, that molasses has merit but I'll never believe that molasses is better than eating the cane as it is grown. I won't believe that brewer's yeast is better than barley or rye or hops.

It is my aim, with my eating, to eat as wide a variety as possible of wholesome, naturally grown vegetable foods. I do not believe that a high protein diet is of benefit to mankind. In fact, it can be readily proven that a high protein diet can cause many serious ailments. I think the man who talks about a high protein diet has something to sell . . . something on which he is making a good profit.

Now I am not impunging upon the integrity or qualifications of any of the nutritionists or those who do these things but I am suggesting that you investigate and do a little considering and brain exercise. I will further grant that most of these well known names have contributed greatly to the welfare of mankind . . . and I mean that honestly and sincerely. I know that many or most of these authors and lecturers have been responsible for starting hundreds of thousands of people, and perhaps millions, on the road to good health via the natural food route.

However, this does not alter the fact that they are not always right and nobody is. But my main object at this time is to bring home to you very forcibly that I do not believe there are any 'miracle' foods.

115

CHAPTER

21

FOOD SUPPLEMENTATION

I do not advise the use of supplementation of foods nor do I use supplements myself. I admit that I have on a few occasions taken vitamin C tablets from natural sources. This was when travelling and I felt that I was not getting adequate supplies of good raw vegetables and I took the vitamin C specifically to take up the slack. It is my sincere belief that we should get our nutrients from our food without resorting to the taking of food supplements or vitamin pills or tablets. However, I also realize that not 1% of the people of America get the proper nutrients from their food. This is a positive, clinically established fact. Therefore, the use of supplements is either pardonable, justifiable or even necessary.

Back to my own case. I go to a lot of trouble to get proper food and in the proper preparation of that food I must have the cooperation of my wife and the other members of my household if I am to eat according to my knowledge and convictions. All the other members of my household take vitamin supplements for the simple reason that they eat many foods that I will not partake of. They use maple syrup, they use some bakery bread, they use pork products, they use a fair amount of meat. They do not consume the large quantities of raw vegetables and fruits and grains that I consume. Some of them drink an occasional cup of coffee and one of them smokes an occasional cigarette. They also partake of small quantities of alcoholic beverages and some fried foods.

Therefore, I consider the supplementation of their diet advisable or essential although I do not direct their diet program and assume no responsibility for it whatsoever. I do know that they have had (all three members) much better health since they have eaten at my table than they did before and all of them are in comparative good health. Let me express it this way. They eat probably 75% of the same food that I do. The big difference is in the other 25%.

I do not permit any chemicalized food in my home. The only canned foods that I allow in my home are sardines, salmon and some Chinese vegetables from China. Some coarse salt and many herbs are used. I do not, as I mentioned, use any form of food supplementation nor do I ever intend to and I do not consider food supplementation necessary or advisable except when you admittedly do not have a proper diet or do not try to follow a proper diet.

I have visited with and travelled with various well-known, renowned nutritionists and nutritional counselors and I was appalled at the enormous number of supplements that they partook of at, or before, each meal. Among them are my friends Beatrice Trum Hunter, Betty Lee Morales and the Rodales. I feel that the use of supplementation is a direct admission that they do not eat correctly or they do not even attempt to eat correctly. Now this is not a matter of character assasination because I still regard these famous fine people as good friends but it does indicate a great divergence in viewpoint. The reason stated by some of my friends for the use of supplements is that they are not sure that they get the proper nutrients in the food because they are not positive that it is

118

organically grown or they are not sure of the sources. Therefore, the use of supplementation is, according to them, fully justified in this manner.

My contention is that they can't be one whit more certain of the organic source of their supplements than they can be of the food that they buy. In fact, if they grew their own food at least they'd be sure of the source and of its 100% organic content.

I realize that in most cases we cannot grow all of our own food because of climatic restrictions. However, I consider the argument fallacious . . . to use supplements because they are not sure of the organic content of their food does not hold water in my book. This feeling I have clearly and frequently enunciated to my friends.

Realizing full well that 99% of the people of America or of the world do not have a proper diet nor do they make any attempt to get a proper diet, I must in fairness justify the use of concentrated food supplementation. If you realize, and you should realize, that you don't get a proper diet then supplementation of food is advisable and essential.

Now I have made discreet enquiries concerning the natural versus synthetic content of most vitamins and I've learned that no matter what claims are made, few if any vitamin supplements on the market are 100% organic and if they are not 100% organic then I say let's forget the whole matter. If it's a watered-down version then who knows how much water was used? I want no part of a deal of that nature. So then I say, "Let's not fool ourselves. There is no such thing to my knowledge as a 100% organic content supplement or vitamin".

However, in spite of this I still believe that there is justification in vitamin or food supplementation. I base my findings upon 15 or more years of observation and those who use supplements, and who have comparatively the same diet as neighbours or friends or relatives who do not use supplements, definitely do enjoy better health. I see examples of this every single

119

day of my life. Therefore, I stand firm and state, "I do not believe that any person who wants to follow a proper way of living should use concentrated food supplements or vitamins. On the other hand, I qualify again and state that because 99% of the people in the world do not have a proper diet food supplementation is fully justifiable and should be done by 99% of the people of the world".

CHAPTER

22

FOOD PASTEURIZATION IS SYNONYMOUS WITH DESTRUCTION

I have opposed pasteurization since I was knee high to a grasshopper. Surely when I was ten years old I didn't know much about chemistry or nutrition or health, but I did feel that pasteurization was not good. Now it may be supposed that I heard it discussed in my childhood and from that I formed my opinion or dislike or opposition to pasteurization. But I swear this is not true . . . I do not recall ever hearing it discussed in my childhood, except as a great benefit to mankind which was widely publicized when pasteurization was introduced. But somehow I didn't feel that I wanted any part of pasteurization.

Pasteurization did not come into actual effect when I was ten years old but it had already been mooted and was used in some quarters. It was not until about five or ten years later that it came into wide use and then it became compulsory a little later on.

121

Then where would I get my opposition to pasteurization at that age? I don't know but aren't there some things we know inherently? Aren't there some things which our subconscious mind warns us about? I think this is true.

As a child I never liked vegetables but I instinctively ate them . . . yes, even the ones I didn't like. And a strange thing was that I would invariably consume them before my meal. I sort of wanted to get them done with and out of the way so I could enjoy the other food. What I actually was doing was eating the good food first and fortifying myself and then eating the cooked crap after. But I didn't realize this, as I say, and it was done instinctively.

Now I'm not trying to give you any song and dance that I had some powers or special guidance, because that's pure and simple humbug. I was no better and no worse, I hope, than the average kid in the neighborhood.

Anyway, since my childhood I have opposed the use of pasteurization and have managed to build up a pile of evidence indicating that pasteurization is harmful. But how strange . . . it was not until my 62nd year that I had conclusive proof that pasteurization was not only harmful but that it was foisted upon an unsuspecting public just so some people could get rich.

From a chemical food journal to which I subscribe, I learned all about this new sanitary milk. Now they no longer just pasteurize it but they heat it to about 246 degrees in a flash and then the milk will keep practically forever. Very convenient for those who want it or who profit from it.

But in this article telling of the great merit of this sanitary or sterilized milk, the writer let the cat out of the bag. He said, "We know that pasteurization destroys about 30% of the nutrients in milk." Of course he intimated that his process didn't do such a thing! But the point is that they, the food technologists, admitted that through all these years they knew that pasteurization destroyed 30% of the nutrients. Imagine what that means to the millions upon millions of children who were raised on pasteurized milk. The implication is staggering!

In other words, the processors, in cahoots with the government, knew that they were harming our children . . . but that didn't matter, because there was money to be made in pasteurized milk and they were going to have that money. And we all know they made it . . . and plenty.

One of the important things that you must realize about pasteurized milk is that the pasteurization process was never intended for food. Remember, when Pasteur was called into the wine industry in France, the wine was turning sour. Now in my opinion, wine — that is, commercial wine — is not a food and pasteurization may be right or legitimate for wine. But it was not and is not now the right thing for milk or any food product.

The reason milk was pasteurized in the first place was because it was claimed that milk is supposed to carry certain germs or bacteria which caused or were said to cause disease in human beings. Now this is a debatable point but the fact is that the true reason for the pasteurization of milk in my opinion was commercialization, although they would make you believe it was for sanitation, health and the prevention of disease. If there are any other reasons for the pasteurization of milk then I have not been informed of these reasons. Pasteurization definitely slows down the souring process. Proper refrigeration slows down the process even better.

The argument that the pasteurization of milk increases its keeping qualities is not borne out by the evidence. Well, for your information, let me tell you that if you looked in the American Encyclopedia you will find that at the turn of the century the Americans had an exhibit at the World's Fair and they supplied it with fresh milk. Imagine fresh milk from America being sold in Paris and we didn't have airplanes and we didn't even have fast steamers in those days. Yet the milk left America and reached Paris in pure, wholesome and sweet condition. How was this miracle performed? Very easily . . . by simple refrigeration. And if you don't believe me, I beg you to check the American Encyclopedia and see whether or not I am telling you the truth. This, I wish to remind you, was at the turn of the century. Therefore, the excuse of not being able to keep milk sweet is pure hokum.

Pasteurization for sanitation means one thing . . . that we are afraid the milk is dirty and therefore we pasteurize it. Well, as for me, I don't want dirty milk whether it is pasteurized or otherwise. If the milk is dirty then I don't want it. Pasteurization enables dairies to sell rotten, dirty and polluted milk and it enables them to handle it with impunity. It also enables them to sell milk loaded with antibiotics and other drugs and chemicals. But they are not concerned about giving the public a good wholesome and healthful product. If they were, they wouldn't serve either pasteurized, homogenized or sterilized milk. The only milk that is fit to drink is wholesome, fresh milk without any treatment whatsoever.

Surely, you know that pasteurization does not improve the nutrient value of milk. In fact, even a child knows that it seriously impairs the nutrient value of milk.

So what our politicians or board of health is trying to tell us is, "We can't give you clean milk from healthy animals. Therefore, we are taking the best milk we can get — dirty, filthy, germ-laden or otherwise — and we're pasteurizing it so it will not do you any harm."

If you or anyone else — scientist, medical doctor, health officer — can deny what I have said here, I challenge you to do so. I have spent hundreds of hours threshing out the matter of milk and pasteurization. Oh, yes, I have had the bogey of tuberculosis thrown at me and that is one of the reasons milk was pasteurized because it carried the tuberculosis bacillus from tubercular cows and brought it into man. Well, in the first place, it has never been positively proven that bovine tuberculosis can be passed on to man. But whether or not milk causes tuberculosis is neither here nor there. I don't want milk from tubercular cows under any circumstances and neither do you.

124

CHAPTER

23

YOU HAVE BEEN POISONED

I knew a man, quite a good friend of mine and much older than I, who was intelligent, full of life, generous and a lot of fun. The thing I recall about him most was that he carried a little roll of candy in his pocket at all times and I don't know whether he called them tummies, dummies or yummies but they were some sort of an ant-acid pill or something which he just popped into his mouth after every meal. He used to swear by them. He said they gave him relief from or prevented some pains in his stomach.

I had a father-in-law, who between meals and after meals and before meals, used to burp up deep cavernous belches that seemed to come from the bowels of the earth and came up in blasts like something from Dantes inferno. He'd feel so good after every belch while everybody else felt sick to their stomachs. But he was the boss of the household and everybody — at least the sons-in-law — sort of

125

said something like 'Gesuntheit' but actually under their breath they probably said 'I hope you choke, you bloody old hog'. He too, was always taking milk of magnesia and pills of some kind . . . he was never without them.

Well, I could go on and give you another 50 or 60 examples like this that I have noticed in my life apart from the casual people I knew who always took these ant-acids or whatever they are called.

I have never resorted to any of these disruption pacifiers although in my youth I took an occasional dose of bicarbonate of soda. But, strange to relate, I always resented the fact that I had to take some sort of medication to correct stomach problems.

Of course, everybody said it was a stomach disorder or something was wrong with your stomach, or you had a stomach upset or something didn't agree with you. Never, but never, never did anyone suggest that it was some lousy, contemptible, despicable imitation food that you ate. No, it was always something wrong with your stomach as though you were gifted with a weak alimentary tract or organs.

This brings to mind the story about the man on an ocean voyage. It was a rough day and the ship was rolling like a ball on a teeter totter. Anyway, he rushed over to the rail that was occupied by most of the ship's passengers doing likewise, bent overboard and let go. A casual observer on the boat, one of the few who had good sea legs and a good constitution enquired, "What's the matter fellow, got a weak stomach?" And this fellow's reply was a classic. He said, "A weak stomach! Why what's the matter? Am I not throwing mine as far as anybody else?"

So wherever we go or wherever people get together or socialize you will hear someone complain that something didn't agree with him or caused a little upset or heart burn or indigestion. Never is it suggested or suspected that something was wrong with the food that was eaten. I want to tell you this, if you have any condition that comes on after you've eaten something — whether it's 15 minutes after or 15 hours after — you've been poisoned. Please believe me, I've experimented with this, I've tried it on myself and on others and I've also investigated and I've reached the conclusion that you could eat practically any food, even in a bad state of decomposition even to putrefaction without having anything wrong or go haywire with your stomach. If it doesn't agree with you you'll probably vomit it up within a few minutes or if it manages to get down into your alimentary tract you'll probably get rid of it in diarrhoea because the human anatomy has the ways and means of handling things that are wrong when they are natural and no chemicals are involved.

When chemicals are involved your body's reaction is entirely different. It doesn't know how to handle the chemicals and therefore you get cramps and you get irritations and pains and gurglings and 101 different things. It's because your body's processes are thrown into a tail-spin. The body doesn't know whether to expel this item or to store it or what to do with it and in many cases, too many cases, it is a fact that these poisonous chemicals (food additives) are cumulative. So the body builds up these various harmful chemicals because it doesn't know how to handle or excrete them, then when it builds up to a fairly high dosage you run into a disease or sickness or even death.

What I'm trying to convey to you is that when you get a reaction from eating some food, almost invariably because it contains some chemical additive, you have been actually poisoned. There are various degrees of food poisoning from minor to serious . . . luckily most are minor and the upset clears up on its own in a few hours or a day or two. However, when you get enough or build up a big enough dose of something it's liable to kill you or at least necessitate surgery or drastic purgative measures and that is absolutely true. So whenever you have the slightest disorder resulting from food you can be sure that a food additive is to blame and you've been poisoned to a lesser or greater degree.

If you need an ant-acid pill or if you need tums or a laxative or something else I tell you again, you've been poisoned and you've no right to inflict this kind of food or food chemicals upon your body.

I've learned that practically all food additives give me a reaction. Now the reaction may be a minor one or it may be a major one. Some of them create sharp distress and it can take many and various forms. If I get a reaction of any kind to any food I know that I've been poisoned.

One of the things that has affected me more than most is benzoate of soda. For your enlightenment "benzoate of soda" finds its way into many, many foods. Usually, it is demanded by the food and drug that this be put on the label but I am absolutely certain that in many instances it is not put on the label and we don't know we're getting it. You understand it is virtually impossible to know when you've ingested chemicals. While many foods have the chemical additives listed on the label there are also as many or more that have nothing marked on the label because the government and the food processors have entered into an agreement whereby the processors can put various stipulated chemical additives (poisons) into food without anything being put on the label. This agreement is referred to as "standards of identity".

This is great stuff for the food processors and for the government but it plays hell with the anatomy of human beings and the great benefactors of all this are the medical profession, the hospitals and the undertakers. I'm not joking a bit, I'm dead serious. Undoubtedly these food chemicals kill hundreds of thousands of people but very, very seldom is a food or a food additive blamed for the evil that it causes. So I'm talking to you as man to man and I'm telling you in the most emphatic terms at my command that the ingestion of normal proper wholesome foods will cause you no disturbance, no trouble, no after effects . . . if you do get after effects it is because you've been poisoned.

Now I can hear you just getting ready to throw a bad nasty curve at me by saying, "I know I've eaten different fruits and different vegetable and they've caused me a great deal of discomfort.

For example, cucumbers just about slay me". And my argument is that it isn't the cucumber. Either you take drugs, I mean medical drugs or you smoke or you drink liquor or drink a lot of coffee or you use other substances that affect your gastro-intestinal bacterial flora and therefore you have distress. But if you ate the cucumber and did not use the products mentioned you would, after two or three times eating this specific food, have no discomfort and you'd be able to eat all you like. I fully realize that if you over-eat, for example, on sour apples or other unripe fruit, or if you eat a couple of quarts of strawberries every day you are apt to break out into a rash or hives or some other disorder. I point this out to prove that you can over-do anything, including water.

Another very important thing to consider and bear in mind is that practically all of our fruits, vegetables and grains are coated, treated or covered with various harmful deadly chemicals and their residues are apt to cause trouble because it is often virtually impossible to wash off these deadly sprays and dusts. Even the chemical fertilizers can cause trouble. It has been distinctly proven that plants will pick up certain chemicals from the soil. If the soil has been loaded with nitrogen and other chemicals, they are imparted to you through the food you eat. There have been such cases, especially among animals, so we must not minimize the role that chemical sprays and fertilizers play upon the human anatomy and the worst of it is, in most cases you cannot prove or connect the poisoning with the guilty food, because the discomfort comes later. It is not generally recognized and we don't look for the trouble in the food, we look for it in other sources and the real culprits — the chemical fertilizers and the chemical sprays — get away with virtual murder. So back I am to my original theme.

When you have a stomach upset don't say you have bad digestion, that this food is hard to digest ... place the blame right where it belongs on the chemicals found in your food whether added deliberately or by accident.

CHAPTER

24

NO MAN'S LAND OF SCIENCE

I received a letter from a friend and I want to quote part of it verbatim:

"I've been well and can now say I managed to live through four years of so-considered high risk areas for diseases without contracting even minor ailments. In Washington, when I took a physical before state department's release, they wanted a second test because they just couldn't believe anyone could come away from there without at least showing some bugs or amoebas. And I was condemned as very foolish for being so careless as to eat raw vegetables merely by washing with water. This should prove something."

Now that you have read that note — let me fill you in.

In 1963 I took a trip around the world and one of the company of five who accompanied me was a man by the name of Clarence. We picked him up in Addis Ababa, which was where we had arranged to meet. We toured the hinterland of Abyssinia in a land rover with a native driver-interpreter for 15 days and then went on to many other interesting parts of the world. Clarence was a maverick something like Tobe and before long he was rebellious but nothing serious arose. But there were a few little incidents that occasionally made me bristle a bit.

About five or six weeks later, when in Pakistan, we were heading for a state called Swat. This state, evidently, is one of the few that at that time still held its independence, although it was a part of Pakistan.

We came to a check-out point and there was a barrier across the road and the guard asked us for our passports. The others all immediately handed over their passports but I just said, "What do you want my passport for?"

He said, "It's a routine check!"

I said, "I know, but I am in Pakistan and I was checked coming in. What do you have to check for?"

He said, "We are supposed to do this."

I said, "I see no reason to do it whatsoever. I think it is someone asserting his authority like a petty bureaucrat."

He said, "If you don't show us your passport we won't let you through."

I said, "Then you are being high-handed. I am a legitimate traveller from a Commonwealth country and you have no authority to stop me from going on in this country as long as it is Pakistan. Besides, I went through here two years ago and no such high-handed action was inflicted upon me."

The guard said, "You were here two years ago and you didn't need a passport?"

I said, "That's right!"

He asked, "When were you here?"

I said, "In July, 1961."

He disappeared for five minutes and came back with a book and he said, "Can you find your name in here?"

I looked through it and on July 10th, 1961, my name was signed there and I said to him, "There it is!"

He looked and said, "You're right! O.K., you don't need a passport."

Then I heard a remark from behind me, "By God, he was right . . . he was here before!"

I turned and saw it was this chap, Clarence, who had made the remark. I didn't reply but suddenly I realized the cause of my difficulty with Clarence. He thought I was full of crap and everything I told him he didn't believe until this time when what I said was completely borne out. Needless to say, I had no more trouble with Friend Clarence. As a matter of fact, when we spent a few weeks in Hong Kong he had been very, very intolerant and opposed to the Chinese. This had been one of our obstacles . . . I liked the Chinese and maintained stoutly that they were wonderful people and were as good as any people on earth — they were clean, they were reliable, they were friendly, etc. — while he maintained otherwise. As a matter of fact, the first incident that brought about trouble between us was when I wanted to eat in a Chinese restaurant in Addis Ababa and he refused to go. He said they eat rats and they're dirty.

I said, "I have lived with Chinese people ever since I was a kid and they don't eat rats and they're not dirty. They're probably the most reliable people I've ever known in my life and their word is their bond and there is less cheating, thieving, stealing and dishonesty among Chinese than any group in the world."

When we parted in Hong Kong when he was flying back to Alaska he said, "I guess I'll have to revise my thinking about the Chinese and many other things!"

Years went by and I got a letter from Nigeria one day, from this selfsame Clarence. He had evidently taken a position with the American government and was working in Nigeria. He was a top-notch mechanic.

This letter told how he was supposed to eat out of cans and never drink local water and never eat raw vegetables and fruits that were native-grown, without scrupulously washing them in chemicals. He wrote and told me this and my reply was, "If you live on the prescribed diet, you'll wind up being sick and perhaps very sick. And you'll probably come back to America, if you're there very long, either a partial or complete cripple and you'll never be the same again as long as you live."

He said, "What should I do?"

I told him, "Eat all the native foods right from the start, but start them off in minute quantities and gradually increase the tempo. If you want to wash them, then wash them in water only . . . native water, but preferably from a good clear stream or well."

He wrote back and said that his superiors had told him "No" and if he did that he would come down with dysentery — in fact, the worst kind which is amoebic dysentery — or any one of a thousand other horrible, terrible, deadly diseases.

I said, "They're full of baloney! Right from the start eat small quantities of native food, as I told you, and build up your gastro-intestinal bacterial flora so that you can handle anything found in that country."

He wrote back again and said that his superiors didn't like the idea but anyway he was doing it. Then he said to me, "Will you please send me some books that will scientifically prove that what I am doing is right?"

I began to send him books and he built up a fairly extensive library. I sent books on chemistry, biochemistry, biology, physiology as well as books on food, nutrition and health. I think he took a couple of stints on the Nigerian gambit and now has returned to Alaska.

This is the connection, as you will understand, between what I have told you and the quotation from his recent letter.

Yes, the government authorities cannot believe that a man can survive and be healthy and come back from a few years in a backward foreign country without being afflicted by any one of many diseases. I contend that most people come back with these diseases because they tried to live the American style in a country that is not adapted to living American style.

If you live in a large city like New York or London or Tokyo, you need chlorinated water, you need disinfectants, you need pasteurized milk, you need sewage systems, you need shots and injections and vaccinations, because you're living like ants in an ant hill or bees in a beehive. But that is not the way man was intended to live.

If you must breathe the foul air that your neighbor expels, if you must drink the water that your neighbor excretes, then you are violating every principle and every law of nature. Therefore, you must improvise for yourself and find ways and means of survival in the face of these biological violations.

However, you can't take these teeming city principles and invoke them in the wilderness. Tens of thousands of Europeans have gone East and tried to go native and tried to live in the East, on desert islands, paradises, enchanted islands. I've read innumerable

135

accounts of them and practically every one failed because they took sick, and they had to be rushed back to civilization and some of them died. You see, they were trying to live civilized fashion on a tropical island and it just doesn't work. They brought with them first of all, their own foods...the things they liked, the things they enjoyed, and they didn't want to do without them. So they brought oodles and oodles of canned foods, dried foods, packaged foods, dead foods, heavily chemicalized and hydrogenated foods, nutritionless foods...and that was the main reason for their downfall and sickness. Also they brought with them their drugs and their shots and their injections which made things worse.

I recall, when I was being entertained by the King of Swat and we were sitting in his judicial chambers in an earnest discussion, that I somehow told him that I was one of these health nuts and that I drank the water from the Swat River and ate food with the natives. His first remark was, "You'll get dysentery and you'll wind up in a hospital."

I said, "I don't think so. I've been doing it right along all over the world and I haven't wound up that way yet."

Then I expounded my theory about the gastro-intestinal bacterial flora, and he said, "You know what, there was another guy like you here. He was our last political agent, a Dr. Cobb. He had similar ideas and practices and he maintained the same philosophy. And the strangest part of all was he never did get sick and everybody else did."

The king scratched his head and said, "Maybe you've got something! You are not so crazy at that," and then as an after thought "neither was Dr. Cobb."

I know I've got something because I've been following it for 25 years. On that trip around the world where there were five of us, four of them got sick at different times — quite seriously, too — but I remained unscathed except for diarrhoea for one day, due to eating too much raw corn. The only other one who remained healthy most of the time was the female member of the group. She followed most of my practices, much against her will, but she turned out to be the toughest member of the entire party.

Hardly a day goes by that I am not told about someone who got sick with dysentery — or worse — on a trip to Mexico, South America, Asia, various Tropical Islands and elsewhere. And the story runs about the same . . . usually it started as an intestinal disorder. I suggest there is a sound biological basic reason for all this trouble. In our civilized way of life, with the broad regular use of liquor, tobacco, drugs, medicines, plus bacteria-destroying chemical preservatives in foods, our normal protective gastro-intestinal bacterial flora have been killed off so that the body is left defenseless to the onslaught of any "foreign" bacteria. In simple language, I am suggesting that your intestinal tract is almost sterile or close to it and when you get a little different bug — it doesn't have to be a harmful bug at all, but he multiplies rapidly because he has no natural enemies — he takes hold and you are in trouble! And it could be any one of a thousand bugs.

I stress, it is a fact that most civilized ways of living create a rather sterile gastro-intestinal bacterial flora, so even the more or less innocuous types of other germs or bacteria, when they get into your intestinal tract, can play havoc . . . and they usually do. But if you do as I do and as I advise — that is, eat a wide variety of raw foods wherever you go — then there is very little danger of this happening because you have your good healthy bugs there to protect you.

The average conventional American diet consists of about 95% cooked, processed, chemically treated foods and obviously they will contribute nothing to your bacterial flora . . . nor do they require any help from your flora to be digested or assimilated. Raw foods require bacteria for digestion and assimilation and also contribute bacterial flora to your alimentary tract. That is why that bit of lettuce, celery or cabbage can cause you intensive agony, distress, pain and actual suffering. You are simply looking for living bacteria to aid in digesting and assimilating that specific raw food. You have often heard people say, "Why I don't even dare eat a bit of lettuce.

137

Otherwise I suffer excrutiating agony." Or it could be cucumber or some other vegetable or even some fruit. And the reason for this is just as I have outlined.

You can't keep drinking alcohol in any one of its forms, smoking a few packs of cigarettes a day and taking all kinds of drugs and pills, without destroying your microorganisms and your natural enzymes. That is why in hospitals they feed mostly cooked pap . . . so it will not cause distress to any of the patients. Rarely do they offer any salads and if they do there is just a nibble.

I want to stress that eating a nibble or two of raw food is not the answer . . . it is raw food in wide variety regularly.

As soon as I land in a foreign clime I immediately start nibbling on small quantities of their food. I eat in the native eating places wherever possible, but in most cases I buy my own fruits and vegetables and prepare at least one or two of my own meals every day.

Now if you want to travel and not come down with these bugs, you know how to do it!

CHAPTER

25

DON'T EAT PROCESSED FOODS

The food supply of America is at its highest and best level. More foods, better foods and a greater variety of foods are available in America today than ever before in history.

However, this does not mean that Americans are getting this kind of food or that Americans are eating this kind of food. In fact, it is just the opposite. The American people are today eating the worst food and have the worst diet of any people in history. Please do not think that I am exaggerating or that I am off my rocker. I beg of you to pay attention, to listen and then after I've presented my case if you don't care to believe me then investigate for yourself. But everything I say here is absolutely true and can be proven with scientific evidence.

To begin with, most of America's food is produced via

chemical farming methods. Practically the entire supply of dairy products in America is pasteurized which means that most if not all enzymes have been destroyed, rendering the food of doubtful value. Many or most of the nutrients have been impaired or rendered unassimilable by the body. The food processors have, because of their own interests, fragmented and refined most food. This is most noticeable in our bread and other grain products. Grain is probably mankind's best food. I mean by this seeds but seldom if ever do you eat seeds in their whole complete state and it is only in the whole complete state that they are fully nourishing and nutritive.

I want to stress — and make the statement emphatic and positive — that the chemical additives in food, the refining of food and the processing of food are done 100% for the benefit of the processor . . . never for the benefit of the consumer. There is more profit in making processed food the way they make it and that is precisely why it is made in that manner. They are not concerned with its nutritive value, they are not concerned whether it's good or harmful, they are not concerned whether it brings sickness or health . . . they are interested in making as much money as possible from the food which they supply and selling as much as possible. This goes for every manufacturer of food in the U.S.A. and Canada and perhaps elsewhere.

Furthermore, trickery, chicanery, bribes, political maneuvering and other methods are resorted to to keep the public in ignorance concerning the true merits of the food. For example, the food industry works under what is known as the "standards of identity" which means they can use various chemicals and other substances and preservatives in their foods without telling you, the public, about them or listing them on the label. Ice Cream, Coca Cola and other soft drinks, catsup and many, many other products are examples of this terrible abuse and outrage. In other words, the processors and the government through the Food and Drug work out a deal whereby they can include this whole, vast array of chemicals and fragmented foods and these ingredients do not have to show on the label. So therefore, if you are under any illusions that the food supply is safe, that if there is anything harmful in it it has to be on the label, you are making a tragic, terrible error that can cost you and your loved ones your health and even shorten your life.

For years I've said that I don't object to any processor putting any one of the 4,000 chemical substances in food as long as it is clearly so stated on the label. In other words, if the consumer is damn fool enough to use a so-called food with poisons in it then it is his look-out because it is his duty to investigate and read the label and find out what he is eating. I am of the opinion that if all the ingredients are put clearly on the label the processor is relieved of responsibility and it is strictly "caveat emptor" or buyer beware. However, with the standards of identity the poor consumer is not even given that slim chance of knowing the harm in what he is eating.

The fact that no one has challenged me when I made these statements probably a hundred times before indicates that I speak the truth and that it is not a flagrant exaggeration or a lie . . . you can check this out with the American government, the Food and Drug or any other governmental agency. Furthermore, the food processors can manipulate their food products, like for example they manipulate hamburgers and wieners and peanut butter. Peanut butter does not have to be all peanuts, hamburger does not have to be all meat, neither do wieners have to be all meat. Any one of many substances can be added and included in these foods and they still can call them hamburger, wieners, peanut butter, bread, catsup or whatever the case may be. I am of the conviction, for example, that you and I have the right to believe that hamburgers are all meat and that wieners are all meat too. We also have the right to expect that the peanut butter is made out of peanuts and that bread is made out of wheat. But be careful . . . I assure you there are at least a dozen different substances used in the making of these products, apart from the meat or the wheat.

Ice Cream is another of the badly manipulated, supposed food products. Many ice creams do not contain any cream at all. Cheese is another product that is easily manipulated . . . processed cheese is probably the worst offender of all. What it contains frequently

141

shouldn't happen to a dog. I don't have the time or space to go on and show every specific item but it would be well worth your while to investigate.

O.K., let's take my own diet. At home I do very well. I live on mainly grains, vegetables and fruits with some fish and some dairy products and very little meat. In fact, I avoid meat whenever possible. This is fine when I'm home but when I travel — and I do have to travel — there is practically nothing in the restaurants that I can eat and I've tried in hundreds of different places but I can't get anything resembling food. So I resort to a couple of eggs or a salmon or a sardine sandwich. Salads are virtually impossible to get . . . that is a good salad without any junk or as it is called "dressing" on it. So I do have a rough time.

Right here let me also stress the food that you get in most restaurants is not what you think it is at all. If you order chicken soup in the restaurant you think that a chicken was killed yesterday or today and they used it in making soup . . . that's the farthest thing from the truth. In 99% of the cases it comes out of a can and in practically every instance it contains monosodium glutamate which I consider to be a definite poison — only it's a slow poison. All the restaurants use it because it enhances the flavor by acting on your tastebuds and you think it's excellent even if it is just dishwater. Monosodium glutamate activates your tastebuds and you think that it's the elixir from the gods. Well, monosodium glutamate is used in practically every product so they can serve up the worst slop and make you think it's nectar.

Now I didn't believe that the restaurants served these horrible, canned and prepared foods. I was told this many years ago but I just refused to believe this could be true. Anyway, I made the rounds of a few restaurants and with the exception of the bigger and better Chinese restaurants most of the food served in the restaurants today comes out of cans or packages or is prepared in one central point and distributed to the various branches or franchise outlets. So this is my story . . . America has the biggest food supply in the world, they have the best foods in the world, they even have the best system of

142

distribution in the world and yet we eat the worst food of any people in the world, and the most poisoned food of any people in the world.

Please believe me, I speak the absolute truth. I don't care if in telling the truth I hurt the food or any other industry, I seek only to benefit the American people.

One source claims there are 2,112 additives in our food supply, others say the number exceeds 4,000. I'm not sure just how many there are. For example, according to the standards of identity the label says cottage cheese. Here is actually what they are permitted to use: salt, sodium caseinate, ammonium caseinate, calcium caseinate, potassium caseinate, lactose, flavor-producing bacteria, carob bean gum, gum tragacanth, calcium sulfate, furcelleran, gelatin lecithin, sodium alginate, propylene glycol alginate, sodium carboxymethl, cellulose, sugar, dextrose, glycerin, propylene glycol, and dioctyl sodium sulfo-succinate.

So there you have it . . . they are allowed to put 21 different items into the cottage cheese without mentioning it on the label because of the "standards of identity" law. I understand that they can use as many as 33 different preservatives, 33 different food colors and 28 different antioxidants but nobody except the processor of that specific product knows which one or ones were used. It is recognized by top ranking medical authorities that ingestion of chemicals can cause violent attitudes and behavioral symptoms which are referred to as the "pharmacology of violence".

An allergy specialist reported that over 100 patients of his showed sensitivity to flavouring additives alone yet the sufferers could not trace the source of that problem because practically none of the products containing these additives were accurately labelled. I stress that all of these patients were from only one doctor in the United States and from only flavor additives. You can just imagine what the score would be if all doctors and all allergists reported on all chemicals in foods. You can visualize that the report would be staggering, astounding, unbelievable.

143

So there you have it. My advice is to stay away from processed foods at least until the food processors smarten up and serve the public some decent food and name the additives on the label. The only person who can get results is you, Mr. Consumer. You can make good food processors, you can make good Food and Drug Inspectors by standing up and demanding it. I'm grateful that the young people are standing up . . . the old fogeys are too weak or too brain-washed or probably too weakened from so many chemical additives in the foods they have consumed.

CHAPTER

26

WATER

Today in America no one can deny that pure, wholesome water is something hard to come by. I am sure that true pristine water is not available in any urban centre in America. The only pure water I presume would be distilled water but water found in nature is never distilled and as water is one of the most vital components of man's existence a great deal of attention and thought should be given to it.

In this age of pollution our water supply is probably the first important thing that is seriously affected. I don't have to go into detail to bring home my point but I just want to make it clear that water, being of such tremendous importance, deserves our closest scrutiny and thought.

I don't know how long water softeners have been on the

market but I dare say something like 20 or 25 years. They have made tremendous sales growth and now are widely used throughout America. Now I want to make it clear that water softeners are something entirely different from filters. A simple filter is something that will remove particles from the water. It could be dirt, filth, insects and occasionally macro-organisms . . . although it would take a mighty good filter to do that. I've seen the massive debris after a filter has been removed and exposed to view and it's utterly astounding . . . almost unbelievable what is found in a filter from a normal water tap. I do not consider filtering in any way harmful or deleterious to your water but I positively and emphatically warn against using any type or kind of water softener for your drinking water or using water that has been distilled.

In the same breath I want to emphasize that I strongly object to the fluoridation of water as well. Any tampering with our water supply is to be looked upon as harmful or dangerous.

Then too, there has been quite a hue and cry concerning the benefits or the harm of hard water and soft water. Hard water, as we know it, is water that contains minerals and it seems that the harder the water the more minerals it contains. Then there is soft water which is the water as it falls from the heavens as rain.

I want to point out very clearly that both water softeners and water distillers are a ways and means of making money. Both are produced and manufactured by industries and these industries do all in their power to point out the advantages to be gained by using their equipment. So they go about preparing or procuring evidence to support their claims that their equipment is of benefit. I have taken the trouble to investigate and study the facts or data and the promotion they present to sell their equipment.

My reaction is that there is only harm to be found by using water softeners and in drinking or using distilled water.

There is a health group known as "hygienists" who recommend the use of distilled water. I deplore this action especially

146

from a group that is supposed to be enlightened. Yet a great number of their members use distilled water and widely advocate its use. One of the arguments that the distilled water advocates present is that because our water is so badly defiled and polluted distilling is the only answer. I do not accept this. I have good water on my farm at St. Catharines, Ontario, I have good water on my farm in Duncan, British Columbia. Water on my farm in St. Catharines comes from a well 65 feet deep and there is also a well on this farm that is only 20 feet deep. Both produce water of excellent quality and flavor. The water from my farm in British Columbia comes from a stream and while, when there is a storm or after a heavy rainfall the water may be a bit murky or carry silt, generally speaking, the water is fit to drink and we use it without harm of any kind.

No doubt there are wells where the water is of poor quality or polluted but I still believe that much of the water supply coming from wells and springs and streams is still usable where they are not too close to a large city. It doesn't take very long for a stream when it's flowing to clear or purify its water. Therefore, I contend that it is not yet necessary to drink distilled water rather than the water from our wells, springs and streams.

I haven't been able to make up my mind from the evidence that has been presented whether distilled water is preferable to fluoridated water but I would prefer to use neither. If I were faced with an alternative I presume I would accept the distilled water. Probably I would also accept the softened water rather than the fluoridated water if I had a choice. This is because I know for certain that water containing added fluorine is harmful. There are numerous experiments to prove this contention whereas no great amount of work has been done on soft water or distilled water to prove their harm. At least no such experiments have come to my attention.

However, my personal investigations, observations and experiences have clearly indicated that there is harm or question concerning the safety of both distilled and softened water. Basically, I do not understand why people insist upon interfering with the normal processes of nature.

My objection to distilled water, first and foremost, is that it is not found anywhere in nature. Secondly it is actually made by a chemical process. Third, it is void of all extraneous matter and contains no vitamins, minerals or gases. Even rain water as it falls from the sky picks up various components as it passes through the atmosphere.

I refer to distilled water as "hungry water" and suggest (without concrete proof) that it leeches needed elements from the body. I know for a positive fact that if distilled water is put into a steam or hot water boiler or heating system it will cause erosion and eat into the metal in "no time flat". You can check this out with any heating man or "stationary engineer". Ordinary tap water or lake or river water will not react in this manner.

Distilled water has definitely NOT been proven safe for human drinking water no matter what the "paid for" scientists who try to sell distilling apparatus tell you. I am at any time prepared to accept proof of its safety from all sources, but until it is presented I warn "don't use it".

When travelling, people from North America are warned by all authorities not to drink water without first boiling it or treating it with chlorine or some other method. On the many trips that I have made throughout the world I've been warned repeatedly about the grave danger in drinking water from the regular and various sources. Most of the people with whom I travelled took precautions wherever possible or drank bottled water or soft drinks rather than risk the water from the taps or from the streams or the rivers. I at all times drank the water as I found it in nature. I've yet to be harmed by it. Now this does not mean that I would knowingly and willingly drink water from a dirty stream or from a source that was anywhere near filth or pollution. But when I go into the country and I see a stream flowing for a fairly long distance I am not too much afraid to drink that water and I've done it in Mexico, I've done it in Ecuador and Peru. I've done it in Mongolia, Russia, New Guinea, China and practically every country on the face of the globe. I do it in Canada and the United States and in Britain also.

Now I'm not suggesting that the danger of pollution or the polluting of our water supply does not present a genuine danger to our ecology and to our way of life because I know definitely that it does present a threat and a danger. But I still insist that with a bit of common sense and precautions and a bit of investigating you can find lots of good streams and sources of good water throughout America.

Let's put it this way. There are many streams or bodies of water or sources of water that I would not drink but I would definitely use my eyes, my ears and my head concerning the water that I drink no matter where it happens to be.

By the same token I prefer not to drink chlorinated, fluoridated or otherwise treated water in the cities, towns or wherever else it may be.

CHAPTER

27

ANIMAL FOOD

While I am not a 100% vegetarian I am convinced that the vegetarian way of life, followed along the lines of raw vegetables and grains, fruits and nuts is the best and the healthiest way of life for man. There is ample, scientific evidence to prove that a man can remain in perfect health on a strict vegetarian diet. In fact, there is plenty of evidence to indicate that the vegetarian way of life as described above is far better and will keep a man in better health than meat eating. Therefore a chapter on animal foods is important.

We must at the outset recognize that basically our food animals are raised for slaughter. There are also cows and goats that are raised to give milk. In eastern countries sheep are also used for this purpose along with yaks, camels and horses. With the advent of big business it is essential that animals produce the greatest amount of food in the shortest possible time. As soon as a laying hen falls off her high rate of productivity her head comes off. As soon as a cow slips from her high output of milk she is sold down the river or slaughtered. When a steer reaches the proper weight he is slaughtered. The bull is kept for service and the day he outlives his usefulness he is butchered.

Now I cannot quarrel with this argument, if animals are kept for feed purposes. I assume that that is the way it must be. However, there is an aspect that is seldom brought to light that deserves the attention of thinking, sensible, alert individuals. I maintain that somewhere along the line things become tangled up. Granted, we must raise our food animals as economically as possible but we must never lose sight of the fact that we want our food animals to be healthy . . . as healthy as it is possible to have them and that is precisely where we have been fouled up because my studies clearly reveal that in America we do not have any healthy animals.

I go further . . . I suggest that all of the animals that we eat are sick. Even the "domesticated" cattle are hardly ever perfectly healthy. I consider this an astute observation considering it was made about 40 years ago. I have attended many cattle exhibitions, displays and shows and I have seen some mighty fine animals. However, the health of the animal, as far as I know, is judged only by its proportion, its suitability for beef or giving milk or for breeding purposes. Never is a food animal judged by its strength, endurance, and the condition of its vital organs. If it were judged by these standards then none of our food animals would qualify as healthy animals. Examinations after slaughtering clearly indicate that many vital organs are diseased and impaired in practically every slaughtered animal.

At the cattle shows I observed that only the rather stout, fat, well-filled out animals were desired and those were the ones that won all the prizes. Never did a thin or sinewy animal ever win a prize. In fact, they were never even displayed.

It so happens that I have been in Ethiopia where it is claimed they have more cattle than they have in any country in the world.

Maybe it is per capita but in any event I did see more cattle in Ethiopia than I've ever seen anywhere and this I noticed . . . there were no fat cattle to be seen. At first we thought that this indicated that the cattle were not healthy or were not properly fed but soon we realized that that is the proper way for cattle to look . . . not the way ours look. It takes a little bit of thinking to reach this conclusion.

We have been spoiled in America. It is not only a matter of standards. In America we expect our animals to be big, husky, chunky and well filled out but that does not mean that such animals are best. Is it not strange that here in America we recognize the harm in fat people and everybody wants to be thin and slender but when it comes to cattle we want them well filled out and fat? Then again when we go to buy meat everybody wants lean meat. Yet every cook says that you must have fat to make the meat taste right. This thing appears to be nothing short of madness.

Anyone who has ever been a spectator or has taken part in competitions among animals would naturally assume that these splendid looking animals were all healthy but I know different because I know how they are fed and that is the crux of the whole situation. If our animals are not healthy — and I contend they are not healthy — then the trouble lies with the feed or the feeding program. In the first place, practically all of the pasture land in America is chemical fertilizer fed which means clearly and unmistakably that the forage crops grown there are out of balance. It is utterly impossible to have balanced crops on chemically fertilized land. I say utterly impossible and I mean just that. Therefore, the animals that graze such land cannot be adequately nourished.

Practically all of the animals in America before they are marketed are put on a feed lot. That is, they are confined in certain areas and they are fed a prescribed formula to fatten them quickly to make them ready for market and to have them gain as much weight as possible. Now when on a feed lot or on a farm the grass eating animal's food is supplemented to varying degrees with grains or grain mixtures. I have for many years studied these feed mixture formulas

153

whether they apply to chickens for laying or for broilers or to turkeys or to cattle, sheep, hogs or other domesticated animals.

Now I don't know whether the chemical companies own the feed companies or whether the feed companies own the chemical companies but they are definitely interwoven. The entire animal feed industry is dependent upon processors' residues or wastes such as come from the beet sugar refineries, the seed oil refineries or other sources. The waste resulting from these processes literally amounts to millions of tons. These residues, in my opinion, are not even fit to put on the land for fertilizer. The extraction process by means of various chemical solvents plus the obvious fact that the oil has been removed which is by far the most vital part of the seed, means that applying such wastes to your soil would only create serious imbalance on the land.

Here we have these mountains of wastes, big mountains, so they are put to use and turned into money. Now this could not be done without a great deal of maneuvering because let's face it clearly . . . who wants to use or consume wastes? In my opinion it is much worse than garbage because garbage does contain some whole wastes, like for instance the outer leaves of cabbage and the remains of food but these processors' wastes invariably contain only fractioned food substances that can only cause imbalance in whatever ways or means they are used.

However, the chemical and feed companies are or were aware of this so they try to correct the imbalance by adding synthetic chemicals and other wastes like the wastes from meat packing plants to correct the created condition. Researchers, economists, food technologists, agriculturists and others sat down and tried to work out a ways and a means or a formula that might correct this imbalance and thus they came up with these animal feeds that are used by at least 99% of all the farmers in America. Because there is billions of dollars of profit to be found by converting and selling these wastes the corporations can afford to buy their way into our agricultural experimental stations, into our universities and into the very core of our existence and today everyone believes that these

154

formulas are the proper food for our food animals. That is why I say there cannot be a healthy food animal as long as it is fed on these formulas. Granted, there are a few farmers or cattlemen who provide unchemicalized pasture for their animals and who feed their animals only whole grains from organic fields but these are rare exceptions.

It would be interesting for you to visit a milking parlor but make sure you see the whole thing including the laboratory and really it looks like a hospital and that is really what it is. Routine tests are made upon all animals and a wide spectrum of drugs are continually injected into and fed to the animals. In the larger dairy operations a veterinarian team is in attendance or on-call. I know some farmers who went out of the dairy business because they claimed it was virtually impossible to keep their cows healthy and they had to keep replacing them and today a good cow runs at least $500 or better. At the present moment I know a half dozen or more dairymen and they, too, recount that it is a serious problem maintaining their herds in health and I didn't say good health.

I should state here also that the dairy herds are inbred and inbreeding does not contribute to good health in these animals and that is the understatement of the year. I suggest you write to your agricultural experimental station and ask to be sent the feed formulas for any specific animal or for all of them. Then take the time to study and read just what your animals are fed. I think it would be most enlightening and perhaps a bit frightening, too.

At the present moment a serious controversy rages about a product commonly called DES or stilbestrol but properly known as diethylstilbestrol. It is known as an estrogen. Actually the use of this drug was banned more than 10 years ago as an implant in the ears of cattle and in the necks of chickens. At the time of the cranberry scandal the Food and Drug banned its use as an implant or a food so they are now using the same drug but they call it an anti-biotic and not a food ... it is fed as a drug and this makes it O.K. Now they are telling us that because of the banning of DES we will not be able to feed our populations and 50 million of us will starve. It is admitted that the use of DES does make the animal grow faster and

155

it does make him ready for market perhaps 6 weeks to two months before non-diethylstilbestrol fed animals but there is a story here.

Diethylstilbestrol causes a disease akin to a goitre in the animal which make it heavier, and bigger. Furthermore, the animal being actually sick loses its appetite and doesn't eat too much but it passes the American government's very low standards for No. 1 beef and that is why the proponents of this drug say it saves the consumer money. This is a deliberate lie . . . it does not save him money because the gain that is made by the chemical company and the farmer is lost by the housewife when the meat shrinks considerably in the roasting or cooking. So actually the consumer would be greatly benefitted and the cooked weight increased if this insidious, contemptible, disease-creating practice were stopped.

CHAPTER
28

DAIRY PRODUCTS

When I suggest or advocate that dairy products be removed from the human diet I'm challenging Titans and it's a battle that I can't win. However, I'm not looking for victory, I'm only trying to expound truths. When I say dairy products I mean anything that is made from cow's milk . . . pardon me, it could be goat's milk, sheep's milk, yak's milk, camel's milk or mare's milk. Whether you believe it or not, all of these kinds of animal milks are used by the Mongolian people for food. No doubt some are used by various other peoples in the mountain regions of Asia and other parts of the world.

To make my task even more laborious and difficult dairy products have been used for many thousands of years, just how many thousands I do not know . . . but the Bible dates back approximately 5,000 years and I'm sure that it was known even before then . . . how long nobody knows.

I contend that they are not beneficial in any manner, shape or form. The only justification for the use of dairy products in my opinion is the fact that they will sustain life, they will prevent starvation and hunger and perhaps with less harm than many other types of food. I'd say the use of dairy products may be less harmful than eating meat, for example, although I cannot prove this. I'm stating clearly that in my opinion dairy products are not proper or good food for human beings. When we talk of dairy food it is wise to specify just what this encompasses because many people might not recognize that most chocolates contain dairy products and many other foods likewise ... puddings, for example. I'm sure there are many other products on the shelves of the supermarkets that contain milk which the average individual does not generally recognize as containing milk. That milk is convenient and nutritive cannot be denied but milk has an expressed and positive purpose in life and that is to nurture the new infant or the newborn of any species until such time as it can partake of the normal and natural food of that species. That is the specific purpose for which milk was created by nature.

For anyone above the infant stage to consume milk, be it of the same species or other species, is in my opinion wrong and also deleterious to health. That milk as we know it in its various forms is pleasing, delicious, appetizing and satisfying cannot be denied but here we are not dealing with that aspect, we are dealing with milk and dairy products as they pertain to or affect human health.

We must not allow ourselves to be misled by the propaganda machine, mainly supported by the dairy industry which again involves billions of dollars. It influences our government, our researchers, the medical profession and other august bodies including the National Research Council, the Academy of Sciences and such. So the literature that I have is scanned.

I understand that the human being in infancy is provided with a thymus gland whose specific function is to handle the milk that is fed by means of a breast. As the need for milk lessens due to the use of other foods the thymus gland shrinks and in due course changes its function as the infant outgrows its need for or dependence upon milk. Nature provided and intended that milk was to be consumed only direct from the mammary gland. Any other means and method of utilizing milk causes it to have a much impaired value.

It has been conclusively proven that a breast fed baby has a better shaped mouth, better shaped lips and better facial characteristics than a child who was fed or raised on the bottle. I have investigated this, both from the literature available and from personal observation over many, years and found it to be true. Furthermore, I've learned that those who were nurtured from the breast have a much better chance of reaching old age than those who are denied that great privilege.

Through various forms of communication we have been indoctrinated for the past 60 years with the tremendous value of milk. We have literally been swamped and brainwashed to the degree that most people look upon me as a maniac or an ignoramous when I even suggest that milk is not the world's best food. Simple, basic, common sense would clearly indicate that a man has no more right to drink cow's milk than he has to drink cat's milk or pig's milk. Honestly, would you like to drink pig's milk? Then why would you drink a cow's milk or a goat's milk? I have no quarrel with the dairy industry or the dairy farmers but I am interested in truth and in human health and welfare. Now I'm not dealing specifically with aesthetic practices or principles, I'm not dealing with the right or the wrong morally about the drinking of milk ... I'm specifically here interested in milk and its impact upon the health of human beings.

If dairy products were eliminated from the diet of the people of America tomorrow the incidence of heart disease would drop drastically, practically totally. I do not suggest that dairy products are the only cause of heart disease but they are certainly one of the foremost causes. Fresh milk from wholesome, clean, healthy animals is bad enough but pasteurized milk, skim milk, 2% milk ... this is adding insult to injury. The crime is being compounded.

Years ago when I wrote the book "Milk, Friend or Fiend" I

159

brought to the attention of the world a very important thesis and that is that if human beings were fed cow's milk over a period of two or three or more generations the human being would begin to assume the characteristics of the bovine. I contend seriously and scientifically that this must be the end result because the milk of a cow is supposed to turn a calf which weighs 30 or 40 pounds at birth into an animal weighing close to 1,000 pounds at the end of a year whereas human milk is supposed to make a 7 or 8 pound baby at birth into a child weighing approximately 20 pounds in one year and as the ribo-nucleic acid genetic code is contained in our milk it will actually malform the human anatomy into a semi-bovine form. In experiments with children who were heavy milk drinkers and whose parents before them were heavy milk drinkers it was established that the secondary sexual characteristics were masked or altered so that you couldn't distinguish the male body from the female body at around the age of puberty.

There are literally dozens and perhaps hundreds of reasons why human beings should not drink cow's or other milk. I realize I'm depriving you of your ice cream and your sweet cream and your sour cream and your cottage cheese or your cheddar cheese or your 101 other cheeses but if you are seeking health and truth then you have no choice but to give up the eating of dairy products.

I have loved dairy products all my life, I still love them but I treat them with respect and use them only in moderation. I suggest that you do likewise, or better still, give them up completely ... perhaps you have a stronger character and more willpower than I.

160

CHAPTER

29

VEGETABLE VS ANIMAL FATS

Let's have a wee bit of a discussion about oils. Perhaps you refer to them as fats. I think that is the general name . . . fats.

Most of the fat that we use is the fat that comes from animals, known as animal fats . . . butter, cheese, milk, cream, meat and all such things as are derived from the carcasses of animals. Oh, yes, I should also mention fish in this group.

We'll discuss the vegetable fats, those that come from seeds which are the source of most of our oils . . . corn, sunflower, soy bean, safflower, peanut, sesame, walnut, almond, linseed and cotton. To the best of my knowledge and belief, every seed contains a fairly high amount of oil.

Generally speaking, animal fats are considered to be saturated

161

and vegetable oils are said to be unsaturated. It is still a fact that some of the animal fats are not too highly saturated and some of the seed oils like coconut oil are quite highly saturated. But broadly speaking, the seed oils are considered unsaturated.

The term polyunsaturate refers to molecular structure. The molecule of a fatty acid is a chain of carbon atoms with many bonds that join with hydrogen atoms. If all the bonds are attached to hydrogen atoms, the molecule is said to be saturated; if one bond is vacant, it is unsaturated; if more than one is vacant, it is polyunsaturated.

To make animal fats useable or edible we use heat. You might remember the good old days when mother rendered her lard from a hog and tallow from cattle or sheep. In rendering it and making it ready for use you had to use heat. Then when you went to use the fat, whether in frying, cooking or baking, you had to use heat again. So actually before you use fat it has gone through two heatings and from 250 to 450 degrees is used.

I am bold enough to suggest, without offering any clinical or research proof, that if the fats were used without any heating . . . for example, as an Eskimo uses blubber, which is whale fat . . . there would be no health problem arising from the use of such fat. I mean that there would be no heart disease or arteriosclerosis or thrombosis which today we know are caused or contributed to, by animal fats.

I am suggesting that it is the heating of the animal fats that first and foremost brings about the cardiac problems that arise from using saturated fats.

Let's go to the vegetable fats or oils, as we know them. In the olden days they used to get their fats from the seeds by pressure. That is, they would squeeze them until the oil came out. But even with the best methods of pressing you still could never get all or even most of the oil out of the seeds. This was called cold-pressing. They used hydrolic means later and this got more out but it still didn't get it all out and there was a lot of oil left in what remained of the seed.

From a business point of view, this was very uneconomical so they developed a method of heating the seed and then pressing it and they got much more oil out. But business is always looking forward and they found a much better method by using a chemical . . . that is, a solvent. They tried various solvents and of course the yield of oil from the seed was much greater. Now the solvents were many and various but at last the chemical boys came up with a solvent that is referred to as hexane gas.

This hexane gas, when put in with oil under heat, works absolutely like magic. It's a miracle. You put a bit of hexane gas in with chopped up corn or chopped up soy beans and immediately all the oil leaves the seed. I understand they get better than 99% of the oil out of the corn, soy beans or other seed material.

This was good . . . wonderful! It made oils very economical. But what is this hexane gas business?

According to my chemical index, this hexane is the chief constituent of petrol, ether or ligroin. It is a colorless, very volatile liquid, with a faint peculiar odor. It is insoluble in water, miscible with alcohol, chloroform and ether. The lethal concentration for mice in air is about 40,000 parts per million. In other words, it will kill a mouse if there are 40,000 parts per million in the air.

It is used for determining refractive index of minerals and as a filling for thermometers instead of mercury, usually with a blue or red dye. Its human toxicity, it says, may be irritating to the respiratory tract and in high concentration its action is narcotic.

Obviously hexane is a deadly poison. So I hope they can get the hexane out of the oil before it is used. The general method of doing this is to filter off the oil and this leaves the residue of the corn or the soy beans in a vat. Then they apply heat to both the oil and the residue and this supposedly drives off the hexane gas.

Now I am firmly convinced that they drive off most of the hexane but chemical reactions must have occurred. Even a kid who took the first couple of lessons in chemistry knows that a chemical reaction occurred there, heat or no heat. So when you use vegetable oils that were solvent treated you are using oil that has been affected by hexane. And if you used the remaining residue for any purpose which is generally referred to as "meal", for example, soybean meal, it would be residue plus the effects of the hexane.

Can you deny the truth of what I am saying? I am saying that you have combined hexane gas with oil and you get a sort of an oil, but there was a chemical action or reaction and you are getting the end result of that chemical action in both the oil and the residue.

Now after the oil is rendered, if they want to make margarine or something like Crisco or Domestic shortening, then they take that oil that they have made in this manner and they mix it again, under heat, with hydrogen gas and pulverized nickel and you get the hardened Crisco, Domestic shortening or margarine.

Now if you have followed me from the start, you are probably as mixed up as an 80 year old man coming off the merry-go-round. But the fact that I am trying to get home to you is that what originally started as a bit of fat in a seed, which you would get in its entirety and in its natural state if you ate the seed, is now a contaminated, contemptible, chemical concoction . . . and the Lord alone knows what it is. I'm sure no chemist knows and nobody else knows.

I contend — and I have done so now for ten years — that there is not one decent useable oil for human beings on the market on the North American continent.

It is a positive fact that fats and oils are an indispensable part of the human diet. The physiologists tell us that they provide the soluble vitamins and the essential fatty acids of the so-called vitamin F group.

So now I'm going to tell you that animal fats are far, far superior to vegetable fats. Believe me, it actually breaks my heart to say this and I say it for only one reason and that is because it is true. I don't care whether it is lard, or suet or mutton fat. The fact is that these three, without processing, are much superior to the best vegetable oil that you can get anywhere.

Of course, butterfat is superior to any of the above three and it is so far ahead of processed hydrogenated vegetable fat that there really isn't any basis of comparison.

Any individual who uses vegetable oils with an idea of benefitting his body and his health certainly is making a terrible mistake. Please understand that I am thoroughly familiar with the cholesterol story and the blood serum levels and the saturated, unsaturated and poly-unsaturated fat business. In fact, I'm so full of it and so steeped in it that I am slithering around in it.

It has been my bad fortune to take the time and effort required to thoroughly study the oil situation. I have poured over two massive volumes, one entitled "Vegetable Fats And Oils," by Eckey, and another, "Bailey's Industrial Oil And Fat Products," and I don't know how many other papers and studies where oils and fats are discussed and mentioned. Actually, I started out believing and preaching that vegetable oils were a superior product, far superior to animal fats. But when I began to study and investigate I was shocked beyond belief by what I learned.

Please believe me, I could not find one single redeeming feature in vegetable oils. It doesn't make any difference whether you are talking about sunflower oil, safflower oil, soya oil, sesame oil, walnut oil, olive oil, linseed oil, cottonseed oil, or rapeseed oil. It is a vegetable oil and it just isn't worth a tinker's damn.

Please forgive me for blasting your hopes and your dreams, because so many, many people have accepted the fact that vegetable oils were so much superior. This is to me a great tragedy also because it's almost blocked off all avenues of escape or means of living on a proper wholesome, vegetable diet.

But what do you want me to do? Do you want me to lie? However, there is a redeeming feature and I ask you to bear with me a little longer.

It is not that there is anything wrong with vegetable oils, it is what goes wrong and what takes place in the processing. You could find the best oil in the world by chewing a few grains of wheat. Now I've never heard of rye oil, but you can bet the last nickel you own that rye seeds contain lots of good oil. And flaxseed oil . . . why, man that's the best oil ever created, according to the experts.

What I'm aiming to get across to you is that the finest oils in the world are found in vegetables and in grains and in nuts, but it's in the processing that they are slaughtered, murdered, annihilated, corrupted, and adulterated.

To tell you the honest truth, I've tried earnestly to get all the oil I need from seeds and nuts and I find that one must consume a fair quantity to obtain sufficient oils to sustain the body in good health. Grains and nuts must become a permanent part of your diet if you are to receive adequate, proper fat. Root and leaf vegetables do contain good oils but in smaller quantities. Those who do not eat seeds and nuts will end up with serious problems due to lack of assimilable fat.

Rancid oils have long been regarded as a very serious danger in the foods of mankind. Some authorities have expressed the opinion that all rancid oils are carcinogens of the first order.

I neither dispute nor agree but for many years I have wondered and recently my suspicions have been more or less confirmed and I would say that rancid oils are one of the foremost causes of or contributors to cancer in human beings. From what I have learned and seen of oils and their processing, I would agree that there are seldom any oils that are processed before they become rancid.

Granted, all oils go through a reclaiming process . . . that is, by means of refining, deodorizing, bleaching and various other methods. I say you can't bring the dead back to life. If it was rancid to begin with, then all the fancy doctoring will not make it a respectable food product again ever.

Most of the oils used in food in America today are absolutely harmful, carcinogenic substances and if proper research studies were made today, this would be proven. When oils are hydrogenated, it means that one more felony has been compounded and they are even worse than they were before. Therefore, I suggest that oils in the form that they can be purchased in America are not only nutritionally bankrupt but are a positive cause of or contributor to many diseases, including cancer.

Now there's a strange thing I want to relate here. If the oil were rendered by ordinary squeezing or cold pressing and left that way in crude form with the particles in it, well there are factions in those particles that would temporarily prevent the oil from becoming rancid. But nobody would buy crude oil and once the particles are filtered out rancidity begins to set in immediately, even if kept cool.

The mystery to me is how they can sell these cold pressed oils and prevent them from being rancid. They must use some magic that they haven't bothered to tell me about. Further, where, pray tell me, can you get genuine cold pressed oil? I do not know of one single proven source. So-called cold pressed oil to me means only words until proven otherwise.

Now I recall on my visit to Hunza, I wanted to get the oil affair straightened away so I made it a point to ask the Mir if he would get one of his subjects to make some apricot oil while I was there so that I could watch the process. The Mir was kind enough to arrange a demonstration for me.

I was taken to the house of a Hunza woman and I saw her perform the process. She produced a couple of handfuls of apricot kernels, put them into a mortar and mashed them all up with a pestle. When they were all mashed up she put the mass into an iron

167

pan and then put the pan over the heat. I carefully noticed that the pan didn't get very hot because she put her hands into the pan with the macerated apricot kernels and kneaded them just like a baker would do when he kneads dough. With her fingers and knuckles she kept on kneading and kneading and the pan was getting warmer and her fingers were getting warmer and after quite a bit of kneading during which the pan had become good and warm, drops of oil began to drip from her fingers and from the mass of macerated apricot kernels.

I watched the drip, drip, drip and before long she had a few ounces of fresh oil that she poured into a bottle. I examined it. I tasted it. It had an attractive color but it was quite murky and it was the faction in that murkiness that kept it from going rancid.

But even then, they carefully explained to me that it was not good policy to make very much at a time. They just made what they needed for that day and perhaps the next day. Then when they wanted more oil they had to go through the same process again.

Please understand, I do not say that animal oils are good oils or proper oils or that they will benefit your body. I am careful to state that they will do you a lot less harm than will the conventional highly processed vegetable oil that you can buy because most animal fats are not subject to such vicious treatment and monkeying with. I definitely do not advise the use of processed animal fats like lard. If you use animal fat it must be from the meat itself.

The fat that you get when you eat a steak, a pork chop, a stew, or a lamb chop, is much, much better fat than you would get from any vegetable oil that you buy in any store.

Of course if you eat enough fresh grains, seeds, nuts, and perhaps avocados and other vegetables and roots you definitely get all the good oil that you need. That kind of oil would be so far superior to any animal oil, or any processed vegetable oil, that there just is no basis for comparison.

168

Just so that you will know I'm not as crazy as I sound, I want to quote this article verbatim —

"TESTS FAVOR ANIMAL FAT — Recent USDA research has revealed that a lack of dietary iron coupled with the intake of certain vegetable fats can result in the development of enlarged thyroid glands or goiters. The problem was less noticeable when diets included butter, lard, or beef fat.

"The research was conducted by Columbia University scientists who studied rats which were fed iron deficient diets containing 20 percent fat. The fats tested included fresh and mildly oxidized beef fat, chicken fat, butter, lard, cottonseed oil, olive oil, corn oil, and soybean oil.

"The animals' thyroid glands were weighed at the end of the trial to see if the fats had caused any differences in the size of goiters. Rats fed butter, lard and beef fat had the lowest incidence of enlarged thyroids. Olive oil, an unsaturated fat, caused the highest incidence of enlarged goiters. And the proportion of enlarged thyroids was intermediate among rats fed chicken fat, soybean oil, and corn oil."

The truth of the matter is, folks, that in the processing of the vegetable oils, most of them have been turned from a fat into an actual plastic. And dear friends, plastics don't belong in the human body.

Let it be clearly understood I favor the vegetarian way of life and my diet is 95% vegetable, but I clearly state the meat and animal fats are much to be preferred to processed hydrogenated vegetable oils.

In my household I use very little oil. In fact, I prefer to use no oil in any form. You might ask what you can use for frying? Well, you shouldn't fry any food to begin with because frying is definitely, seriously harmful. What can you use for baking? You can use butter. What can you use for cooking? Well, friend, I don't care what you

169

use but don't use oil. If you want to live and be healthy, commerical oil is not for you!

"But the body needs oil!" you argue.

Ah, with that I agree completely. The body needs oil and needs it badly and needs it regularly. So I say to eat nuts, eat grains, eat seeds of any kind, eat avocados and eat carrots. All the root vegetables contain oil.

Oils can be had and you can get them by the means suggested above. If you want to be healthy, use no manufactured oil but get your oil right from the source as nature intended.

CHAPTER

30

ENERGY UNLIMITED

Probably the most frequent complaint that I've heard from people is that they lack energy. Men, women and children of all ages seem to have this common affliction. Some people just assume that it is natural and there is nothing they can do about it and carry on from there never showing a spark of life and just sort of dragging themselves through from day to day.

I came across a lady in New Zealand who told me that every day for years she had just dragged herself on from one day to the next. She was in her early 60's when I met her and she just accepted it as one of these things that she had to live with until she died and there was nothing she could do about it. This was a tragic mistake. A genuine, tragic mistake because the woman didn't have to suffer through all these years. What was even worse was that the woman was an intelligent woman in practically every way ... she raised a

171

family, she had everything to live for and her husband was an influential, wealthy lawyer, they had the most beautiful of homes — everything and yet she just had no energy. The doctor couldn't tell her why and that was the way she lived and she didn't care whether she lived or died. In fact, she told me that she didn't care if she died that night.

Well I want to assure you that this chronic fatigue and lack of pep and energy are definitely not normal and they certainly are not an indication of health. The story I told you is a true story but the big tragedy is that it is multiplied hundreds of thousands of times in America today let alone in Britain and in other advanced nations throughout the world. I'm telling you here and now it doesn't have to be and the remedy, the means of ending this is at hand and it's as simple as eating a handful of living grains. I should also stress that this affects, as I mentioned at the start, people of all ages starting in their teens. Furthermore, let me tell you this. When this happens to you or anyone else you get sick, really sick. Basically you are suffering from malnutrition. Here you've been kidding yourself that you're perfectly well fed because you eat the best and the richest and the most expensive of food.

Allow me to suggest that you may be eating what are normally considered proper foods in wide variety and still you're lethargic and sort of dead to the world from the neck up. Yes, and from the neck down, too.

It is not my intent to try and give you a picture of the way the body acts and reacts to food and about the chemistry of the body and the machine the body is which most doctors and nutritionists try to pawn off on people to prove how smart they are and how much schooling they've had. All they succeed in doing when they finish is beclouding and fogging up the true picture and they haven't convinced you nor themselves of anything.

Listen here, whether you eat three or four meals a day or whether you eat 6 meals a day or only 1 meal a day is of little consequence. It is what you eat. Let's even take it a step further.

172

You can eat all of the right foods . . . even if I told you what foods to eat to give you energy . . . yes, you can eat all of them and still have no energy and still feel as bad as ever.

So let's start at the beginning. The energy foods are carbohydrates. Yes, people who eat lots of proteins seem to do all right too and foods generally contain protein, carbohydrates, fats, minerals and vitamins. All of these names that nutritionists throw at you to impress you are truly meaningless. What you need is live, whole food and that's just what you do not get when you buy commerical food.

Normally speaking if you want energy you eat carbohydrates and grains are among the best of the carbohydrates. So the solution is an easy one, isn't it? Just get lots of grains into your system. But yet if you took and fragmented or refined the carbohydrates and cooked them the chances of getting any genuine energy out of them are remote, if not absolutely nil.

If you are lacking in energy you can restore your vitality and whether or not you ever had any great strength you can be filled with vim. Now let me tell you of my 3-V breakfast cereal.

This formula is based upon the early Bircher-Benner Muesli system. The first time that I tried muesli my remark was, "If I've got to eat stuff like this to be healthy, then I don't want to be healthy!"

I don't expect to be given any laurels for a remark like that. In fact, I'm thoroughly ashamed of that remark. However, I'm not trying to hide it . . . that is what I said and that is what I am telling you that I said.

Of course, it so happened that the party who made this mixture for me at that time didn't practice the best means and methods of preparation and there was no great attempt made to make it palatable. It was supposed to be good for you and that meant, it seems, it didn't have to be appealing or tasty. Nevertheless, my remark was positively not justified. Later, why, I gained some

173

knowledge and experience.

I studied the formula carefully and came up with the rhyme and the reason behind Dr. Bircher-Benner's great introduction. He certainly was away ahead of his time, but it proved that mankind was slow in recognizing its true merit. Actually, from my reading it was the first time a man had recognized the value of raw food in the human diet. Therefore, I began to use it and I still couldn't take it to my breast, so to speak. It was all right and I could eat it but it was a sort of a chore or should I say, a bore.

But I kept saying to myself, "I want health – I want it badly – so I'll have to put up with a bit of food that isn't so appetizing. So what if it doesn't taste so hot?"

Then a more advanced thought occurred to me, "Why not try to make it palatable? You've got access to good food and you know a bit about it, so work on it."

I did just that and I got my wife interested and we began a series of experiments. Every day we tried a new batch for breakfast. Sometimes we added and sometimes we subtracted. Sometimes we put more of this and less of that and other times we put less of this and more of that. Well, after monkeying around for about two years we came up with the answer to what I was seeking . . . (a) 100% nutrition, (b) palatability, (c) availability. In fact it was so good and tasteful to eat that there was a great temptation to overeat. The most important thing about this breakfast food, or 3-V cereal as I call it, is that it fulfills the basic needs of mankind. It is 100% nutrition and the items it contains are generally available anywhere. Therefore, no one need be undernourished, not even the poor.

Now if you were to go out tomorrow to one of the health food stores and buy some of the Bircher-Benner Muesli (it goes under various names) you'll say, "What in blazes was Tobe squawking about when he said it didn't taste good?"

But hold it a jiffy! The package of muesli that you buy is by no means anything like the original Bircher-Benner formula. In the first place, the Bircher-Benner original formula, like my 3-V Cereal, was 100% alive. You can readily understand that if the Bircher-Benner Muesli that you buy in the store was 100% alive then they couldn't keep it on the shelves, simply because it would soon be crawling with various living organisms, especially at store temperatures of 70 and 80 degrees. Even under refrigeration it does not keep well enough.

Now the ingredients contained in the store-bought Bircher-Benner Muesli are excellent but they are dead. In my 3-V cereal, as in the original Bircher-Benner Muesli, they are alive. Besides, most of these mueslis are imported and very expensive. The recipe I will give you will enable you to have a much, much better muesli at a very low price. Ounce for ounce it will cost you even less than any packaged crummy cereal on the market.

Anyway, when I wound up with my 3-V cereal, it contained a lot more than the Bircher-Benner formula. I made the additions and subtractions for definite, positive reasons. To begin with, we are living in America, not in Switzerland, and we have access to a much greater variety of food than they have in Switzerland. We must also recognize that Bircher-Benner, having discovered this about 100 years ago, did not have the benefit of the scientific knowledge that we have today . . . but basically the idea behind the Bircher-Benner Muesli was one of the greatest forward steps in the history of mankind. This is a sincere statement on my part.

I have learned the value of variety. I have learned that soils do become depleted, and most commercial grains are not thoroughly nutritionally balanced. Therefore, I felt that by having a wide selection of different grains from different areas of the country perfect balance could be attained.

One of the big shortcomings that I found in the Bircher-Benner Muesli was the lack of chlorophyll. I have taken the trouble to dig deeply and study the merits of chlorophyll and they are tremendous . . . I should say, earth-shattering. I pondered as to

175

how to get this into a muesli. I found the solution and that's why you find alfalfa herb in the formula.

I learned that the Scotch people had kept alive and virile and mentally alert on a diet that leaned fairly heavily on oats. That is why oats are one of the main ingredients of my cereal. I've also learned that oats are better flavored, creamier and more palatable than most other grains. I also found out that oats lose less in the cooking than most other grains, although this cereal is supposed to be used uncooked.

Then I began to study the ways and means of making it palatable. This was accomplished by adding fresh and dried fruits.

You may wonder why I put so many things together in one formula. The reason, I figured most people would if necessary deign to take this formula for one meal a day so I made it a one shot deal and I put all my eggs in one basket. I calculated that you might tackle my cereal for one meal a day, so I had one chance and I was going to hit as hard as I possibly could, with all my might, with that one blow.

If you are going to make this cereal I don't care where you get the ingredients but my suggestion is that you get them organically grown, if possible. But, organically grown or not, make sure you get them.

Buy the best ingredients that you can. None of them is expensive and if dried fruits are too expensive, buy fresh fruits that are cheaper. If dried peaches or dried apricots are too dear, use more raisins, use more dried apples or dried pears or dates or figs.

I permit the use of a bit of milk, but not much milk is required if you will soak the 3-V cereal overnight. In fact, better still, you can soak a whole batch — enough to last a week — and keep it in the refrigerator. I don't think it will suffer any harm and by having it soaked, a lot of water will be absorbed and you will require very little milk. Better still, do without any milk. I say that again, better still, do without any milk!

I have absolute and positive proof concerning the nutritive and the beneficial value of the 3-V cereal because thousands of people through the years have written or taken the trouble to tell me personally how much they have benefitted from using it.

I am not trying to sell you the cereal. I am giving you the formula. Follow it as closely as possible and use it daily and feed it to your family. Even if you have to persuade, coax, cajole or club your children into taking it, do it for a few days. After that they'll take it on their own and want or demand it.

If I do nothing else in my whole life for my fellow man but teach him the merits of 3-V cereal, I will have earned my reward wherever or whatever that amounts to.

I would like to clarify two points. First, the original Bircher-Benner Muesli contained ground nuts. I deliberately omitted nuts because they go rancid very quickly. Second, I now use and recommend only whole grains — not ground or cracked. I find that by soaking the whole mixture together all of the seeds soften enough to allow grinding and chewing without any great effort. Even hard cereals like barley and rice will soften enough to make them chewable and digestible.

Without boasting or exaggerating, it is the finest, the best balanced, the most nutritious assembled food in the whole world. Be sure no flaked, rolled grains . . . all whole grains.

3-V CEREAL

Oats	10 parts
Barley	2 parts
Wheat	2 parts
Rye	2 parts
Buckwheat	2 parts

Millet	2 parts
Sesame	1 part
Flax	1 part
Alfalfa Herb, Powdered	2 parts
Dried Prunes	2 parts
Dried Raisins	2 parts
Dried Peaches	1 part
Dried Apricots	2 parts
Dried Dates	1 part
Dried Figs	1 part

Total — 15 Ingredients

Cut fruit into small pieces. Thoroughly mix fruits and grains together.

Don't cook or heat . . . just add water — spring or well water preferred . . . let soak overnight.

Add milk, cold or warm (never hot), if desired. Eat 2 to 5 tablespoons every day or at least every other day.

It is most advisable to soak the ingredients because I want to return the water that was originally in the food and this can only be done by allowing it to soak. I get best results and the most satisfying flavor by making enough to last me a week and keeping it in the refrigerator and then every day or every other day taking out the quantity that I want for that meal. Following this recipe alone will correct the condition . . . that is the lack of energy and will provide you with energy, all day and all night, if you want it. Isn't it tragic that most people in the world don't know this simple answer to a very difficult problem?

Right now you're thinking this is just too easy, it is just too simple and best of all it doesn't even cost much money. You can buy the ingredients and mix the whole concoction yourself and it will only cost you pennies for a good big breakfast. Why use it only for breakfast . . . use it for lunch, use it for dinner and you can mix a batch of it to last you a week for less money than it will cost you to buy a big package of those cooked processed cereals that were proven by investigations to contain more energy in the package than in the food. So unless you act upon this suggestion you are depriving yourself of a body full of pep and energy.

When you eat the food outlined in this recipe you are getting 100% nutrition. You are not just getting energy, you're getting practically all of the minerals and vitamins that your body requires to maintain itself in perfect health. I have said for many long years that a handful of grains and a handful of greens can sustain you in perfect health indefinitely provided you don't cook them or process them or chemicalize them.

Now one more point. The best energy food in the world can be knocked into a cocked hat if you drink a lot of booze and if you smoke a lot of cigarettes or cigars or smoke a pipe or take drugs. This food will work if you permit it to work, if you don't interfere with it.

All right, now you've got the answer. Do something about it and be filled with pep all day, every day.

CHAPTER

31

THE MERITS OF SPROUTS

Heavens to Betsy, what can a city dweller do to protect himself against the chemicals in his vegetables? It's bad enough that he gets loads of chemicals in his milk, in his meat, in his fish, in his fruit but he even gets them in his vegetables.

Well, to those of you who do not consume many vegetables, this may not be a problem. But to me, for example, and many of my friends, who eat vegetables as a major part of their diet, these sprays are very, very serious. So what do we do?

Not many people realize just how much danger lies in the deadly sprays in our vegetables, fruits and grains and don't for a minute rest secure in thinking that your meat, eggs and butter are safe. They are definitely unsafe for they are loaded with chemicals, antibiotics, etc. A large portion, if not most, of our vegetables during

181

the winter come from California — the Imperial Valley and many other points. Take a trip down there some day and look things over . . . you'll be surprised, shocked or startled out of your wits at what you see. You will no longer wonder why so many of us get sick . . . you'll wonder how any of us stay alive.

As I tell people, either you've got to buy yourself a farm or a piece of land and grow your own or you will have a hard time remaining alive and in good health. From what I see in the supermarkets we have some of the nicest looking vegetables that were ever grown . . . and they really are nice looking. But just how badly sprayed and poisoned they are is another matter . . . one over which you and I have no control and very little knowledge about. Only the farmer who grew them and sprayed them knows just how badly poisoned they are. Still, we're lucky that many of these poisons or most of them are water-soluble and they do wash off. But if you wash extensively or soak them, you also soak out some or many of the water-soluble nutrients.

However, there is a way to avoid a great deal of this contamination and that is by sprouting. The Chinese have been doing this for I don't know how many thousands of years. Evidently they were the first people to do it and this has been handed down and the western world of recent years has been doing a fair amount themselves. I've been doing it for about 35 years, off and on.

The Chinese use most of their sprouts in making their Chinese foods, which means they are heated . . . although the Chinese do not heat to a high heat and often when you eat in a Chinese restaurant you will find that most of the vegetables are still crisp and flavorful and not cooked right through, which is good.

I would suggest that a sprout is probably the finest form in which a seed can be eaten. By eating sprouts you get practically the full benefit of the seed as well as the benefit of the sprout which contains nutrients not found in the seed itself. A most important consideration about sprouts is the fact that you have control over them. You buy, or better still you grow, your seed which can be mung beans or soy beans, but alfalfa makes mighty good sprouts and practically any seed can be sprouted, such as, beans, peas, garbanzos, lentils and many more. Make sure you get high grade seed . . . with a germination of about 90% or better and don't settle for less. The Chinese, when they buy mung beans, demand 99.99% germination or they won't buy them . . . and they get them. They seldom miss sprouting a bean.

Sprouts are grown indoors and therefore they are subject to no contamination whatsoever. I do not suggest that they wouldn't be better if they were grown outdoors . . . in fact, I think they would . . . but they won't sprout unless you follow a specific procedure. In any event, when you have your sprouts, you are getting something that is completely safe to eat and probably as nourishing as any food that you could find anywhere.

When you eat a lettuce leaf you are eating only the leaf. When you eat a sprout you are getting partially formed leaves as well as the root and the stalk et al.

Sprouts taste good. The best tasting of all, in my opinion, are soy bean sprouts. They are much meatier than the other seeds. But peas, beans and lentils are good and add variety to your sprouting schedule.

The nutritional value of sprouts ranks among the best of foods and therefore you can safely consume fair quantities every single day with great benefit to your health. You can eat them just as they are, you can use them in salads or you can use them in cooking. But it is best to eat them raw and fresh. For winter use they are hard to beat.

METHODS OF SPROUTING

Sprouting is easy. No special paraphernalia whatsoever is required. It is not an exaggeration to say, "You take care of your sprouts and your sprouts will take care of you."

Only the highest quality seeds should be used for sprouting. Because of my lifetime of experience with plants and seeds, I stress the importance of using only seed-quality mung beans and other seeds for sprouting purposes. It may sound rather strange when I say to buy only seed-quality seeds so please allow me to explain.

When you buy beans or peas or rice or barley or other grains or seeds in your food market, these seeds are usually food-quality seeds. There are no rules, laws or regulations governing the viability or germination of seeds sold for food purposes. However, when it comes to seeds for growing purposes, then the Department of Agriculture has strict regulations concerning their viability or germination. Here I will give you figures as they are laid down by the Department of Agriculture of the Dominion of Canada. All seeds sold throughout the country must have a viability or germination ability above the minimum specified. This selfsame procedure, with some variation, is demanded throughout the United States, too.

Minimum Percentage Germination

1.	Artichoke	75
2.	Asparagus	75
3.	Cardoon	55
4.	Carrot (cultivated)	60
5.	Celeriac	60
6.	Celery	55
7.	Celtus	75
8.	Chervil	75
9.	Chicory (cultivated)	65
10.	Chives	65
11.	Cornsalad	75
12.	Cress, garden	75
13.	Cress, water	35
14.	Dandelion (cultivated)	55
15.	Dill	50
16.	Eggplant	65
17.	Endive	65
18.	Leek	65

19.	Lettuce	70
20.	Okra	55
21.	Onion	75
22.	Parsley	55
23.	Parsnip	60
24.	Pepper	65
25.	Rampion	55
26.	Rhubarb	65
27.	Sage	50
28.	Salsify	75
29.	Savory	50
30.	Sorrel (cultivated)	65
31.	Spinach	65
32.	Spinach, New Zealand	50
33.	Thyme	50
34.	Tobacco	75
35.	Tomato	75

I stress that these figures are minimum and usually the germination percentages are actually much higher. A good grade of mung beans for sprouting should have a minimum germination of 90 per cent — accept no less.

Therefore, when you buy seed-quality seeds you must get high germination. So I stress again that the seeds or the peas or the beans sold in the food stores are of a much lower grade and much lower germination than seed quality seeds.

Now there is one very vital thing that you must watch in buying seed-quality seeds and that is, many of them are treated with various compounds, usually mercury compounds. Now why these seeds are treated is quite a long story but the fact is that they are treated with dangerous and harmful deadly chemicals. So when you buy seeds be sure that they are thoroughly washed.

Food-quality seeds are generally untreated and most of the mung beans sold throughout America are untreated, but you must protect yourself and I would emphasize thorough washing.

185

Now, take alfalfa seeds. Most of the alfalfa that is used for seeding purposes throughout America is highly treated with various chemicals. So, either be sure you buy seeds that have not been treated or make sure you wash them time and time again to make sure that all of the harmful, deadly chemicals have been removed.

Here is a list of the various vessels or containers used in sprouting:

1. Large 10-gal. earthenware crock
2. Bath tub
3. Clay flower pot, unglazed
4. Sprouting trays
5. Any glass jar
6. Sprouting kit
7. Butter dish
8. Red clay flower pot saucer
9. Sink strainer
10. Soup or tea leaf strainer
11. Coffee percolator
12. Cloth or towel
13. Paper towel
14. Sponges
15. Blotting paper used in germination tests
16. Petri dishes
17. Any plate, platter, crock, dish, jar, bottle or wide-mouthed jug

METHODS

First and foremost, be sure to thoroughly wash the seeds. I usually rinse them a minimum of three times before allowing them to soak.

(1) Here I will describe the Chinese method. This is used by the largest Chinese restaurant in Toronto. This restaurant serves thousands of people daily and they use enormous quantities of mung beans. They also supply mung beans to the wholesale trade. I would

rank their method Number One among all methods known and the results they get are ample conclusive proof that this is by far the best method that has yet been discovered.

I am sure that if anyone cared to take the trouble they could go down to one of the larger Chinese restaurants and would be shown the technique right on the spot.

So we start with the highest quality beans that can be purchased. This organization buys them by the carload. They use 15-gallon crocks. Approximately 1/5 of the crock is filled with mung beans. Then hot water is poured over them, filling the crock brimful. Now this is not boiling water, but hot water. This is allowed to stand overnight.

In the morning the excess water is drained off and a wetted down reed mat is placed over the damp mung beans.

The seeds are rinsed every 3 hours but even after the first night's soaking in good warm water an appreciable change has taken place in the seeds. They are much fatter, or plumper, it seems. By the next day, that is 48 hours afterwards, you can see the swelling and the signs on the seed that it is ready to burst. On the third day the sprouts are usually visible. The fourth day shows root growth and sprouting.

Here is a sample of the actual procedure:

Wed. 4 P.M. — Soak 2 3/4 lbs. mung beans in warm water, 85-90 degrees, in a clean galvanized garbage pail or crock. Leave overnight.

Thurs. A.M. — Pour off water. Then transfer the 2 3/4 lbs. of swollen beans into clean 15-gal. crock. This only fills 1/4 of the crock. Lay soaked reed mat on top of beans for dampness and humidity. On top of crock place a fairly tight fitting wooden lid. Noticeable swelling takes place.

187

Thurs., Fri., Sat. — Beans must be dampened every 3 hours. Maintain temperature at 74 degrees.

Friday — Sprouts appear. Crock now 1/2 full.

Sat. — Sprouts 1/2" or more long. Crock 3/4 full.

Sun. — Crock solid full. Dumped into cold water bath. Fished out with a net, then put into clean bushel baskets for delivery to stores and restaurants. They will now keep under refrigeration for another 6 or 7 days.

One pound of dry beans makes six pounds of sprouts.

The same procedure can be followed for other kinds of seeds.

I have given close details concerning this method because it is simple and effective. By the 5th or the 6th day, the crock is practically brimful with a tight, solid mass of roots and sprouts. They are scrupulously clean, they have gained tremendously in size and weight and are crisp and crunchy, wholesome and delicious.

While I have listed numerous means and methods of sprouting, with slightly varying procedures, I see no reason why the above simple method cannot be followed in all cases. If you want fancy dishes or if you want to play around with it and have fun, that's a different story, but this direct, simple, wholesome, clean and botherless method is the best of all.

(2) Here is an excellent method where only small quantities of soy beans, mung beans or other seeds are sprouted.

Put beans or seeds in a quart fruit jar or any glass jar. Cover with water and soak overnight. The next morning, drain off the excess water. Invert jar, using a piece of muslin or better still, a piece of copper or galvanized screening to cover the mouth. Rest the jar on two small pieces of wood to allow circulation of air.

Keep in the dark for 2 or 3 days, by means of a heavy paper bag inverted over the jar. Sprinkle a little water on the beans every day or better still, a few times a day, to insure a good supply of moisture. In 3 to 4 days the sprouts should be ready for eating . . . raw, cooked or in salads.

Now I cannot testify that the Chinese method would be suitable for all other types of seeds, but I have found that it works equally well for mung beans and alfalfa. I feel confident that it will work with most other kinds of seeds, too.

I must warn you that soy beans are defintely not as easy to sprout as mung beans.

My friend, Gil Watkins, of Madeira Beach, Florida, gives these methods for sprouting:

(3) Use a wide mouth gallon jar with perforated lid or nylon net. Use mung beans, alfalfa, fenugreek, etc.

Soak 3 oz. of mung beans or fenugreek seeds for 24 hours or alfalfa seeds, 1 ounce, for 4 hours. Then drain and spread the seeds around the jar that is now lying on its side. Twenty-four hours later soak for 15 minutes and drain. Twenty-four hours later do it again. Twenty-four hours later they are ready to eat or refrigerate.

(4) His other method is to take a 3 qt. tin can and perforate the bottom. Put about 3 ounces of mung beans or fenugreek seeds in the can. Set the can in a larger container of water, covering the seeds for 24 hours. Drain and place about a double thickness of terry cloth or towelling on the seeds. Keep it on the back of the sink and every time you get near it, run water on it to keep the cloth moist and to filter out any mould that might start.

He also gives these excellent salad dressings for your sprouts:

1. Two tablespoons of sesame, peanut or safflower oil and 1 tablespoon of cider vinegar.

189

2. 1/3 blackstrap molasses
   1/3 cider vinegar
   1/3 tupelo honey

(5) Here is the sprouting method as given by the U.S. Department of Agriculture in their bulletin No. 534:

"A year-round fresh vegetable that may be used raw or cooked can be obtained by sprouting soybeans in a flower pot or strainer. Peking, Cayuga, and Otootan are good varieties for sprouting because they germinate quickly and uniformly. Other varieties, however, can be used satisfactorily for this purpose.

"One-fourth pound (one-half cup) of dry beans of some varieties weighs about a pound when sprouted and may make as much as 5 to 6 cups of sprouts. Other varieties may yield only 2 to 3 cups. Flower pots 6 to 7 inches in diameter at the top and 6 1/2 to 7 inches high are large enough to allow for the expansion in volume. Rustproof wire netting or cheesecloth can be used to cover the hole in the bottom of the pot to prevent the beans from falling through and at the same time allows for drainage.

"Sort the dried soybeans, discarding shriveled and dead-looking ones. Wash the good beans thoroughly; then soak them overnight in 1 1/2 cups of lukewarm water. In the morning drain the beans, put them in the flower pot, and cover them with dampened cheesecloth. Put a piece of damp cardboard over the top of the pot and weight it down. Keep the pot in a dark place at about 78 to 80 degrees F.

"Three times a day pour water over the soybeans, draining it off immediately. Take care not to break the tender sprouts as they appear. Each evening sprinkle the beans with chlorinated lime solution to keep down mold growth and bacterial spoilage. The solution is made by dissolving 1 teaspoon of calcium hypochlorite in 3 gallons of water. This amount will treat 5 to 6 pounds of dry beans and may be stored to use with successive sproutings.

"Soybean sprouts are ready to use when they are 2 to 3 inches long. Both beans and sprouts are eaten. The loose skins may be removed by washing thoroughly. Sprouts can be served raw in salads, or they can be cooked in various ways or used in such dishes as omelets, stews, fricassees, or chop suey. They are very tender and lose their crispness if put into hot dishes more than a few minutes before serving."

It is advisable when sprouting grains like wheat, oats and rye that one should not wait until the sprouts become long. It is generally conceded that short sprouts for grains are advisable. They are at their best when the sprout is about the same size as the seed . . . that is, double its original size from seed to sprout. When they are allowed to grow too long they suffer in quality. Many seeds, including sunflower, will become bitter if they are allowed to grow too long.

When the sprouts have attained the right size, keep them in the refrigerator and they will remain in good condition for many days. Some people remove or cast aside the original seed or the seed coating. I prefer to eat the whole, complete sprouted seed and I would recommend it to those of you who read this book. Why fragment your food? I also believe that by wasting the original coating you are wasting some of the valuable nutrients.

It is an accepted fact that the chlorophyll content of the sprouts may be increased by exposing the sprouts to some sunlight a short time before serving.

To get best results from your sprouts it is advisable to have plenty of heat. A controlled heat of 70-80 degrees would be ideal. During the fall and winter, when the weather is apt to be cool and some homes are not too warm, it is best to put the sprouts in a location where they can be given added warmth; for example, by means of an electric light bulb. Try to keep the temperature above 70 degrees for best results. Always be sure to keep the sprouts in darkness to simulate the conditions the seeds would get if they were underground.

After they have been sprouted, if they are allowed some light, it will increase the various nutritional constituents. Where the atmosphere is hot and dry it is advisable to water more frequently. Do not allow your sprouts to dehydrate. Withholding water will definitely cut down the rate of development of growth of the sprouts. However, too much water will in most cases cause decay and other troubles.

It is important to remember that the utensils, the cloths, the paper, the blotters or whatever else is used in the sprouting of your various seeds should be kept washed and rinsed and thoroughly aired after each sprouting. Then they should be put out into the open air. This will prevent any mould or fungus from gaining a foothold. I suggest that interchangeable cloths and papers and towels and blotters be used. They should be exposed to the air and the sunlight in between uses. This will prevent failures and deter the growth of disease organisms and give bigger, better and more flavorful sprouts.

Sometimes when sprouting seeds you will find that the seeds do not germinate or that they begin to rot or ferment or mould. It is usually due to one of these causes:

(a) Seeds are old or have been improperly stored, thus low germination.
(b) Too much water.
(c) Insufficient water.
(d) Too cold.
(e) Too much light.
(f) Lack of air.

While it would seem, from the information that I give in this chapter, that you may have problems or troubles in growing sprouts, I want to assure you that I seldom, if ever, run into any trouble in growing sprouts. In fact, I can't recall when I have encountered any difficulty.

The basic requirements are:

(a) Viable seeds.

(b) Proper amount of moisture. Remember, keep seeds moist but not soggy wet.

(c) Proper degree of heat or controlled temperature.

The quantities that I advise for beginners is a teaspoonful of small seeds like alfalfa or mustard, a tablespoonful of the larger seeds like mung beans, and 1/2 cup of the larger seeds like beans or peas. After one or two trials you will learn the ropes and know the quantities to use.

Where the local supply of water has been heavily chlorinated or treated with other chemicals such as fluorides, this may definitely inhibit the growth of your sprouts. However, we hope and trust that there usually is insufficient of these chemicals to prevent the sprouting of seeds . . . but it can happen.

(6) In my own work in sprouting I follow the Chinese method but I do not rinse the seeds every three hours or even every day. All I do is sprinkle water upon them and make sure they are damp and covered with the paper towel in place of the mats and with a cloth towel over the top . . . and I have never had a failure.

I describe the art of sprouting in the following manner: "See nature at work. Procure good seeds, add water, air, warmth and a covering to stimulate soil conditions and then watch nature perform See the miracle of growth at work . . . and it is perfection. See nature combine living matter with water and air and extract the elements from the atmosphere and develop a new, living, expanding, growing organism."

I do not advise the use of chlorinated lime solution or any other inorganic chemical. Regular rinsing with clean water will prevent the formation of undesirable moulds and organisms.

CHAPTER

32

SEAWEEDS ARE GOOD VEGETABLES

A few things you should know about seaweeds. There are four genera that you should be acquainted with.

No. 1 Kelp (Fucus Vesiculosis).

No. 2 Dulse (Rhodomenia palmata).

No. 3 Laver (Porphyra Laciniata).

No. 4 Another Laver (Ulva Latissima).

Of the four, Kelp is the best known and the most widely used. But in my humble opinion, it is the poorest, the least nutritious and the most processed.

195

Dulse is the tastiest and the most nutritious and very widely known, but not known as well as kelp.

Dulse is a bright red leaf with deeply divided fronds. It is found off the coast of Scotland and Ireland and both species of Laver are also found in the seas around Scotland and Ireland and South Wales.

Dulse and the two Lavers are said to contain significant quantities of Vitamin B-12, which vegetarians are said to be deficient in.

In England the Ulva Latissima Laver is stewed and then covered with lemon juice and is highly esteemed. This is known as the green Laver.

The Porphyra Laciniata Laver has a curious purple color and is also stewed and fixed with lemon. It is considered both pleasing and nutritious.

Dulse is the only one that is eaten just as it is . . . plucked from the ocean and dried. Now I rate Dulse as the finest of all the seaweeds, especially from the viewpoint of nutrition.

Kelp is usually highly processed before it can be used. It is sold throughout America. Both the Porphyra and the Ulva are usually cooked but the Dulse is usually eaten just as nature made it. The only change is that it is dried so it can be handled and shipped.

Therefore, none of its valuable nutrients are lost. So for health's sake, eat Dulse. It tastes very salty, but I have noticed a peculiar thing about Dulse. It will not make you thirsty. Now this is unusual but I assure you it is absolutely true.

Furthermore, the salt found in Dulse is, in my own opinion, not only assimilable but completely utilizable by the body processes. Therefore, the body can derive all the benefits from it.

I consider Dulse one of the finest forms of natural, unprocessed organic foods.

It is claimed that seaweeds contain more elements than any land-grown food.

CHAPTER 33

THE TRUTH ABOUT SOY PRODUCTS

I am the first man and probably the only man in America or in the world who objects to the use of soy products in the diet of human beings or animals. Here I beg of you to note that I said soy products and I did not say soy beans.

Ninety per cent of all the soy products made, at least in America, are made from waste products left after the oil has been extracted from the soy beans by means of the hexane gas treatment. It is referred to as soy bean meal or soy meal or soy protein or hydrolyzed soy protein or vegetable protein and it probably has many other names as well. But the fact remains that they are all soy or soy bean products, or more accurately, soy bean residues or wastes.

About five years ago I openly and viciously attacked soy bean

199

products. I received a letter from one of the largest processors of vegetarian foods which is controlled by a religious movement and they took strong and emphatic exception to my denunciation of the soy products. They went to great lengths to point out how wonderful their products were. I wrote back and told them that if they would boldly and clearly state that their soy products were made from the whole bean, without any treatment, then I would retract my statements. But they did not reply and therefore I must assume that their products are made from the wastes of the soy beans and are not true soy bean products.

I was also attacked and challenged by other manufacturers and processors of soy products but not one single one of these people who attacked me would go on record as stating that their products were made from the whole soy bean.

The reason I knew that their products were made from the waste products of the soy bean was because the waste product is comparatively low in price whereas the whole soy bean is much more expensive and it requires more processing. Therefore, any company that attempted to make soy products from the whole soy beans would not be able to compete against the lower costing products. And I presume they feel that the public would not pay the increased price for the healthful instead of harmful soy products. I contend they are wrong on all counts.

However, there is a little more flavor to this story that I would like to tell you about. In order to justify the use of this horrible, destructive, harmful waste product called soy products in various forms, they have even concocted a story that tells you that the raw soy bean will cause sickness and death. What I am telling you may come as a surprise but it is 100% true and can be certified by anyone who is willing to investigate.

There are two research projects, with the accompanying documentations that positively prove that untreated or raw soy beans contain an enzyme inhibitor that will kill you or do you serious harm.

I came across this evidence about 15 years ago but instead of being frightened away from the soy beans, I made it a point to eat them. I did not believe that nature concocted a bean to poison people and animals, so I tried eating a few beans and more beans and then lots of soy beans, without cooking, and I lived to tell the tale. Therefore, I knew that these research projects were phoney somehow and the people who peddled that story were deliberate bold-faced liars and subsequent investigations have doubly or triply proven this assertion. I also tried the whole raw soy bean eating on a few of my friends. They, too, are still alive.

During the past few years, because of my statements made everywhere, one of these experimental stations, at least, has done some work with raw soy beans and nobody has died. So they are beginning — at least, this one institution — to re-evaluate their thinking about the merits of raw soy beans.

Now if you are at all intelligent or you have one ounce of brains in your bean, you'll be wondering what's all this about? What rhyme or reason would anyone have to pass on a story about raw soy beans causing you harm or killing you? It doesn't make sense. At least, it doesn't make sense on the surface.

However, there are some smart boys around and some of those big business outfits are pretty smart. So listen to me while I tell you the story . . . the true story and the whole story, so help me, God! No, I don't believe in taking oaths. My word is my bond and what I tell you is the truth and I don't have to take an oath to prove it to you. For those of you who don't know me, I'm taking this oath, because that might impress you that I really am speaking the truth.

The soy bean industry — that is, from the grower to the processor, the distributor and the exporter — is one of the greatest, the most important industries in America. In fact, if I am not seriously mistaken, soy beans are America's foremost agricultural crop . . . worth a billion dollars or more annually. Soy beans in various forms are used in many, many other products besides food.

Soy bean oil is very widely used . . . probably one of the most important vegetable oils in America or in the world. I don't know whether there is more soy bean oil sold than corn oil, but I'm telling you, there is a lot of soy bean oil sold.

Well, soy bean oil comes from the soy beans so you can imagine that there are virtually mountains of leftover soy residues after the oil has been taken out. So the question is, "What are they going to do with those mountains of remains of extracted soy beans?"

That's it, the smart boys found a market for it. In fact, they have found many, many, many markets for it . . . too many markets, for often they are hard pressed to supply the demand. But they had to prove that it was O.K. Therefore they concocted the story that the whole raw soy bean will kill you and the residue is wonderful food. Soy bean residues have been used for many long years as food for animals, apart from their use as human food, especially for babies.

Now you can well understand that if soy bean residues were no good and harmful, after a few years the farmer who feeds it to his animals would quickly recognize this and he would stop using it. So the chemical boys came up with a good solution. They sell these soy bean residues as a wonderful food for the animals and then they tell you to supplement this mineral and other nutrient deficient waste with certain synthetic chemicals to balance up what they have removed. And that is what is done in the animal food industry throughout America.

The same applies to the residues left from the beet sugar industry and the corn industry and other industries as well. The residues go mainly into making animal feed and then they have to add synthetic supplements to make up for what they have extracted. But in spite of this — or as I say because of this — animals get sick and die.

However, as most animals are only fed for a short period, the harmful results do not turn up in about 90% of the cases. It's only when you are dealing with animals such as cows that are kept for milking purposes that the sickness and ill health become apparent. That's why any herd of cattle requires a flock of veterinarians to look after them and keep shooting shots and vitamins into them.

The removal of the oil is not the most harmful thing that can happen to the soy bean. The animal might live and get by on the remainder. But the fact is that the present day method of extracting the oil is done through the use of a solvent and the solvent most widely used is known as hexane gas. This is a deadly, caustic, stinking petroleum product that is much more smelly than gasoline. When placed in a vat along with chopped up soy beans under heat, it removes 99.99% of the oil almost instantaneously. That is why it is used, even though it is harmful. Then they syphon off the oil loaded with hexane gas and then heat the residue and the oil to drive off the hexane gas. But as any jackass would know you could never ever get rid of the harmful effects of the hexane gas and its various chemical combinations.

Now I want to impress you with the fact that these soy bean products have no connection whatsoever with good wholesome, decent soy beans. Soy beans can be made into many nutritional, healthful, satisfying vegetarian products and you should use them. But don't buy any product that is made from soy bean residues . . . and at least 90% of all the soy bean products sold throughout America are made from soy bean residues that have been treated with hexane gas and are harmful to man and beast.

CHAPTER

34

GELATIN, PROTEIN AND STERILITY

If there is one so-called food on earth that has caused more trouble than any other food on earth, that so-called food is gelatin. I actually shudder when people call it food because it isn't a food in any sense of the word. To me it is a rank toxic substance . . . a poison. I say to you, with all sincerity, that gelatin has started more infants and children on their way to sickness and untimely death than any other substance on earth which is used as food.

I know of no language suitable to convey my feelings about this substance known as gelatin but to begin with I'm going to quote in toto from the Columbia Encyclopedia as to the meaning or origin of gelatin:

"Gelatin — glutinous material or animal jelly obtained from the supporting structures (e.g., hoofs, bones, and tendons) of vertebrate animals by the action of boiling water or dilute acid. The process of manufacture is a complex one which involves removing foreign substances, boiling the material (usually in distilled water in aluminum vessels) to prevent contamination, and purifying it of all chemicals used in freeing the gelatin from the connective tissues. The final product in its purest form is brittle, transparent, colorless, tasteless, and odorless and has the distinguishing property of dissolving in hot water and congealing when cold.

"In contact with cold water it takes up from 5 to 10 times its own weight and swells to an elastic, transparent mass. Gelatin, being readily digested and absorbed, is a good food for children and invalids. It is important in fine cookery as a vehicle for other materials, in the form of jellied soups, molded meats and salads, and frozen desserts. Preparations of it are used in the home manufacture of jam, jellies, and preserves to insure jellification of fruit juices. It is used in the drying and preserving of fruits and meats, in the glazing of coffee, and in the preparation of powdered milk and other powdered foods. Bakeries use it in making meringues, eclairs, and other delicacies. In confectionery making it is used as the basis of taffy, nougat, marshmallows, and fondant. Ice-cream manufacture employs it to maintain a permanent emulsion of other ingredients and thus to give body to the finished product. Added to cows' milk for the feeding of babies it prevents the formation of large curds. In scientific processes gelatin is widely employed, being used in electrotyping, photography, waterproofing, and dyeing and in coating microscopic slides. It is used as a culture medium for bacteriological research and also to make coatings for pills and capsules, court plaster, and some surgical dressings. It affords a base for ointments and pastes, such as toothpaste; it is an emulsifying agent useful in making liquid combinations and various sprays. In its less pure forms gelatin is known as glue and size. Vegetable gelatin, or AGAR, is derived from East Indian seaweeds."

Actually this should be sufficient for any human being with a gram of intelligence to never permit gelatin in his home or on his table, but I'll go beyond and I'll try to leave out my personal feelings and treat the matter in a more or less scientific manner.

Now I'll quote from a paper called "Gelatin . . . How It's Made":

"Collagen is the basic source of gelatin. Many animal tissues contain collagen, including pigskin, tanner's stock, and ossein. Pigskins arrive at the gelatin plant in a frozen condition. They are frozen just after removal at the packing house. Ossein is bone tissue — dried cattle bones — remaining after decalcification with mineral acids.

"Calf skins unsuitable for leather comprise tanner's stock. Such skins usually undergo a preliminary lime treatment before leaving the tannery and are available in an as-is condition or dry."

"Cone mills water-wash all types of stock before chemical treatment. After the preliminary washing, tanner's stock and osscin receives a soaking in 5% milk of lime slurry for 30 to 90 days. That softens the stock and dissolves a great deal of the non-collagen proteins."

"After liming, the stock again enters the wash mills where water removes the excess alkali, and a strong acid such as hydrochloric neutralizes the remaining lime. After this step, the stock is soft, light in color, relatively low in salt content, and has picked up about 3 to 5 times its weight in water."

Then the pigskins and other materials are cooked and various substances added until the product is ready to be dried and made into what we know as gelatin. I could give you this in much greater detail but I think you get the point.

Gelatin is recognized as being what is known as a very lop-sided protein. I have heard various individuals, yes, even scientists and medical doctors and nutritionists, say that gelatin was a valuable protein . . . or some call it a protein sparer. Obviously people who talk in this manner and boost the value and sale of protein have never in their lives made even a cursory study of the subject or the product.

207

For those who believe that gelatin is a valuable protein, here is the actual score with regard to the essential amino acids comparing the protein of gelatin with that of casein which is milk and gliadin which is wheat and zein which is corn:

	Gelatin	Casein	Gliadin	Zein
Alanine	0.6	1.50	2.00	13.39
Tyrosene	0.0	4.50	1.50	3.35
Tryptophane	0.0	1.50	1.00	0.00
Cystine	0.0	.06	.45	?
Histidine	0.4	2.50	1.84	.82
Phenylalaline	1.0	3.20	2.35	6.55
Valine	1.0	7.20	3.34	1.88
Arginine	9.3	3.81	3.16	1.55
Leucine	9.2	9.35	6.62	19.55
Lysine	7.61	6.00	.92	0.00
Methionine	0.00	3.40	2.10	?

From the above we learn that gelatin contains no tyrosene, tryptophane, cystine or methionine and I could find no record that gelatin contains any threonine or isoleucine.

It is my desire to point out to you that I have made a very careful, deliberate, painstaking study of gelatin and I must admit that I am completely baffled as to how gelatin ever became an object of food or diet. Its history, its background and its chemical composition are so bad, so horrible and so unbelievably rotten that I cannot understand how it became so popular and so widely used. However, I must admit that when millions or billions of dollars are at stake some crazy, insane and unbelievable things happen. I am sorry to say that even reputable researchers and scientists have occasional good words to say for gelatin and my only explanation for this is that they, too, did not bother to investigate or study the true background of gelatin.

Well, so far you have the dissertation from the Columbia Encyclopedia and you have the references from the article "Gelatin . . . How It's Made." Now I presume you demand irrefutable scientific proof and it is up to me to produce it or back down. You might say, "Stop playing upon our sympathies and provide proof. Sympathies don't go with scientists". So I'll go ahead.

Macrae and associates, in the course of their studies on "The Nutritive Value of Yeast Protein," examined the supplementary value of yeast protein, casein and gelatin for maize protein in the nutrition of the pig. They obtained negative results with gelatin, confirming the earlier finding of McCollum, Simmonds and Pitz.

Voit and the other investigators had demonstrated that gelatin did not act as a complete protein and could not completely replace protein substance. But thus far the fundamental reason for the failure of gelatin completely to replace protein material had not been revealed.

With the coming of the World War, gelatin as a food once more was brought to the front and Homberger recommended its extensive introduction in the diet of the masses. In the meantime, further research work on the subject was in progress. Osborne and Mendel, experimenting on rats, found that gelatin was inadequate as the sole source of protein but when half of the gelatin was replaced by casein or gliadin satisfactory results were obtained. Totani, in 1916, was unable to secure favorable results when his gelatin was supplemented by tyrosine, tryptophane and cystine. He also found, contrary to practically all other investigators, that the gelatin appeared to be badly absorbed.

Proudfit: "Gelatin, composed entirely of protein, lacks several of the essential amino acids and cannot be used alone to supply either the growth or maintenance needs of the body. It is not without its uses in nutrition, however, for this form of protein may be used to fill part of the protein quota if supplemented with other proteins. In special diets (liquid) gelatin water and jellied broths are valuable adjuncts. As jellied soups, salads, and desserts, gelatin may be used to advantage to lend color and variety to the daily menu . . . "

Frank investigated the course of metabolism in gelatin

feeding, comparing gelatin with casein in both long and short term feeding experiments. He found gelatin to be fully as well absorbed as the casein in the short term experiments and even better absorbed in the long term feeding tests as these progressed. The Nitrogen balance was positive with the gelatin feeding but the test animals (rats) lost weight, slowly at first but more rapidly as the experimental feeding period was lengthened. When the gelatin was replaced by casein the weight loss was arrested.

Richter, working with rats, studied the nutritional value of some common carbohydrates, fats and proteins by the single food choice method, employing a diet which contained only one of the above. Survival time on gelatin averaged 11 days as compared with 38 and 32 days on two different samples of casein, but the rats ate only small amounts of gelatin. The author noted: "In general, the rats on proteins lived much longer than would have been expected from the caloric value of the ingested foodstuffs."

Block and Boiling, reporting on "Nutritional Opportunities with Amino Acids," pointed out that: "The low nutritive value of gelatin, as mentioned by Prout 100 years ago, is evident from its amino acid composition. Gelatin is deficient in, or almost devoid of histidine, tyrosine, tryptophane, phenylalanine, cystine, methionine, threonine, leucine, isoleucine, and valine. Thus of the 13 amino acids discussed in this paper, gelatin is amply supplied with only arginine and abundantly with only glycine."

In an article sponsored by the Council on Foods and Nutrition of the American Medical Association, Turner dealt with "Selection of Protein Containing Foods to Meet Protein Requirements." Discussing high protein diets she observed that: " . . . Gelatin also may be incorporated in significant amounts in hot beverages or soups."

After more than a century of investigation a definite place has not been established for gelatin as a food or nutrient. Gelatin today is accepted in the following light:

1. It does not serve as a complete protein but may act as an important supplement to other proteins.

2. It has great protein-sparing ability.

3. It possesses considerable nutritive value and is a valuable addition to the diet.

Moreover, discrepancies in the reports of different investigators can probably be accounted for by variations in the gelatin employed, a factor which will be considered at length in the closing pages of this review. Von Noorden, as noted in Fitch's "Dietotherapy," believed that "the variable composition of gelatin is but one of the reasons why it is so ill adapted for the building up of protein."

In infant feeding Gregor showed that gelatin was completely utilized by the infant and considered it of value because of its protein-sparing ability. However, he observed intestinal disturbances when large amounts of gelatin were fed.

Elterich, Boyd and Neff reviewed the literature in relation to the nutritive value of gelatin and its place in infant feeding and presented their own experiments along the latter lines. They worked with a small number of children, feeding them "a relatively large amount of gelatin over a fairly long period of time . . . " The same infants were employed throughout the test, the feeding periods being divided into successive gelatin periods and non-gelatin periods; 100 calories or 4 level tablespoons of gelatin were employed during the gelatin period. (Four level tablespoons of powdered gelatin are approximately one ounce by weight.)

These investigators were unable to find any accelerated growth as a result of gelatin feeding although they did not observe any unfavorable consequences of the large amounts of gelatin employed. They considered that gelatin "may be a food factor in certain unusual allergic infants, where the ingestion of either breast or cow's milk cannot be tolerated."

The Council on Foods of the American Medical Association reviewed briefly some of the later work described above and concluded that: "The claim that gelatin is an aid in the digestion of milk, however, is in the opinion of the Council not established." This was in line with an earlier decision rendered, in 1932, by the same body (then known as the Committee on Foods) to the effect that:

"There is no satisfactory evidence that gelatin increases the digestibility of milk or milk products. Such claims are not permissible."

Lautz conducted an **in vitro** investigation of the effect on peptic digestion of artificial feeding as used for American infants. Gelatin was included among the additions studied and resulted in the production of a thick mixture the effect of which was "to depress the peptic digestion both of the protein taken as a whole and of the milk protein taken separately."

When we consider the possible variations in the character of the gelatins utilized in these studies it is remarkable that results were, for the most part, so consistently favorable. Much of the controversial data in the above literature may be reconciled by a careful study of the experimental procedures followed. Such a study reveals that successful results have almost always followed the use of relatively small amounts of gelatin (1 to 2 teaspoons per day or about 5 to 6 grams) in the milk formula, while failure has accompanied the employment of excessive doses of one ounce of gelatin per day. It is significant, further, that the most enthusiastic reports have come from those investigators who were working with inadequately nourished infants, that is, with infants whose diets needed supplementing or changing. As might be expected, adequately nourished normal infants did not respond as definitely to the addition of gelatin to their diets.

Remember, these are the proponents of gelatin who are trying to sell gelatin who are doing the talking here. But they're also hanging themselves.

"Gelatin feeding has a striking influence upon the curve of pigment regeneration and red cell formation. Gelatin added to a sugar diet will usually cause a sharp rise in the curve of pigment regeneration. This rise is not as marked as after meat feeding. It usually reaches its maximum after two to four weeks, and then may show a fall coincident with malnutrition which may develop after prolonged gelatin feeding . . . "

Several investigators have noted increases in renal weight after gelatin feeding, particularly when large doses are supplied to the test animals. Wilson reported that: "Gelatin tends to produce a more marked increase in kidney weight than either caseinogen or liver." The MacKays noted that the protein intake was one of the most important factors determining the weight of the kidneys in albino rats and observed that gelatin provides a much larger increased renal weight than any other protein fed. While the kidneys were damaged when gelatin was the sole source of protein, when casein was added to the gelatin diets no renal damage was observed. Kruse and associates, in their investigations on the nutritive deficiencies of gelatin, observed that their animals "all showed renal lesions at autopsy, even those with satisfactory growth records."

Hogan and Ritchie observed the development of anemia, growth failure and death in animals, caused by the addition of deaminized casein to a diet containing gelatin and gliadin as the previously adequate source of protein. Deaminized casein plus casein did not result in anemia.

Fertility and related problems have also received attention. Evans and Bishop, in a study of "The relations between Fertility and Nutrition," employed gelatin and casein in a diet deficient in Vitamin A for as long as 200 days without physiological ill effects detectable in oestrous. Cunningham and Hopkirk, in New Zealand, studied dietary protein in relation to sterility and were able to render male rats sterile either by feeding diets of excessively high protein content (65 to 82%) or by feeding diets containing 15% to 18% protein, but in which the protein was largely derived from maize or maize and gelatin. They considered the latter effect to be due to a deficiency in some of the essential amino acids, advancing the hypothesis that the tests require a liberal supply of such amino acids.

You will note that they considered that the condition was brought about by the deficiency of some of the essential amino acids. This is a logical viewpoint, as shown by the chart that I have given which proves that gelatin is deficient in most of the essential amino acids. It is simple to understand that such a product taken as food can cause a tremendous imbalance in the amino acids and common sense would indicate that a well balanced diet is required if one is to maintain sexual virility. I wish to stress that a heavy protein diet caused sterility in rats and this would be especially bad if the protein was an imbalanced one.

Maison's results were entirely negative. The work ability of his subjects was still increasing when gelatin was administered after five weeks of training and continued to increase during the gelatin period. No improvement in training was effected by gelatin and its omission did not result in any decrease of the ability of the muscles, contrary to the results obtained by Ray and co-workers. On subjects trained for a full year the gelatin produced no improvement nor was there any decrease of ability after the gelatin was discontinued. Maison considered that Ray's subjects were inadequately trained and also postulated that a psychic effect might be involved.

Karpovich reported on experiments which he conducted in conjunction with Pestrecov where they found no effect of gelatin upon the working capacity of muscle. To take the psychological factor into account they administered farina "under the guise of 'concentrated gelatin' " with "a noticeable 'stimulating' effect." Karpovich concluded: "It may be stated positively that addition of gelatin to a normal diet does not act as a special source of extra power, nor does it increase endurance."

On the whole, therefore, while we are not yet able to assign to gelatin a definitely favorable influence upon muscular activity, a study of the reports indicates that gelatin probably has some beneficial effect, at least upon certain individuals. Just how great this effect is and just what percentage and type of individuals are benefitted, remains to be determined by future investigations.

To those with high blood pressure, those who have heart trouble and those who fear heart trouble in the future, I say look out for gelatin. I suggest that no one with a heart condition even touch gelatin. It appears that gelatin is a powerful blood coagulant.

The hemostatic action of gelatin was the first therapeutic property of this substance to be recognized, its use in this capacity going back to the turn of the century or earlier as noted by Homberger, Ono, and Dutton. The latter author also noted that Dastre and Floresco, as far back as 1896, had "found that gelatin, when injected intravenously in dogs, shortens the coagulation time of the blood." Moll, in 1903, recommended the employment of gelatin before operations "where a great loss of blood is feared."

During the early years of the twentieth century when gelatin was being extensively used as a hemostatic agent, several isolated cases of infection after its subcutaneous administration were reported, and in a few cases tetanus appeared, followed by death. Doerfler traced the infections to the use of impure gelatin and improper sterilization of the same and pointed out that Krug and Kuhn had demanded "that the gelatin itself be prepared from gelatin-yielding tissues which are fresh and healthy." Doerfler's ultimate findings were to the effect that when sterile gelatin was employed it was very efficient as a hemostatic agent and was to be highly recommended for that purpose.

"Gelatin may be used clinically wherever it is desired to increase the coagulability of the blood. For instance, it is sometimes of service in the treatment of aneurisms. Its most frequent employment, however, is in the treatment of various hemorrhages, especially when from those areas which cannot be reached by local measures, as the lungs, or kidneys; it has, however, been used also as a local application to check bleeding, especially in gastric ulcers. It is employed often with good effect, although not always successful, in the treatment of blood dyscrasias, as haemophilia and purpura

215

haemorrhagica . . . "

Kugelmass conducted an extensive series of investigations relating to the management of hemorrhagic problems in infancy and childhood. In a report rendered early in 1932 he stated: " . . . I have found indirectly that **the administration of 3 per cent gelatin solution devised for recovery from birth shock has reduced clotting time more rapidly than even blood infection.** Gelatin solution administered hourly after birth for three days has reduced the average clotting time from fifteen minutes to three minutes in over a hundred newborns. And the clotting time in intra-cranial injury complicated by hemorrhagic disease has been more strikingly diminished since the routine use of 3 per cent gelatin solution."

"The administration of gelatin arrests bleeding by condensing platelets on the vascular bed. From 20 to 40 cc. may be injected intravenously in 10 per cent solution, or it may be fed in 10 per cent solution, either directly, sweetened and flavored with vanilla and mixed with milk, or as a jelly, which may be kept on ice for two days."

Dutton pointed out that: "Gelatin-glucose-saline solution, in quantities over 50 cc., is contraindicated in uncompensated cardiac valve lesions; in cardiac dilation or myasthenia; in degeneration of the myocardium; in arteriosclerosis with hypertension; in pulmonary congestion or edema; in all cases in which the kidney is not able to respond to stimulation; in uremia with salt retention; and in the presence of dropsy."

Bayliss referred to the danger of tetanus spores in the gelatin and noted that the necessary sterilization resulted in the loss of a great part of the viscosity of the gelatin solution. He pointed out, further, that: "Another unwelcome property of gelatin is that of causing intra-vascular clotting." Also, "In cold weather, the setting to jelly in the tubes and cannulae, if a block occurs, may become inconvenient."

"Apart from a somewhat increased salivation observed directly

216

after the injection of the larger doses of gelatin solution, there were no symptomatic reactions of any kind . . . " Hueper reported that "the intravenous injection of solutions of gum arabic, ovalbumin and gelatin elicit in the blood a complex of cellular and plasmatic reactions characteristic of macromolecular hematic disturbances . . . " All three substances apparently caused "a clogging of the glomerular filtration membranes when present in excessive amounts in the blood, and thereby elicit degenerative and proliferative changes in the glomeruli." The changes produced in the plasma of the animals treated with these substances were "accompanied by the appearance of degenerative and proliferative reactions in arterial walls," which, in the case of the foreign proteins, were of the sclerosing type.

The same investigators, associated with Koop and co-workers, reported on studies concerned with the toxicity and elimination of gelatin. They found no evidence of either liver damage or impairment of kidney function after the intravenous administration of gelatin. Gelatin per se was not pyrogenic in the dog, while repeated infusions varying in amount, number and frequency failed to produce allergic reactions. Sedimentation rates and clotting times were increased but returned to normal as the gelatin left the blood. Diuresis and relatively rapid excretion of the gelatin occurred, decreasing 6 hours following infusion, but not all of the gelatin which disappeared from the blood was accounted for by urinary excretion. "Plasma proteins fell rapidly after infusion and were replaced at about the same rate at which gelatin disappeared from the blood. Gelatin was present in only minute quantities after 5 days."

In the normal dog, repeated infusions of gelatin over long periods of time were not accompanied by demonstrable tissue damage, except for capillary hemorrhages in the adrenal glands which were visible for only 48 hours after the infusion. In those animals where gelatin was given as a blood replacement there was evidence of protein leakage in the kidney tubules and minor degeneration in liver and kidney in 24 hours. These changes, only slightly more marked with gelatin than with plasma, were apparently reversible."

Robscheit-Robbins, Miller and Whipple investigated the

usefulness of gelatin as a plasma protein substitute and its toxicity when administered intravenously. In summarizing their results, they stated: "Gelatin given by vein to doubly depleted dogs (anemic and hypoproteinemic) gives no immediate toxic response, no anaphylactoid reactions, and may contribute something to the building of new hemoglobin and plasma protein." Experimental evidence was obtained that "**gelatin may be toxic** when given by vein in moderate dosage over a one to two week period. The condition in such dogs deteriorates and death may follow or the return to normal is slow and there is definite impairment of the capacity of the dog to form blood proteins in these experiments." The authors noted that gelatin escapes freely through the kidney, and this reaction in a diseased or damaged kidney might be harmful. Rapid loss of weight was observed in the two week gelatin injection experiments.

In its 1936 report, the Council on Foods of the American Medical Association did not recognize as allowable the claim that gelatin is of value as a source of aminoacetic acid in the treatment of some of the myopathies. It was pointed out that gelatin was deficient in certain essential amino acids and the Council considered that gelatin had no special significance as a source of amino acids in the diet.

CHAPTER

35

COLD AND HOT DRINKS

Ever since I was a young man I have seen the fallacy in the hot and cold drink affair. Somebody would come in on a cold night and say, "Give me a hot drink to warm me up" and in the summer time I heard "Boy, am I thirsty? Is it ever hot outside! Give me a nice cold drink to cool me off". Of course you've heard something similar most of your life, too.

Now I can't say why I felt there was some false reasoning or something fishy in this affair but I did. I knew that the human body has a thermal control system of its own. I thought it had a mighty good one, too, and I was not deceived. Then the thought sort of haunted me that man among all creatures on the face of the earth is the only one who drinks his beverages at a temperature different from that of normal air or water. Animals, of course, drink their water in the winter at winter temperature and in the summer at

219

summer temperature, so the water is, generally speaking, at normal atmospheric temperature.

You know and I know that we have sweat glands in our bodies and I don't think that the sweat glands have any greater purpose in creation than to maintain the balance of heat and cold in the body. There are other functions of the sweat glands; for example, excreting salt and cooling down the body due to evaporization of the exuded sweat. But apart from these examples I haven't yet learned that there are other positive functional purposes for the exudation of moisture from the body. I do know that excessive sweating causes loss of weight because boxers and others who have to meet a weight deadline usually wrap themselves in warm clothes and do running, skipping or other physical work to cause sweating so that they will lose weight. The more they sweat the more weight they lose. But I feel that this is foolish reasoning because if you don't put the water that weighs pounds into your system then you don't have to excrete it to lose pounds. Why put the extra burden upon your kidneys and upon your excretory or sweat glands?

Now let's take a simple example. We're hot, the temperature outside is in the 90's or close to 100 and we are sweating and someone says, "We're losing a lot of water by sweat and we have to replenish it so let's have a nice cool drink". Of course some people don't like it cool, they like it downright cold . . . in fact, ice cold with ice floating around in it. So the body is at its normal temperature of 98.6 and then we drink a cooling glass of water that is slightly above the freezing point, say 36 or 34 degrees. So here we have it, the liquid being poured into your body is at 34 and your body is at 98.6 and the atmospheric temperature is 98. That's quite a clash isn't it?

Your body mechanisms go to work immediately and say "We're having real cold poured into us and we've got to bring the temperature up quickly". So your body starts to race to bring your temperature up and the cold drink is going to bring it down . . . now you see you have forces pulling apart. Now I'm not fooling, this is common sense. The more cold you pour into your body the more

220

heat your body generates to maintain its equilibrium.

So now we reverse the situation. It's a cold winter day with the temperature nearly zero degrees and we've been outside and we're all chilled. So we stand in a booth somewhere and drink a cup of hot coffee or toddy or whatever it may be whose temperature is very close to the boiling point, say 210 degrees or even 200 degrees. So again, we have an outside temperature of 0 degrees, we have a body temperature of 98.6 and we have a hot drink at 200 degrees. So here your body is again fighting to bring that boiling liquid down from 200 or so to 98.6. You can imagine the load it's putting on your body functions.

O.K., you may say this is all theoretical but I claim it's plain, simple horse sense. You're suddenly giving your body a dandy workout. Whether or not your body appreciates it I'm not prepared to say but I am suggesting that you do a little bit of common sense thinking. Why impose these burdens upon the body? Some people do it all the time. It is my sincere belief that food or drink should be taken into the body at as close to body temperature or atmospheric temperature as humanly possible, for all considerations.

Anyway, I want to tell you about some research work done by a Dr. James S. Feurig who was the Director of the Olan Health Centre located in Michigan State University. He suggests that the summer colds go hand in hand with cool drinks. "When it gets hot then people swing to iced tea, ice water and other cold drinks and then in a day or so they may notice that they have a sore throat. What happens is that the prolonged cold cools the throat membranes and this drops resistance so that it is easier for an organism to take hold and come on."

You'll notce that Dr. Feurig does not say anything about the body's thermal control system. My suggestion is that he hasn't thought of that yet. Give him time, his thinking apparatus is just a little slow, due to drinking ice cold water when the temperature of the body is at 98.6.

CHAPTER

36

JUICES

It is essential that a person who wants to be knowledgable on health know something about live vegetable and fruit juices. Let no one tell you that carrot juice is better than carrots or that orange juice is better than oranges or that apple juice is better than apples, or that any juice on earth is better than the vegetable or the fruit itself.

The only advantage that juice has over the fruit or vegetable itself is the fact that you can take juices in larger quantities and in greater concentrations than you can the fruit or vegetable itself.

There are millions of people in America and countless millions throughout the world who have never had their proper share of decent vegetables and fruits. So it stands to reason that their bodies have been depleted of the elements contained in these fruits, which their bodies sorely lack and they are probably, or almost invariably, suffering from a condition due to the lack of these nutrients.

So when a healer comes across someone who is sick because of a deficiency of any one or many of these nutrients, he justifies the use of juices because of the great amount that can be ingested pleasantly, and often with startling effect.

As you well know, I am not a healer. You also should know that I oppose practically every form of healing on earth. I condone naturopathic healing. I don't support it or recommend it, I condone it as being the least harmful, or perhaps of greater help than any other form of healing known to man.

I must frankly admit that on literally hundreds of occasions I have seen the tremendous benefits derived from the use of fresh vegetable and fruit juices.

So let's get the matter clear and straight without danger of error or misunderstanding. I contend that the fruit or the vegetable in total is far superior in nutritional value than only the juice. In other words, the whole is always superior, nutrition-wise, to the fragment.

The use of juices in varying quantities is justified to correct deficiencies caused by years of depletion. There is another very vital factor about juices, or should I say juice therapy, and that is the simple fact that it is very seldom or almost impossible, for anyone to be adversely affected or harmed by the ingestion of even large quantities of fresh juices.

Now let's say you are going to use juices if you feel it is necessary or important to your health. In the first place vegetable juices, in my opinion, are far superior nutrition-wise to the fruit juices.

I will grant at the outset that fruit juices taste better, are more appetizing and more delectable than vegetable juices. The only vegetable juice of my wide acquaintance that tastes pleasant and appealing is carrot juice. All other vegetable juices, to the best of my knowledge and belief, are either barely acceptable or utterly distasteful.

Still you can make some very pleasant juices by mixing various vegetables. You can add beet, celery, parsley and other juices to carrot juice and still make it taste pleasant and palatable.

Practically everyone is acquainted with tomato juice and it is highly esteemed and very palatable and tasteful. However, I must tell you the truth. Tomato juice in its pure natural form is tasteless, if not distasteful. Try it and see. You'll realize I speak the truth. The kind that you usually buy in cans that tastes so good, contains some, or a great deal of, seasoning. I suggest a great deal. So it's the seasoning or the herbs that are added that make it taste pleasant, not the juice itself. Let it be understood that I unalterably oppose, from a strictly nutritional viewpoint, the addition of salt, pepper, sugar or any other flavoring or improving agent. If you do add anything it will definitely harm the true natural product.

Because fruit juices taste better they are more widely used than vegetable juices. But again I stress it — if you are seeking health and taking juices to benefit your health, then please accept my word for it that vegetable juices are more nutritious.

I am reluctant to sing too highly the praises of any food or substance, but I have seen more people get well and derive benefits from vegetable juices than I have seen from any therapeutic measure of my acquaintance and knowledge.

Now, you may ask, "Why are vegetable juices more nutritious than fruit juices? So, we'll take a carrot and class it with an apple. You wash the carrot and you run it through the juicing machine and the wise person will also include some of the leaves of the carrot. In it you get as close to the perfect juice as is humanly possible.

Now you run the apple through. To begin with, no one would dream of running the seeds of the apple through so they usually take out the seeds. So there with one swoop you have removed probably the most nutritious part of the apple. There was nothing to remove with a carrot — all of it went through the juicer — and in the juice will be found most of its food value. But if you have eliminated the apple seeds you are being short changed.

The same holds true for peach juice, pear juice, orange juice, plum juice. The point I am trying to stress is that when you make juice, you are getting in the juice a fragmented product to begin with because you are losing some of the vital factors that remain in the pulp and cannot be extracted by a juicer.

If the seed of the fruit is utilized along with the fruit, then its nutritional value will be equal to that of a complete vegetable.

For example, when you make celery juice, you use the whole stalk and the leaves and if the roots were clean and scrubbed, they could be used too. The same holds true for a beet. For optimum nutrition you should also use the beet leaves and where you are using leafy vegetables, by using the entire leaves you are getting close to optimum nutrition.

Please believe me, I have no animosity towards fruit nor am I trying to deprive you of something that is tasty and delectable but I feel you are interested in the truth as it affects your health and therefore I am telling you the truth.

Another reason why juices are so beneficial and widely used is that many people, especially when they reach past middle age or get beyond 50 and 60, have either poor teeth or plates and therefore the eating of hard vegetables like carrots or beets is practically ruled out. I consider shredded vegetables inferior to fresh juice because of oxidation losses.

Therefore, the juices play a vital part in helping these people regain or maintain their health.

When making juices, it is important that you are aware of the fact that the only juices fit to drink or use are fresh juices. You cannot make juices for the next meal in advance. Many people I know do make a quart of juice to last them for the whole day. This is wrong. They are defeating their own purpose because much of the nutrient value of the juice is lost by oxidation, even if kept in a closed container in the refrigerator.

If you need juices, if you are taking them to benefit your health, then, in heavens name, make fresh juice each time you take it.

Juicing machines are readily available. There are various kinds and types. Some people advise the hydraulic or pressure system of making juices. Others use the rotary juicers. It is claimed that the press juicers are better but I cannot see the particular advantage over the centrifugal juice making machine.

Of course, their argument is that in whirling the fruit or the vegetable about and getting the juice that way, some oxidation takes place. With this I have to agree, but on the other hand trituration is slower but perhaps it is better. The juicing machines of the trituration type are much more expensive and require more effort because first you have to grind up the vegetable to a pulp and then press out the juice.

Even if this machine is superior, and I grant that this may be possible but it is not proven, the extra effort and the time consumed nullifys its advantages.

But whichever way you get your juice, it is much better to get it than to be without it if you are deficient in the vitamins that the juice contains.

If you are suffering from any condition, try juices. First of all, they cannot harm you. In fact, there are few on this earth who would not benefit from their use. Besides, fresh fruit and vegetable juice is quite pleasant to take. It is low in cost, much lower than medical fees and drugs and will probably clear up your condition

227

much better and faster.

CHAPTER

37

EVERYBODY LOVES SWEETS

The most common and most widely used sweetener in the world of course is plain ordinary white sugar, properly called Saccharum Officinarum. There is also raw sugar, brown sugar, yellow sugar, turbinado sugar, clean raw sugar, Demerara sugar and others which are products from the sugar cane. Then there is blackstrap molasses, Barbados molasses, sorghum molasses and other types of molasses.

Sorghum is similar to sugar cane and is called sugar sorghum. It is properly called Holcus sorghum and yields a honey-like syrup. This plant is also known as broom corn.

One of the best known and most liked sweeteners of all is maple syrup. Then I must add one of the most widely used of all sweetening agents in industry is glucose also known as corn syrup, grape sugar, corn sugar, dextrose, dextro monosaccharide, D-glucose monosaccharide, glucoin, dextropur, dextrosol, C6H12O6. A sweetener that is not often mentioned and is one of the best is dates; and dates are usually reasonably priced and if purchased in quantities the price is quite low. There are really very few sweeteners on the market that are better than dates.

Carob, commonly known as St. John's Bread or Buxer, properly called Cerotonia Siliqua, is a sweetener with a chocolate flavor. Licorice, properly called Glycorrhiza Glabra, is also very sweet and is frequently used in medicines, for making drinks and beverages and confectionery.

The two best sweeteners in my opinion are honey and dates. You may be surprised to note that I do not recommend maple syrup, even the best maple syrup, as a sweetener — evidence indicates that it is not as good as honey or dates. My reason for avoiding maple syrup is first, because of the high heat required to boil it down to its proper consistency and also the fact that in most sugar bushes where the maple syrup is made from the maple trees they use pellets containing formaldehyde or a similar poison. Formaldehyde is a deadly poison. It is what is used by the undertakers to embalm a body. In the sugar bush it is used to keep open the hole from which the syrup is drained from the tree. Otherwise, nature tends to plug it up to prevent the tree from literally bleeding to death. So therefore, your maple syrup is permeated with formaldehyde and when it is boiled down the water boils out but the formaldehyde becomes more concentrated. Therefore I can't see the use of maple syrup as a good sweetening agent or food.

I recommend honey and use a lot of honey. In fact, it is our main sweetener but some knowledgable people claim honey is food for bees not for man. It is a positive fact that honey does contain many vitamins and minerals and if it can sustain and maintain the life of a busy insect like the bee then it must be a reasonably good food.

Now let's discuss honey. Honey is a food and contains food factors, vitamins and minerals. Often this is disputed but it is an

230

absolute proven scientific fact and can be verified in the United States Government Handbook No.8. Honey supplies quantities of iron, copper, phosphorous, silica, calcium, magnesium, potassium, sodium and other minerals. Honey contains the following vitamins — thiamin (B1), riboflavin (B2), Ascorbic acid (C), peridoxine (B6), pantothenic acid, nicotenic acid (Niacin). Honey also contains vitamin K, the blood-clotting factor.

These enlightened individuals refer to honey as bee vomit. I can't agree with that belief but nevertheless I must concede that honey is food for bees. Honey is claimed to have healing values and this can be scientifically established.

Saccharin is still widely used in America as a sweetening agent. I consider it as harmful, every bit as harmful as the cyclamates which were recently banned by the Food and Drug Administration. By actual comparison with the synthetic sweeteners common white sugar becomes a good food or a good product.

If you need a sweetening agent I strongly urge you to use dates and or honey. Pasteurized honey should never be used. The best honey to eat is comb honey.

Here is an explanation of the various sugars:

Beet sugar is sucrose from sugar beets.

Blood sugar is the carbohydrate found in the blood.

Cane sugar is sucrose obtained from sugar cane.

Fruit sugar is levulose or fructose.

Grape sugar is glucose or dextrose.

Inert sugar is a sugar consisting of one molecule of glucose and one of fructose resulting from the hydrolysis of sucrose.

Malt sugar is maltose.

Milk sugar is lactose.

CHAPTER

38

ABOUT GLUCOSE

Every day over the radio there used to be a program sponsored by one of the largest manufacturers of glucose (corn syrup) in Canada. They used various pretty adjectives to describe it, to make you and others believe it had special merit or value. This form of advertising is, in my opinion, downright criminal. The program was distinctly beamed at young people ... boys, girls and youths.

The term glucose has a very wide meaning. It covers an enormous amount of ground.

According to the dictionary we find "A form of sugar occurring in fruits and honey; a syrup containing natural glucose and other ingredients; a main source of energy for living organisms; occurs naturally and in the free state in fruits and in other parts of plants."

Glucose is also known as dextrose, grape sugar and diabetic sugar. It is widely distributed in nature, occurring in the blood of all animals in small quantities, usually about 0.1%, and more abundantly in fruits and plant juices, where it is usually associated with fructose and sucrose. It is especially abundant in grapes, of which it often constitutes 20% of the total weight or more than half of the solid matter. Sweet corn, onions and unripe potatoes are among the common vegetables containing considerable amounts of glucose. Glucose is also obtained from many other carbohydrates through the means of hydrolysis, either by acids or by enzymes as in natural digestion, and thus becomes a principal form in which the carbohydrate of the food enters into the process of nutrition.

From this description you will gather, as I have gathered, that glucose is many and varied things and occurs in many forms and in many fruits and other substances in nature. Adhering strictly to the scientific term, it could be any one of many substances, synthetic or natural. But you will note that in the original interpretation of the word glucose it said, "A form of sugar occurring in fruits and honey." As someone interested in food and being a believer in nature, I would maintain strongly that glucose is only a substance in fruits and honey.

Now let us deal with something else . . . the important part of this discussion . . . and that is glucose as it is found on the shelves of our supermarkets and as it is consumed by the general public.

In a healthy body the glucose of the blood is constantly being burned and replaced. Ordinarily any surplus of glucose absorbed from the digestive tract is converted into glycogen which is readily reconvertible into glucose. Thus, while other carbohydrates occur in food in greater quantity, glucose occupies a very prominent place, partly because it is more widely distributed than any other carbohydrate, being a normal constituent of both plants and animals, and partly because it is the form in which most of the carbohydrate material of the food comes actually into the service of the body tissues. It is estimated that over half the energy manifested in the human body is derived from the oxidation of glucose.

It is not to be inferred from the foregoing statement that the body obtains the energy of glucose by oxidizing it directly or such. There is abundant evidence of intermediary metabolism but conflicting views as to its details.

Now let's talk about the manufacture of starch, glucose and dextrin.

Starch is usually prepared commercially from corn or potatoes, by a mechanical process of grinding and washing. The suspension of pure starch in water is thus obtained; by allowing it to settle slowly, the impurities are deposited first and may be removed. A microscopic examination of starch will reveal the source of the material, as the granules are characteristic of the plant from which they come. Starch is used in laundry work, in cooking, in the manufacturer of pastes, and in the preparation of dextrins and glucose.

The hydrolysis of starch to glucose is carried out on a very large manufacturing scale. A few per cent of hydrochloric acid is used as the catalyst and after the completion of the hydrolysis this is carefully neutralized. The evaporation of the glucose solution thus prepared yields thick syrupy solutions which are widely sold as sweetening materials for domestic use and in the manufacture of candy.

According to the best scientific information that I can find there are 16 different kinds of glucose. This was discovered by Emil Fischer who applied the work of van't Hoff to his sugars. Back in 1893 he produced 11 different kinds of the total of 16 that were possible. The study of glucose and the sugars is said to constitute one of the most largely studied branches of organic chemistry.

It is claimed that hard candies are composed of about 70% glucose and the balance is sucrose and water. A certain spokesman for the corn syrup industry has this to say in defence of his product.

"Now let us stop right here and fuss and fume a little over

the good people who fear glucose because it is 'a chemical product'. Let us see how much more of a chemical glucose is than cane sugar. Glucose is made from corn and the solution is treated with a mild acid to split off the simple sugar from the starch. The cane sugar is extracted from cane or beets and the solution is treated with an alkali to remove the organic acids. This is the chief difference in the processes and if, so far as the manufacture goes, glucose is a dangerous chemical while sucrose or cane sugar is not, then we might as well come to the conclusion that caustic lime is edible while vinegar is a poison."

Of course, this was written by someone in the employ of the chemical industry and I'll let you judge its merits for yourself. I believe it's best to let a man hang himself!

So there we have it . . . we have a fairly comprehensive story of what glucose really is. Note that the apologist is quite perturbed that sugar is not attacked or maligned and only his product, glucose. Actually, I have made no comparisons but if it is comparisons that he wants then I would say sugar is a bad, harmful, contemptible product but glucose, judging from the information at my disposal, is much worse, much more harmful and much more contemptible.

But hold! The whole truth has not yet been told. We know, for example, that glucose is made from starch but now let's find out from what starch is made.

Generally starch is made from corn in the United States, from potatoes in Europe and from arrowroot in the West Indies. The process consists of destroying the cell tissues, usually by mechanical means, and then washing out the starch and drying it carefully. By further treatment with a dilute acid and by heating it is converted into glucose or grape or corn sugar or corn syrup.

Starch occurs as white granules in nearly all plants. Starch granules from different plants differ greatly in size and shape. The food value of cereals and many other vegetable foods is due primarily to the starch which is present in them. For example, rice is about

236

75% starch, corn 50% and potatoes 20%. This starch is hydrolyzed to maltose and then glucose in the process of digestion in the animal body. The liver then converts the glucose to a polysaccharide known as glycogen. This substance is very similar to starch. Indirectly, its combustion furnishes the heat and energy necessary for the life of the higher animals.

Dr. Martha Jones, medical consultant in nutrition to Hawaiian sugar planters, was appalled at the 300 deaths per year among employees' babies. She decided to do something about it. By changing from corn syrup and refined sugar as baby formula carbohydrate to natural unrefined sugar-cane syrup, the next year went by without a single fatality among the same families.

There was an experiment conducted by Lukans and Kahan. They did this experiment at the University of Pennsylvania and they tried all forms of sugar and fed them to cats. And it appears from their research that only one form — glucose — caused diabetes in these animals.

My feeling against glucose goes back many years. I fed glucose to my first-born because the advertisements, the diet sheets, the government and all such agencies told us that it was a wonderful food, wonderful for children and so low in price. They said it was clean and wholesome and pleasing. I feel now that the feeding of glucose to my child was a factor in her ill health and ultimate death. Now I do not suggest that it was the only cause or the specific cause but I do feel that it was a factor. I was sold a bill of goods by these various agencies and I'm trying to prevent all those who will listen from having this happen to them.

I admit that the evidence in my personal case against glucose is not positive, only circumstantial. My own feeling is that it is a commercial chemical monstrosity. I have also been informed that much of the starch is made from the corn stalks and not the corn . . . and also from sawdust. The chemists will tell you that this makes no difference but I suggest that you get the glucose your body needs, wherever possible, from whole wholesome foods and not from residues.

I want to stress another factor. I am willing to stake my reputation that the starch used for making corn syrup or glucose is not made from the kernels of the corn but from the residues left after the chemical treatment by a solvent and the extraction of the oil. Therefore the starch is made from residues after chemical treatment and then glucose is made in turn from this.

I contend that glucose so manufactured cannot be called a food in any form or manner. It is a chemically treated mass made from chemically treated and solvent treated corn residues.

If glucose was used only by the older people — by men and women — well, it wouldn't bother me so much because a mature grown person is supposed to have some intelligence. But most of the corn syrup is eaten by infants and growing boys and girls. Therefore, I suggest that they are in grave danger and are being continually harmed by this chemical substance at a time when they should be getting good whole food to build their bodies for the future.

You can readily understand that this residue or glucose would be a very low cost item. What it really is, is converted, chemically treated garbage. Therefore, it is low in price and when they put it in a nice can with a pretty colorful label, they can get a high price for it and make an enormous profit. So they can spend vast sums of money advertising it over the radio and television and through the other advertising media. Also, they can afford to pay hockey, baseball and other sports stars high fees for testimonials.

When there is good honey to be purchased at only a little more than this monstrosity called glucose or corn syrup, why any sane-thinking, informed parent would buy corn syrup or glucose for use by his family is beyond my understanding. Oh, yes, I know they make very attractive cans and they also have spouts and gadgets of a very elegant nature and they make it very convenient, but I suggest that it is a harmful substance . . . in simple words, a slow poison, and maybe not so slow at that. Further, I have yet to see it on any shelf in a store or supermarket as glucose.

I suggest that the guilty culprit is not glucose as found in fruits and honey but synthetic glucose. Glucose is or can be involved in the following conditions: Increased Glucose — Acromegaly, Adrenal Tumors, Cortical or Medullary Tumors, Diabetes Mellitis, Hemochromatosis, Hyperthyroidism, Intercranial pressure. Decreased Glucose — Addison's disease, Adenoma or Carcinoma of the Islets of Langerhans, Cretinism, Hyperinsulinism, Hypopituitarism, Hypothyroidism, Insulin Shock, Muscular Dystrophy and Myxedema.

Please friends, take heed and feed your children honey or even despicable sugar rather than harmful, health-destroying corn syrup or glucose, no matter how wonderful the athletes, writers and the sports announcers as well as many famous sports personalities tell you it is.

I don't think the sports people would be happy to know that they are leading children to sickness and disease. Someone should tell them the truth . . . or would the big money blind them to the truth?

CHAPTER

39

FOOD POISONING . . . NO, CHEMICAL POISONING

Are you concerned about salmonella, botulism or staphylococci poisoning? If you are, let me reassure you that if you eat proper, wholesome, natural, unchemically treated food, you are in no danger whatsoever. Let those worry who eat all these packaged, frozen, treated and prepared foods and attend banquets, dinners and parties for they have good cause to worry.

Well, whether you believe it or not, it is a fact that mild food poisoning is becoming a common occurrence and I maintain that the modern methods of food processing are the guilty culprits. The more complicated the processing of food becomes, the graver the danger of food poisoning by salmonella, clostridium (botulism) and staphylococci. No, it is not because they operate in filthy, dirty or unscientific establishments because the contrary is the truth. I believe that most of the food in America is sterile clean and probably that is the root of the trouble.

Let's take an example. My studies reveal that clostridium botulinum is as much a part of the scene in America as aphids or flies or mosquitoes. They are ubiquitous. In fact, as a kid, when you ate your mouthful or so of dirt, you probably got a heck of a lot bigger dose of botulism that you will ever get out of a poisoned food, yet the poisoned food with botulism will kill you. Why? It's really very simple.

Clostridium in its native habitat in the soil everywhere is innocuous and wouldn't even hurt a little microbe, because it is surrounded in its native habitat with thousands and millions of other bacteria that keep it in check. And because it is everywhere, it finds its way into food. For example, if an apple or a peach touched the ground, it would probably have spores of the clostridium on it. Or if the food packer touched the earth and then handled some food, he'd probably wind up with clostridium on his hands and on the food. So there you have it . . . it's everywhere.

But clostridium has one peculiar characteristic. Its spores are extremely hard to kill. So when they boil, cook or sterilize the food, if it isn't raised to a very high degree of temperature, some of the spores of the clostridium remain unharmed and they are probably the only ones that remain unharmed because all the others have been killed. So this clostridium begins to grow and grow and multiply and because it doesn't have any of its natural enemies, it becomes murderous and when you eat a couple of bites of food containing it . . . wow, you're in for real trouble! You get clostridium poisoning. So I'm telling you, it's not because the processors are dirty or are not careful . . . it's because clostridium spores are hard to kill.

The safest and best way to avoid clostridium poisoning, staphylococci and salmonella, is to eat natural raw wholesome unchemicalized foods and then you can become chummy with all of them and remain in good health and have a long life.

Probably these three items are also more resistant to the

242

chemical preservatives that are added, just as they are resistant to heat, and the chemical additives or preservatives kill the other stuff but leave these free to continue on the rampage.

The National Academy of Science Committee on Food Microbiology cites surveys which demonstrate that salmonella organisms are present in 17% of raw poultry, 24% to 54% of commercial egg products and 4% to 58% of the raw pork tested. Coagulace positive staphylococci have been demonstrated in about 20% of the cheddar cheese from retail markets and clostridium perfringens in about 70% of the raw meat, poultry and fish sampled in Wisconsin.

CHAPTER

40

THE B12 STORY

I want to discuss with you here and now the vitamin known as B-12. I am picking this one vitamin out of a whole host of vitamins for a discussion for a very positive definite reason.

Scientists and nutritionists throughout the world stress most emphatically that an individual on a vegetarian diet starves for vitamin B-12, claiming you cannot get it in foods of vegetable origin.

Please let me emphasize at the outset that I have studied the matter rather broadly, most thoroughly and my conclusions are that while the scientists are not lying, they are certainly ill-informed.

On the basis of medical check-ups and investigations, it is clearly manifest that vegetarians do suffer from a vitamin B-12 deficiency. Now, I contend that it is wrong for the scientific body and nutritionists to assume that because vegetarians who do not eat meat and potatoes and gravy and animal products, suffer from a deficiency of vitamin B-12, that vitamin B-12 is not found in foods of vegetable origin.

There is not a shadow of doubt that vitamin B-12 is found in adequate quantities in foods of vegetable origin. I'll name one to begin with . . . Dulse. Adequate quantities of B-12 are found in Dulse. I can add, furthermore, that all seeds contain Vitamin B-12.

So if all seeds contain vitamin B-12, why should any vegetarian be deficient in that vitamin? Let us for the sake of argument say that vitamin B-12 is found in fair quantities in buckwheat. Well, vegetarians who eat buckwheat should in this way be adequately supplied with vitamin B-12. But, there is a big but there, two things might happen. The vitamin B-12 might be destroyed in the cooking, or they may be eating other processed, chemicalized foods that destroy the vitamin B-12 that they get from the grain.

For a moment let us discuss vegetarians. It has been my experience that people who follow the vegetarian way of life are imbued with the sentiment that life is precious and holy — whether it be the life of a rabbit, a calf, or a bull. Therefore they want no part of foods that come from taking the lives of these innocent animals. I applaud them for their principles and their zeal. However, by actual experience I have found that most vegetarians, in their attempts to avoid any foods containing animal matter, eat some of the most atrocious foods on earth. They eat the most concocted, the most processed, the most chemically treated, the most abominable foods known to mankind. But as long as it doesn't contain animal matter it is O.K.

I realize that many vegetarians will be annoyed and angry with my statement but I again stress I am only stating what is absolutely true. I have followed vegetarian menus for 15 years. I read vegetarian magazines assiduously — practically all of them. I am associated with, I work with many vegetarians and I have friends who are vegetarians. They are the finest of people. They have the finest

246

principles on earth, but the diet of 90% of all vegetarians is in my opinion, nothing short of abominable, be they in America, Great Britain, India or elsewhere.

The crap that they eat is worse than the combination of southern fried chicken, hamburgers, hotdogs, French fries, cola drinks, beer and liquor. Therefore, just because a vegetarian is deficient in Vitamin B-12 does not mean that the food of vegetarian origin is deficient in vitamin B-12.

Come on now ... those of you who have been spreading this untrue story prove me wrong or stop this nonsense.

CHAPTER

41

LET'S TALK ABOUT VITAMINS

This is a subject about which much, very much has been written. I do not intend to belabor the topic but I do have some important things to tell.

G. Bunge, the great physiologist, a truly great scientist, was a pioneer in the field of vitamins before the turn of the century, long before the name Vitamin was coined by Casimir Funk in 1912. Bunge conducted a laboratory and had a group of co-workers or students working with him and I think he was one of the earliest men who did work with what we know now as vitamins. If anyone deserved the Nobel Prize, it was Bunge. But he's pretty well forgotten by now . . . in fact, you'd have one heck of a time digging up any good informaion concerning his work . . . but I suspect his is the foremost work in the field. However, I've had a rough time getting any data about him and his work and I have searched high and low but for some strange reason he is not mentioned in any encyclopedia.

Anyway, he had some mighty good workers and I think I have mentioned the names of two of them . . . Lunin and Socin. I'm not even positive about the correct spelling of their names.

They were busy isolating food factors and feeding them to various animals in experiments and they were always trying to extract and isolate the factors that really were important . . . just like the drug companies today try to extract the vital part and then synthesize it and that's how they make all their drugs.

Well, the boys in his laboratory came up with a finding and that was that no matter how they tried, the isolated factors when fed to the animals just didn't work as well as the whole food. And they bluntly admitted that there was something there in the whole food that invariably worked better than the purely isolated substances.

I've come across, on different occasions, the names of these researchers — Bunge, Socin and Lunin — in different ways. However, each time it was in relation to the fact that they were unable to solve the mystery but somehow there was something in the whole food that brought better results than when the factors were isolated.

Today they have isolated the vitamins and they have become big, big business. So far in the B vitamins alone they have isolated 21 factors each supposedly performing a specific function in the health of man. Science and the chemical industry are already looking forward to the time, as they say, in the near future when man will sustain himself in perfect health by the swallowing of a few pleasant-tasting vitamin pills.

No matter what they tell you about the value of vitamins, I want to assure you that whole, wholesome food is best and there is no other way to maintain or earn good health.

Hold it! Don't jump to any conclusions. I am not saying that vitamins are no good . . . I would be a fool if I did say so because vitamins have proven their merit in countless numbers of cases. What I am saying is that the whole complete food is still better than the isolated vitamin. Of course most people will not eat the whole food but they will slip a couple of vitamin pills into their faces . . . and that's better than nothing. In fact, it's proving satisfactory as many will attest.

Now the American government or should I say, the Food and Drug Administration or the Department of Health, has some peculiar ways and habits. They accept some vitamins and they won't accept others. Actually they have stated that some of the vitamins do not exist and that some that they do believe exist have not been proven of value or necessary in the human diet so they refuse to acknowledge them. They just put a blindfold on their eyes and say they can't see and they want everybody to play at being blind and therefore they believe that no one should be allowed to make, sell or use them. Please believe me, this is a true statement and this has been going on for many years.

There is one thing that I want to be careful to warn you about and that is the difference between synthetic and natural vitamins. Even though some supposedly great scientists repeatedly tell you that the synthetic is as good as the natural, don't you buy that bill of goods. What they are trying to tell you is that a dead fish is as good as a living fish or that a chemist knows as much as nature. It does so happen that some of the synthetic vitamins perform almost as well as some of the natural vitamins and vitamin C is such an example. From tests that have been made they cannot prove that synthetic vitamin C is inferior to natural vitamin C . . . but I would still buy the natural vitamin C every time. I have seen them both in action. I say stick to the natural and avoid the synthetic.

I also know that natural vitamins will seldom if ever cause an over-balance or a toxic condition but synthetic vitamins can easily be taken to excess. It would appear to me that the body has the ability and the means to slough off any natural vitamins that it doesn't require, whereas with the synthetic vitamins the body evidently loses that ability and can get itself into serious trouble with an

251

over-abundance of synthetic vitamins.

I have made myself unpopular with most of the health stores in America by my utterances claiming that we should get our vitamins from our food and nothing will ever make me change my mind. I sincerely believe that we should get our vitamins and our nourishment from the food that we eat. However, I do realize that sometimes, in fact too often under present conditions, it is difficult to do. I also realize that some people just will not eat the proper foods. In such cases natural vitamins can be the means of maintaining one's health or even saving one's life. And I do not deny that vitamins have their distinct and necessary place in our society.

Here I am giving you a list of all the known vitamins up until the time this book goes to press and I'm also giving you the foods in which these vitamins can be found.

VITAMIN A

Vitamin A is referred to as the Antixerophthalmic, Anti-infective, Arerophtol vitamin.

Vitamin A is fat soluble and is formed from precursors in the body from yellow pigments of plants. It is essential for normal growth and development and the development and integrity of the epithelial tissue and for normal development of the bones and teeth. Vitamin A is stored in the liver. The conversion of carotene to Vitamin A occurs in the liver by the action of an enzyme called carotinose.

Purpose: Vitamin A promotes resistance to disease and to healthy functioning of nasal cavities, eyes, ears, sinuses, respiratory and urinary tracts and intestinal flora. It is associated and works in conjunction with vitamins B, C and D.

Sources: Vitamin A is found in lucerne, carrots, lettuce, spinach, soybeans, fruits, oilseeds, fish, milk, butter and eggs.

252

VITAMIN B COMPLEX

Vitamin B comprises a large group of water soluble vitamins which include Thiamin (B1), Riboflavin (B2), Niacin (nicotinic acid), Pantothenic acid (B5), Pyridoxine (B6), Adenylic acid (B8), Biotin, Inosital, Choline, P-aminobenzoic acid (PABA), Cyanocobalamine (B12), Folic acid, Pangamic acid (B15), Amygdalin (B17) and Laetrile.

Purpose: Vitamin B contributes to the following — growth, appetite, lactation, gastrointestinal, endocrine and nervous system. It is of value in marasmus and lymphocytosis. It assists appetite, brings down sugar levels in diabetes, improves biliary action. Also, of value in tuberculosis. Vitamin B is essential in carbohydrate metabolism. Vitamin B is not destroyed by regular cooking or heat.

Sources: Fresh whole grains, seeds, fruits, nuts and green vegetables supply all the B vitamins in abundance. Also, Brewers yeast, eggs, liver, fish, poultry and milk.

VITAMIN C

Vitamin C is referred to as Ascorbic acid and the Antiscorbutic factor. It is probably the best known and the most controversial of vitamins.

Purpose: A deficiency of vitamin C causes scurvy, imperfect prenatal skeletal formations, caries of the teeth, defective teeth, pyorrhea, anorexia, anemia, malnutrition, bone damage, degeneration of cells, blood vessels and other organs and tissue. It is necessary for practically every function of the body. Vitamin C is claimed to be vital in treating and preventing the common cold.

Sources: Vitamin C is found in all vegetables, especially the green leafy ones, and in fruits. Turnips are a good source.

VITAMIN D

Vitamin D is also known as the Antirichitic or Calcifying vitamin. It is essential in calcium and phosphorus metabolism and for normal development of bones and teeth.

Purpose: Vitamin D is involved in the utilization of calcium and phosphorus in blood and bone building. A deficiency of this vitamin causes rickets. Exposure to the sun synthesizes vitamin D in the body. Vitamin D is a specific in the treatment of infantile rickets, infantile tetany and softening of the bones. It is also important in normal growth and mineralization of teeth and skeleton.

Sources: The best source of vitamin D is exposure to the sun and the elements. It is poorly represented in food. The only good sources are whole milk and dairy products, fish, eggs and drippings. Green vegetables, sad to say, do not supply this vitamin. Even the milk and eggs must come from animals that were exposed to the sun and air.

VITAMIN E

Vitamin E is referred to as the Antisterility, Antidystrophic, Alpha, Beta, Gamma-Tocopherol vitamin.

Vitamin E is the term used when referring to this vitamin in general as it is found in foods. Alpha-Tocopherol is the most biologically active of several closely related substances all of which have the same properties as vitamin E. Thus, while alpha-Tocopherol strictly means one distinct substance, vitamin E may mean alpha-Tocopherol or a mixture of vitamin E and various other similar substances. Tocopherol is a combination of two Greek words . . . tokos — childbirth, pherein — to carry.

Vitamin E is fat soluble and stable to heat.

Purpose: A deficiency of vitamin E is involved in the following conditions — endocrine system dystrophy, pregnancy

254

problems, kidney malfunction, impaired growth, muscular degeneration, metabolic changes and nervous system.

Sources: Vitamin E is found in seeds, seed germ oils, kale, parsley, beans, peas, alfalfa and lettuce.

VITAMIN F

Vitamin F is referred to as Linacidin, Linobion and the Essential Unsaturated Fatty Acids (EUFA).

This vitamin is also in dispute. The American Medical Association does not recognize its existence. Bicknell and Prescott state that an essential unsaturated fatty acid deficiency is probably one of the causes of infantile eczema. The essential unsaturated fatty acids are Linoleic acid, Linolenic acid and Arachidonic acid.

Purpose: Vitamin F is of great value in the treatment of Eczema. Also useful in burns and wounds and in tuberculosis.

Sources: Vitamin F is found in vegetable and seed fats and human milk. Margarine is definitely useless as a source of essential unsaturated fatty acids.

VITAMIN G

Riboflavin was once known as vitamin G but is now obsolete.

VITAMIN H

Biotin was once known as vitamin H but is now obsolete.

VITAMIN K

Vitamin K is referred to as the Prothrombin factor, the Anti-hemorrhagic and Oil soluble vitamin.

Purpose: Vitamin K aids blood coagulation and is necessary

for formation of prothrombin. A deficiency of vitamin K reduces blood-clotting time and causes hemorrhages.

Sources: Vitamin K is found in alfalfa, rye, wheat, oats, fish meal and fats.

VITAMIN L

Vitamin L factors are presumably necessary for lactation in rats.

VITAMIN M

Folic acid was once known as vitamin M but is now obsolete.

VITAMIN P

Vitamin P is also known as Citrin and also as the Permeability factor. It is said to be associated with vitamin C but more effective in the treatment of increased vascular permeability than vitamin C. Its acceptability as a vitamin is disputed although it was postulated in 1936 by the Nobel Prize winner, Szent-Gyorgyi and his associates.

Purpose: Vitamin P is effective in diseases marked by increased capillary permeability. It helps prevent bleeding, and black and blue marks caused by injury or blows. Also of value in preventing scurvy.

Sources: Vitamin P is found in Hungarian red peppers, citrus fruits, black currants, rose hips and parsley.

VITAMIN T

Vitamin T is referred to as Tegotin, Termitin, Torutilin, Temina. The factor T is Goetsch's Vitamin.

Purpose: A complex of growth promoting substances.

Sources: Vitamin T is obtained from termites, roaches, yeasts and fungi.

VITAMIN U

Vitamin U is referred to as Cabagin and Ardesyl.

Purpose: Vitamin U is helpful in the growth of chicks. Also, proven useful in peptic ulcer. Vitamin U is the anti-ulcer vitamin.

Sources: Vitamin U is found in cabbage leaves and other green vegetables.

I consider the study and the proper practical use of vitamins to be the foremost advance that mankind has made since the flood. By making full use of our present knowledge of vitamins and by making sure that this knowledge is correctly applied in our diet, millions that are now sick can be brought back to health. Yes, and what is even more important, millions of young and yet unborn can be prevented from becoming sick. You, as an individual, if you are suffering from any condition, can find your way back to health with better than 90% accuracy if you will study the knowledge on vitamins and apply it properly.

Back in the 30's two groups of researchers undertook the study of vitamins in depth and applied this knowledge clinically and the result was two volumes of the greatest contributions to the health of man ever researched and published. One was "Vitamins And Medicine" by Bicknell and Prescott, the other was "Vitamins and Their Clinical Applications" by Stepp, Kuhnau and Schroeder. The Bicknell and Prescott work was done and published in Britain; the Stepp, Kuhnau and Schroeder work was done and published in Germany. It has been translated into English.

Copies of both of these books are extremely hard to get but to anyone who is interested in nutrition and health, these are probably the most valuable books on earth.

The amount of study, reading and research that went into these two volumes is truly unbelievable. The researchers most assuredly deserved the highest honors and tribute for their work but they didn't get it. Do you know why? I'll bet you can guess. These works if properly applied would destroy the healing professions.

When you go through "Vitamins And Medicine" by Bicknell and Prescott you will see that at the end of each vitamin chapter they give you the research experiment that they read and studied to get the information. This work will absolutely astound you. Here I will give you the count of the actual number of research projects studied for each vitamin. Vitamin A — 453, Vitamin B Complex — 380, Vitamin B — 953, Vitamin C — 1093, Riboflavin — 310, Nicotinic Acid — 303, Vitamin D — 262, Vitamin E — 260, Vitamin F — 73, Vitamin K — 388, Vitamin P — 67. They practically proved how the disease was caused and how the disease could be corrected or cured by replacing or adding the required vitamin.

With such a book at your command, you can almost control your life and the lives of others around you. The amount of nutritional and health knowledge contained in these volumes staggers the imagination.

I somehow feel that the medical profession deeply resented the publication of these two books and the fact that they could be purchased by laymen. But they are both out of print now and they would be very costly to reprint . . . but if you are lucky, you may be able to find yourself a copy somewhere. And if you do find them you'll never get over their value and the prodigious amount of work that went into them.

Well, that's my story about vitamins!

CHAPTER

42

WHY I DON'T BELIEVE IN CURES

Please now understand that this does not mean that people who are sick or ill or diseased do not or cannot get well. It just means that I do not believe in the generally accepted term 'cure'. Perhaps it's just a matter of semantics or interpretation or perhaps it is that the word 'cure' has become a bad word because it has been abused and over-used. Perhaps it is because people who use the word 'cure' have been persecuted because they exaggerated or made many unfilled promises. Whatever the reason I try to avoid the word 'cure' . . . chiefly because of its many questionable connotations.

I'd rather say someone had a certain disease and he became well again or his body overcame the condition or that he regained his health. Even when I was a young lad the word cure kept cropping up everywhere. The barkers, 'con' men or Indian medicine doctors and other forms of healers or nostrum peddlers used the word cure so often that it began to have an evil suggestion or a bad smell about it. There were herbal cures, there were snake cures, there were animal cures and witch doctor cures and there were diet cures and water cures and urine cures and sitzbath cures. There were cures by the laying of hands, there were cures by faith healers. The only time that I can honestly use the word cure is when discussing the action of the body when it has been inflicted with a disease or a condition. I say that the body has the ability to cure itself. Only in this one sense do I freely accept the word cure.

Actually I could use the word 'remedy' in place of cure but remedies somehow seem to be connected with a type of treatment or a drug or a herb or a potion. In the dictionary we read that a cure is a healing or the act of healing or the restoration to health from disease. Also, a remedy for disease; a restorative or that which heals. Also, soundness from a wound. Furthermore, I sincerely maintain that no doctor or healer of any kind or sort can cure anybody or anything. That tremendous privilege is vested only in the human body itself.

Furthermore, no drug that was ever concocted or created ever cured anything or anybody of anything.

For example, I have known hundreds of people who had had clinically established cancer and they told me they were cured and to all outward appearances it had disappeared but I know cancer is an irreversible pathology. Therefore I always suggested that it was a remission or that the onset had been stopped or the cancer had been conquered. I contend the same holds true for other conditions be it heart disease, arthritis or diabetes.

I'm not denying that there are many methods of healing that bring satisfactory results and change from a state of sickness to a state of being well and I'm sure that nothing will prevent people from stating that 'I was sick and I was cured' but I prefer not to use the word in that sense and I advocate a way of life and a way of living and eating and drinking that makes the term cure obsolete and meaningless. If you are not sick then you don't have to be cured.

Basically, I would assume that the reason I dislike the word cure is that it implies that one has been sick because in order to be cured you must be sick or unwell. Therefore, by maintaining a condition of health or well being a cure is totally unnecessary and the word never need be used. Perhaps it would be right to say that we should live so that the word cure would be unnecessary in our vocabulary.

CHAPTER

43

DO WE NEED HEALERS?

From what I have seen of the healing arts or professions through my lifetime, I have the feeling that most healers think or believe that they were ordained by God to become healers, so that they might heal and benefit and cure the sick and the suffering and the ailing. And they sort of do it by the divine right . . . that is, they were given the power and the instructions to heal the sick.

Now this could include medical men, surgeons, osteopaths, chiropractors, homeopaths, naturopaths, spiritual healers, faith healers and perhaps a voodoo doctor or any other form of healer. I again maintain that practically every one of them thinks that he has been given his gift by the good Lord himself.

Frankly I believe that the Creator, Jehovah, the Ruler, shunned healers as we are taught to shun Satan. If Jehovah sanctioned healing, he would have been admitting that he was a very poor workman and didn't know how to create healthy beings . . . and this Jehovah does not do or would not do or countenance.

Of course it is your right and privilege to believe that healers are great and wonderful and that they are ordained to do healing and that they perform a valuable function. On the other hand, I am of the school of thought that believes if you are so stupid and so blind that you don't know how to look after the wonderful, glorious body that the Lord gave you, then it is better that you fade out of this existence or be destroyed.

I am not unmindful of the fact that many children are born imperfect . . . that is, with congenital defects, over which the offspring has no control. For these I have the deepest and most profound sympathy and wish with all my being that I could help them or better still, prevent these things from happening.

Nothing will make me believe that the Lord Jehovah creates healers to repair the damage and blunders that he performs in creating life.

I have walked through the forests and the woodlands and along the roadsides and the highways and by-ways but I have never yet seen an animal that died a natural death. I have on two occasions seen a squirrel that was dead and in both of these cases the squirrel had sought to leap from one tree to another at a fairly great height and somehow missed its footing and crashed to its death on the ground.

Now it could have been that the squirrels were poisoned by sprays or dusts or other harmful pesticides and insecticides and this weakened their mentality or the functioning of their organs. Nevertheless, these are the only two cases that I have ever come across in my whole life.

It is a fact that there are experts on horses and cows and sheep and hogs and elephants who will tell you what they believe to be the average life span of these creatures. Well, I am asking you, "How does a horseman know the average life of a horse?" If you said a domesticated horse or a race horse, then probably he could give you a fairly accurate answer. But who would be able to give you this answer about a wild bronco in the wilds or an elephant who roams the veldt? It is absolutely impossible for anyone to know the age of any creature in the wilds . . . and this goes for all the animals on the face of the earth. We don't even know how long a rat lives. We do know how long rats live in captivity but we're not talking about animals in captivity . . . we're talking about animals in their own native grounds.

I know it is claimed that the closest counterpart to a human being, the gorilla, has a short life span. They seldom reach 30 years of age and most of them, I understand, do not get beyond the twenties. But perhaps this is due to the fact that they are shot and killed or hounded to death by man. I would need a great deal more proof to accept the thesis or theory that a gorilla does not attain an age of more than 20 or 30.

I doubt if there are places left in this world today where any gorillas roam free from molesting capture, destruction and murder by human beings. Moreover, I am convinced that if man uses the intelligence that the Maker gave him he certainly should be able to do a lot more for himself in attaining years of life than a gorilla or for that matter, any other creature on earth.

I maintain that sickness and disease are entirely man-made. I do not believe that we get malaria and yellow fever from a mosquito. I do not believe that we get rabies from the bite of an animal. I do not believe that we catch a cold. But I firmly believe that the human body can to an unknown degree practically maintain itself in perpetuity as long as the biological laws are fulfilled and biological requirements are met.

No greater proof of this statement can be given than the experiment conducted by Dr. Alexis Carrel who kept the tissue from the heart of a chicken alive for more than 34 years and it was as strong after 34 years as it was the first day. And he terminated the experiment because he felt there was nothing further to be proved. He scientifically and conclusively proved in the laboratory that a living organism could be maintained in good condition in perpetuity.

So I ask, why should a human being need a healer? Why should he be sick and ailing and lead but a short miserable existence?

Admittedly, I cannot suggest when man got off the track because everything that I read tells me that man has been sick and ailing and suffering and seeking help for thousands upon thousands of years. Nowhere are we shown or given the cause and the reason for man's fall from grace.

Where and when did sickness arise? Where and when did health depart? Why does health depart and sickness appear on the scene?

Up until a few years ago we did not know the answer but today we know positively the why's and the wherefore's. There are men today who are well past 100 years of age. In Russia they claim there are many more than in America. But even in America we still have a few thousand people who are more than 100 years old . . . some of them 135 years of age. If they can do it then we all can do it . . . and some of us can do better, too.

The ages of Methuselah and Seth and Noah and Adam are given in the Bible. If you do not wish to accept these ages as they are given in the Bible, that is your privilege and I will not try to force them down your throat. But if so many other things are true and are so proven, as stated in the Bible, then why would we dispute the ages of these old patriarchs? After all, the Bible doesn't try to tell you that everybody lived to this age. So if Methuselah did it, then why not you and I?

I don't think that we can do it . . . I'm sure we can't . . . but we can make it so that our children and our grandchildren and our great-grandchildren can do it. In fact, I know it can be done and it is not difficult or impossible. It just means getting back to nature and following in toto her teachings. We simply have to accept and follow carefully all biological laws and principles.

We have the intelligence and we have the ability, but do we have the will?

The healers have great and wonderful things going for them. No wonder they are so highly esteemed and respected. No wonder they make so much money. No wonder people follow them like sheep. Again I say, they have so many things going for them.

It seems as though all is fair in love and war and in the healing arts. Some people go to a doctor because he talks to them. It's so nice. I've known women who go to doctors because they like being probed into and being examined.

Now don't get mad at me and don't become hostile if you happen to be a nice girl. I'm relating what actually does happen from my experience and I'm not just slinging mud at the medical profession or at girls and women because a heck of a lot of people love going to a chiropractor for the jerks and manoeuvres that they get at the hands of the chiropractor.

For certain I know many people who love going to a masseur or to manipulative professionals who use massage, rubbing and laying of hands as part of their treatment.

I have visited medical doctors, chiropractors and masseurs and some of the most pleasant experiences and best results I have obtained were from these healers. A masseur of my acquaintance who also knew a little bit about healing and nursing and who was also a good psychologist had a most wide and loyal following. It is true, he had the best practice of any man for miles around — in fact he could never handle all the people who wanted to come to him. On my visits to this good manipulative healer I liked what he was doing to me.

I'm not trying to tell you what percentage of people go to these people because they like going there and because they like the kind of treatments they get. I'm just relating this in a broad, general manner.

There are reasons why certain people go to certain practitioners. Let's leave it at that.

Years ago a very close friend of mine, who was a great respected and beloved physician, told me that a large proportion of his women patients came only for the examination and that the longer the examination lasted, the better they liked it. He charged them higher fees and gave them longer examinations because he, too, was a psychologist.

I have known women who were very religious and they would not violate any principle of their religion. They were sex starved but they went to their doctor regularly and received the obstetrical and gynecological treatments and examinations — some no doubt reached an orgasm during the treatment. But this is perfectly legal and not violating any religious principle or practice and their conscience was clear. But they requested regular treatments by their beloved physician.

This does not necessarily mean it had to be a physician. It could be other healers as well.

Today I know medical doctors and perhaps most chiropractors are too busy to go through with this nonsense, at least so I think and prefer to believe. But don't forget for a moment or ignore the fact that what I said is true.

The story is told that Chinese medicine was run on a little different basis than medicine is practiced in the Western world today. In China the doctor received his payment as long as his patient was well and when the patient got sick, the doctor lost his pay.

Strange? Ridiculous? Unusual? No! Evidently the Chinese

evolved that system of payment to the healers after going through what we are going through with our healers today.

Please understand that I am not saying that China practices this form of payment today because it would not be true. When I was in China in 1963 and 1971 the healer received his conventional fees for treating, whether it was traditional or modern medicine.

Sickness today, as I have stated on various occasions, is the biggest industry in America. I say this without fear of contradiction. Yet, it could be turned into the smallest and most inconsequential industry in America if sane, sensible rules were followed.

How? By simply following the ancient Chinese method of payment. Today, the less the doctor is able to cure you the more business he has and the more profit he makes. Do you deny that this statement is 100% correct?

If, on the other hand, the physician is very successful and succeeds in curing every patient he will have to depend on new business continually. Well, maybe in this golden age of medicine there is enough new business but the proven fact is that a doctor makes most of his money from repeat business. Just like the chain store and the jeweller and the candle stick maker . . . the doctor makes his money from repeat business.

I'm a sort of an industrialist myself because for the past 45 years I have hired help. I still hire help. Well, 42 years ago in those depression years, specifically 1929, 30 and such, I was in business and whenever an employee was injured the government compensation took over. They paid his medical bills and they also paid him about 2/3 of his wages.

Way back then when good paying patients were scarcer than hen's teeth the doctors clung to these compensation cases like a blind man clung to his one eye and he had them come back as frequently as he could and as long as he could. There were occasions when I had to tell the employee that unless he got back to work soon I would

269

replace him with another employee. This invariably brought results.

If the employee came back with the statement, which often he did, that the doctor said he couldn't go back to work yet, I would tell him, "Then let the doctor give you a job". This, almost infallibly, worked and the employee got back to work lickety-split.

Now I daresay the same or a similar situation exists throughout America today. The doctor wants that patient coming back as often as he can get him. He doesn't even look at the patient probably, the nurse does it all and he sends in the top dollar bill to the Board. That's what the medical profession are doing right now with Medicare and such and if I'm lying let the medical profession come over and punch me in the nose. They know and you know that I'm not lying . . . so no punch in the nose for me.

In any event, the day is coming and coming fast, when we will all realize that we can't pay the doctor when we are sick. He'll only get paid when we are well. And then boy, there won't be much sickness in America. You know, common sense indicates this. If a man makes money because you are sick, it is absolutely stupid and senile for him to make you well . . . as though he could make you well even if he tried.

But it is in his interest to keep you sick, to keep you coming back again, and again, and again. Practically every business in America is based upon repeat business and the medical profession is no different. Industry works the same gimmick only we know it as "built in obsolescence". Therefore, we have to take the medical profession out of business. We've got to pay them a good salary, a big salary, whatever they are worth, to keep us healthy, not to keep us sick. And when that gets home to the populace, lo and behold, we'll have healthy people once again.

No, it's not just that the medical men don't make you well. They and the drug corporations keep you sick and their drugs make you sicker and you make no mistake about that.

Let's talk about making you well. Hold it, better we forget it. Nobody can make you well. If you are sick and you want to get well the only person, the only person on earth who can make you well is you. Oh sure, the doctor can administer drugs and he can also perform surgery on you, but your own body is the only thing on earth that can make you well.

The medical profession is the sickest group of people in our entire economic system. This is not an idle statement. It's an absolute fact. Therefore, how can you expect people to make you well who can't make themselves well?

Apart from what I have said being a proven fact, I have also established it most clearly in my own association with medical men and I challenge you to do likewise and you will reach the same conclusion as I have reached. Also this is borne out by statistics.

Staying well is the simplest and most natural function in human life. It is so. It must be so, otherwise all of our animals in their native habitat would be sick. If left alone without man's administrations they are well. The only time that animals get sick is when a human being interferes with them or when they run short of food because of too much multiplication or because of some accident.

What I'm trying to say is that in nature an animal is well and if the lowest form of life on earth knows how to stay well, then surely a man should know how to stay well.

What I'm trying to say is that if nature is left to her own design she will make and keep you well.

Now animals do not stand in nature's path and impede her work and functions but man does. Man eats unnatural food and consumes unnatural drink. In order to be well, in order to stay well, in order to get well, you must allow nature to function unimpeded.

Animals know what to eat instinctively. Human beings have

271

long lost that ability. Therefore, man must be taught what to eat and how to eat to be in good health.

Unfortunately, today we live in a profit system world where everybody wants to make money or a profit. Therefore, many lures are put in our way. If it were not for these lures you would probably get along all right by eating food that nature intended you to eat. But because of the dollar sign which is the big incentive you are taught and told what to eat so that somebody will make a lot of money, but it will not make or keep you well.

So it is very important that you gain knowledge if you are going to stay well. You must learn not to impede nature in her efforts in any way to obtain best results with your health. This makes knowledge about what to eat of prime importance. You must acquire proper, sane living habits.

Today, good health must be bought through study, through inquiry, through trial and error. Still good health is available to all for the asking but they must be sure to ask the right party.

It may come as a surprise to some people to learn that the medical profession is not the only profession that performs healing. When I was a young man, going back almost 50 years or so, I considered the medical profession the only healing profession. We did occasionally hear of a chiropractor whom we regarded with suspicion or doubt. I don't think I ever heard of a naturopath at that time. I did hear of herbal physicians but I never heard of an osteopath or a faith healer or a homeopathic physician.

It must be admitted that even today the medical profession has practically a monopoly on the healing art in America. In some of the States the osteopathic profession has been taken in or taken over by the medical profession. It is my prediction that within a decade or more they will also take over the chiropractic profession, and I also predict that the chiropractic profession will go over willingly, even though there appears to be a great deal of animosity betwixt them now.

As to the merits of the various healing arts it is difficult to make an analysis without prejudice creeping in. I admit that I have been browned off on the medical profession and unfortunately I do not think that the chiropractic profession is built upon firm ground . . . not that the medical profession has anything firmer to rely upon. But I am making no comparisons because comparisons are generally odious. I have investigated homeopathy and the best I can say for it is that I consider it much less harmful than medicine.

Osteopathy I consider as sort of an in-between or a mongrel, between medicine and chiropractic. Faith healing I know little or nothing about and I doubt if anyone else knows much more. I have read extensively about faith healing and still continue to read extensively and I do know for a positive fact that they have produced a great number or probably even thousands of remarkable cures or remissions. That is more remarkable when we recognize that it is done spontaneously so I keep my hands off faith healing. It's something that is greater than I can handle and while I do not forthrightly recommend it, I sure as shooting do not oppose it. I admit it is beyond, far beyond any competence that I might possess. I must further admit that I would not hesitate one moment to advise, recommend it or use it myself if the need arose if natural healing methods failed or where people do not have the strength of character to follow the abstemious way of living that I recommend.

I consider herbalism valuable for those who would like some form of healing but wish to avoid the dangers in medicine. I prefer to look upon herbs as nutritional factors of foods and as such they are acceptable. Where herbalism is practiced without any hocus pocus or abracadabra I would accept it as a sensible, practical form of healing.

Now what is left is naturopathy. If I'd ever favor any form of healing it would be naturopathy but naturopathy has one serious drawback . . . there are too many interpretations as to just what naturopathy is. The naturopathy that I accept is that field of natural healing that deals only with the functions and the prerogatives of nature. The body must be permitted to do its healing on its own. The only interference that is justifiable is the elimination of all

273

causative factors, that the road may be cleared so that nature can do its work unhampered, unimpaired and unobstructed. I do not even condone massage or friction except for the comfort that it may give. It is my opinion that a naturopathic physician should practice his art by clearing away or eliminating all causative factors or obstructions. Only natural food, natural water and natural air are to be used in the practice of naturopathy.

Granted, this may not be applicable in cases of accident. The broken leg will obviously not heal properly until it is put back into place, and I doubt if naturopathic physicians are trained to handle such cases. Here I am now referring to accidents, industrial, motor-car or such induced accidents. But apart from accidents, naturopathy from the surface appears to be the simplest and most natural form of healing but it is not really as simple as it sounds or appears.

In most cases when people seek out a naturopathic physician it is after all other avenues have failed or have been closed and in many cases the damage that has been done is irreparable or at least the damage is deeply engrained or deeply rooted. Therefore, it is hardly fair to judge naturopaths by the kind and class of patient they treat. For example, other healers get many simple conditions as well as some serious, many of which clear up on their own in spite of drugs and manipulations. But the poor naturopath, he gets practically only those which the other healers have given up on or those that are fearful of drugs, surgery and radiation bombs. Still, because of the tremendous power inherent in nature — remissions, improvements and even cures, as they are called, do take place.

I must here relate a story that is absolutely true. A well known political figure in the city of Toronto became ill. He was hospitalized, he was treated and looked after by the best physicians and surgeons available in America. He did not make good progress. In fact, his condition worsened. He was put on practically all the known drugs by his specialists. Anyway, it came the week-end and all his specialists were gone on vacations or sprees or whatever it was and then his condition became critical. The head hospital physician was called and he tried to contact the big shot specialists but they were all away and he had to make a decision on his own. He instructed the nursing staff to remove all medication. Come Monday morning all the big shots were back and found their patient in a greatly improved condition.

Now this is a true story, I swear to it, and it was told to me by the hospital physician. There is no healing agent on the face of the earth that even remotely comes close to mother nature, if left to do her job and her work without shackles.

CHAPTER

44

EARLY DIAGNOSIS — RIGHT OR WRONG

Does early diagnosis increase your life span or does it shorten it? I'll bet some of you will catch your breath with this one, because no one that I know of has ever raised this nasty, disturbing question.

I was married when I was twenty-one and my first-born child was born eleven months later. This was back 45 years ago. Yes, and even in those days they urged you to have a check-up for cancer and I was among the first to suggest to my wife that she go and have a check-up. She did this faithfully for more than ten years. As time went on the routine became more detailed and complicated but they only charged $10 or $15 or $20 in those days for an examination and she religiously went through with it every year.

Now I am relating this background so that you will understand that I have a fairly profound acquaintance with this early detection and early diagnosis business. In those days they did a biopsy and took X rays and they had a few other procedures. Today they are greatly expanded in scope and when you get a check-up they take you through a whole series of tests and examinations.

Back in those days I was convinced that if they found cancer in its early stages then it could be cured. Even today this is the generally accepted belief or impression that you get. No doubt this is the belief or impression that you have.

Now the examples that I am citing here are not the least bit new or unusual and I feel certain that most of my readers will have encountered similar experiences at one time or another, or even often, in their lives.

My oldest brother, to my knowledge, never knew a sick day in his life until he was about 55 or 56 years of age, in spite of the fact that he was quite stout. Then one day he was prevailed upon by his family to go for a physical check-up. He argued and said, "I feel fine so why should I go for a physical?"

Well, his wife and his family had heard the story over the radio and they read about it and everybody passed on the word that everybody should have a physical examination and that is the only way one can detect disease early and keep you healthy. So they prevailed upon my brother to go and have a physical examination.

After a series of exhaustive tests, they found that he had sugar and from that day till the day he died, ten years later, he never enjoyed another single day of good health.

Now this is a situation with which I was on intimate terms, because I saw him practically every day of my life. He lived close by.

A while back I read a story in the newspaper. I have the clipping somewhere but at the moment I can't lay my hands on it. But it told a story like this . . .

A man was crossing the street when he was struck down by a speeding motorist and killed. An autopsy was performed and to the surprise of the pathologist, he found that the man had an advanced case of cirrhosis of the liver, among many other diseases. The pathologist couldn't understand how this man could be out walking in the street and this puzzled him. He investigated and he queried the man's wife and family and friends about this individual. They all stoutly maintained that the man had been in perfect health and that he had claimed he was in perfect health. He had been active in business and in his social life and he had never complained of any illness. And had he not been struck down probably no one would have discovered that he had any disease — let alone so many diseases, including cirrhosis of the liver.

Now I've known at least twenty cases of people who went into the hospital for a routine check-up and there it was discovered that they had cancer. Some of these never ever got out of the hospital again. I'm sure you've heard the story how someone went for a check-up, they opened him up and closed him up again, and then he died a few days later or a few weeks later. Who knows, maybe you haven't heard of such things. But if I haven't heard of fifty — that's a low estimate — then I've never heard of one. I hear of them all the time . . . even today.

Some of these men and women I knew imtimately and they never complained of being ill. This was a routine check-up either for insurance or because their family wanted them to have a check-up. Right at this present moment there is one of my friends in the hospital with leukemia. It was discovered by accident and I'm sure he will never leave the hospital. The people that benefit the most from early diagnosis are the M.D.'s and the medical services.

Then there was the case of my oldest daughter. She went for a routine physical check-up and they discovered that she had a rather high white blood count. So they asked her to come back again in a month and then in another month and then another month. About the fourth or fifth time that she went back they asked if she would permit them to make a bone marrow test. She agreed against my stout opposition. And from the day that they made the bone marrow test she went downhill and she only lasted about three and a half years, then they buried her.

Now I contend and I will swear on a stack of Bibles that she did not die of leukemia ... she died from chemical poisoning. I maintain that if she had never had a physical or that check-up, she probably would have been alive today. I firmly believe that the bone marrow test can be a cause of or contributor to leukemia.

My oldest son, who is a physician, came in to visit his sister and we had a very serious discussion. I was opposed, at that time, very strongly to the drug that was being administered to her. 'Twas a drug called Myleran and I told my son that they shouldn't be giving her that drug and couldn't he request that it be stopped. He said that he had no authority to interfere in this case and he maintained that the drug was of benefit.

I said, "Be specific! Of what benefit is it?"

He replied. "It is preventing her spleen from enlarging."

I maintained that it was shortening her life and he then told me that in tests made with this drug in a New York hospital they found that this drug did not increase the life span of the individuals as compared with those who did not take the drug and had leukemia. But, he maintained, it prevented the swelling of the spleen and made the patients more comfortable ... especially the women who did not like to have their abdomens swollen.

I pressed him and I said, "Then you admit that it did not lengthen the life span?"

"Yes," he said.

"Will you admit that it shortened their lives?" I asked.

To this he would not agree.

"But you admitted that it did not increase their life span," I said. "From what I have seen and lived with, I maintain that it shortens the life span . . . in fact, I know damn well it does!"

That was the end of the discussion. Neither one of us could get anywhere with the other. In any event, when my child died, I felt that she did not die of leukemia . . . she died from chemical poisoning.

Therefore, while I have no proof to offer except the things that I have seen and heard and read and have been told about, I maintain defiantly and definitely that early detection shortens the life. You can accept it or disregard it or think as you like.

Do not run off with the idea that I am suggesting that you should avoid or run away from truth, because that is not so. I am forming my opinion from observations and experiences over a period of more than fifty years.

Another punch in my argument is this question. "Even when the disease is discovered, what can the medical profession do about it?" For example, for cancer they perform butchering surgery and burn you with radiation; for heart conditions they thin your blood and cause kidney and other derangements; for diabetes they make you an insulin cripple for the rest of your life; for arthritis they load you with aspirin or cortisone which make you even sicker. Where are the benefits? They never really cure anything. If you are lucky enough to get well in spite of their treatments, they take the credit whereas nature did the healing.

If something goes wrong with your health stop, think and think some more . . . then act by correcting your crimes against nature and your body. Go out and get knowledge from the most reliable honest sources available and you can correct your condition and get well.

CHAPTER

45

WHY M.D.'S ALWAYS SAY FOOD IS NOT A FACTOR

Because I specifically state that you are what you eat and that food is a factor in health and disease, I am allergic when a physician or a healer goes out of his way to specify that food is not a factor in disease.

Through the years I have figured out that about nine physicians out of ten deliberately go out of their way to emphasize the fact that you don't have to worry about what you eat, that food will not cause ulcers or heart conditions or cancer or diabetes or arthritis or practically any of the other diseases known to mankind. Very rarely you will meet a physician who might say that food could be responsible or involved.

Now I've always wondered why physicians were so outspoken and so emphatic about food not being a factor in disease. A little bit of thinking would have cleared up the situation without too much trouble. You remember the bit of witticism that Mark Twain told folks, "The more they told me about their honesty, the quicker I counted my silverware."

First of all, I understand that up until ten or more years ago only one medical school in all America offered a course in nutrition as part of the medical training. And from the information I have it was only a rudimentary course. I understand that today they do teach something about nutrition in a few of the medical schools.

So to begin with the doctor wouldn't know whether or not food was a factor in health . . . not having studied it. You can readily understand that when a man spends four or five or six years studying anatomy, pathology, physiology, histology, materia medica and kindred subjects, he would know little or nothing about health, nutrition or the properties of food. So from that point of view alone it is easy to understand that a doctor could not see any connection between food and disease.

Then too, the drug houses that disseminate a tremendous amount of literature have an overwhelming effect on what the physician reads or learns. It is by means of their detail men, as they are called, that most medical men learn about the new drugs and you can be sure that food and its merits are not discussed.

Within the past few years I have had a number of relatives, friends and close acquaintances who became ill and some died. You can believe me that I tried to bring home the message that if they changed their diet it would be to their benefit and they could get well or that the food they were eating was causing their trouble. Because of my insistance they would raise the food issue with their doctor and in practically every instance, as I recall, it was brought back to me that their doctor told them that food was not a factor and even pooh-poohed the idea. Thus they continued on their same contemptible disease-causing diet . . . that is, eating anything they wanted to eat.

In these instances all the major diseases were involved. One or more of my circle of friends had cancer, arthritis, heart disease, ulcers or diabetes. Each of these sick people told the doctor that someone had told them that they should change their diet and that food — that is, wrong food — was causing their trouble. In every instance my relatives or my friends, who were the afflicted ones, took the trouble to tell me that the doctor said I was nuts, ignorant or not acquainted with the true facts and that food played no part in his particular affliction.

So far two of them have died, one is on the critical list and one of them seems to have proven me wrong. I hope he continues to prove me wrong.

If the medical profession accepted my views or as I see it, the truth — that food is the prime factor in disease — then they would quickly put themselves out of business. I maintain most emphatically that if everyone had even the semblance of a proper diet, the hospitals would be empty and the physicians would be on the dole . . . and that would be a horrible condition, say the physicians, but I say it would be wonderful.

So I guess those of you who rely on medical advice will pay no attention to the food you eat, the liquor, coffee, tea or cocoa you drink, or the cigarettes you smoke, but you'll go merrily along your way . . . enjoying your sickness and being fussed over by the hospital attendants. They'll treat you kindly and mercifully but before you're much older they'll bury you. And that will prove, according to medical science and medical practice, that food has no relationship whatsoever with disease.

CHAPTER 46

DO HERBS HAVE A PLACE IN NATURAL HEALING?

Although I have written a book on herbs called "Proven Herbal Remedies" which has sold more than 80,000 hard bound copies I am not a herbalist nor do I advocate the herbal system of healing. By the same token I do not knock or advise against the herbal system of healing. If the herbalists used most of their herbs in their natural form without boiling, stewing or the making of tinctures or treating them in other ways I could go along with herbalism very well. Basically, to me herbs and herbalism would be a wonderful method of healing if the herbs were utilized in their natural state. Let me state clearly that I consider herbs used as foods to be of great benefit. I believe that herbs as food are nature's medicine. Thus, in my opinion they are of great nutritive value.

I feel, furthermore, that many of our well known and most popular and beneficial herbs should be broadly used in our diet.

Therefore, in truth I'm not at variance with the herbalists ... I only quarrel with them concerning the mode and method of utilization. I am convinced that herbalism is the oldest healing system on earth and if it were not for the fact that the herbs are boiled and concocted I would consider it the finest healing system on earth. If we would just take the selfsame herbs and serve them up or break them up or mix them up without boiling or damaging them in any way they could be very, very effective in relieving many diseases or conditions that afflict the human body.

No one who has bothered to investigate can deny the effectiveness and the miraculous remedial powers of many of our proven herbs. There really is no mystery concerning the effectiveness of herbs. They are food and they correct deficiences in a way that probably few other methods can equal.

Do you realize that there are in the world not many more than 300 different kinds of food plants, that is those that are generally used in the diets of people throughout the world? If you go to any marketplace in America you'll be hard-pressed to find more than 100 different horticultural food items. When we realize that there are well over a quarter of a million known varieties of plants in the horticultural encyclopedias and that only about 300 of them are used as food, it seems pitiful or tragic. This illustrates how hide-bound man is and how loathe he is to deviate from his normal ways and how unwilling he is to investigate and try different foods.

I've learned, for example, that a man will change his religion, he'll change his spouse, he'll change his friends, he'll change his politics but he won't change his eating habits ... even though it would be to his benefit.

In my book "Proven Herbal Remedies" I list 400 different plants or herbs. With few exceptions I consider them of nutritive value ... some greater, some lesser ... but the reason for the great effectiveness of herbs is that the nutrients or the vitamins or the minerals contained in many of these herbs are not readily found in the normal articles of food, especially cooked foods where the vitamins and minerals have been either lost or rendered unassimilable.

During my lifetime I have witnessed the magic of herbs. I've known herbs to correct conditions in a manner that no medicine or drug could ever hope to match. I stress that most herbs are food whereas most drugs and medicines are poison. Now this doesn't mean that I do not recognize that there are some poisonous herbs, herbs that if taken as food or even taken internally as medicine would cause serious trouble, sickness or even death. There are many herbs that are supposed to be used only for external purposes as a poultice.

It must be recognized that there are still a number of herbs that are used by the medical profession. They obviously use them because they have not as yet found any drug that could take their place . . . as though any drug could ever take the place of the natural therapeutic benefits of the beneficial herbs. I contend that the chicf reason that the medical profession has practically abandoned the use of herbs is because drugs are ever so much more profitable and so easy to handle and dispense. Besides, the patient can't go into his garden or to the woodlands and pluck drugs like he could herbs. Furthermore, it is rather difficult for a doctor to prescribe a herbal medicine and charge you $10.00 or $20.00 as he does for drugs. Herbs just don't readily lend themselves to high prices and profiteering like miracle drugs. And there are new miracle drugs practically every day while through the back door they bury yesterday's miracle drugs. Let's be sensible, there is big, big money in miracle drugs but herbs are as old as time itself. They charge ridiculously high prices for drugs and as their justification for this legal robbery they tell you that they had to spend a lot of money on research, whereas it doesn't cost any money to look into a herbal encyclopedia.

Admitted, today I am science oriented or science conscious. Still, if I had a condition that required treatment and I was offered a choice of a herbal treatment or a drug treatment I would, without any hesitation whatsoever, take the herbal treatment. The reason? There would be little or no danger in taking the herbal treatment even if it did me no good but the drug may cause some or serious irreparable damage to my body even if it did me no good. So the choice is a simple one, a logical one and a safe one. I'll trust a herb any time over a drug. I suggest that you examine the matter carefully.

CHAPTER 47

WE LOOK INTO FASTING

It is indeed surprising that in this day and age of excellent communications most of the world's population know nothing about fasting. Admittedly, many people — Catholics, Moslems and Jews — know fasting as a religious observance.

Obviously the great religions of the world thought that fasting had merit, otherwise it wouldn't have been prescribed as a religious observance. I know that among certain faiths — for example, the Jews — fasting is observed as a means of showing deep feeling or in times of critical situations. I would say that a fast is supposed to indicate a keen feeling or loss or a situation where the very heart and soul of a man is involved.

It is related that Christ, John the Baptist and Moses fasted for forty days each. Terrence McSweeney, the Mayor of Cork in Ireland, fasted for 74 days before he died.

Let me differentiate between what various people believe is fasting. The Jews, for example, deem a fast to be the total abstinence from food and water. They fast on Yom Kippur, the day of Atonement which is the holiest of holy days, when every man, woman and youth over 13 is expected to fast for a minimum of 24 hours, usually after the evening meal before sundown until sundown the following day, and the usual observance is that they never wash nor preen themselves, drink water or partake of food during that period.

The Moslem observance of fasting is that they abstain from food during the month of Ramadan but it calls only for fasting during the day but they can and do eat in the evenings.

Protestants have generally abandoned any form of fasting. The Roman Catholics fast from food before receiving communion. They also follow various other fasting observances like no flesh meat on Fridays and abstaining from certain foods during Lent.

No doubt other religious groups do some fasting but I am not acquainted with the way or manner in which they do it.

Many people go on a fast, as they call it, when they take no solid food but drink water, juices and perhaps tea and other liquids. This actually is a widely used method of fasting.

However, the kind of fasting to which I have positive reference is total fasting of all food for a given period, but water is taken in amounts as required. If you do undertake a total fast it is definitely advised that water must be taken to keep the body from dehydrating. This is generally referred to as therapeutic fasting.

I have been acquainted with this system of fasting for at least 25 years, but it is only in the past 15 years that I have begun to appreciate its virtues. Admitted, the believers in this method of therapeutic fasting are only a very small group. It appears that the medical profession, up until recently, was unalterably opposed to the practice of fasting as a therapeutic measure. Yet strange to relate, it was the medical doctors who were leaders in this field as a means of regaining health.

From my information many or even most of the first teachers and those who practised fasting were qualified medical men. However, they were derided, insulted, embarassed and shamed by the rest of the profession. It appears that these men possessed the intelligence, experience and knowledge to lead the way in a field that shows tremendous merit in healing.

I was directed to read some literature on fasting many years ago and while I was impressed with the results they claimed they achieved, I was dubious or should I say skeptical. But as I went along through the years I came across many people who swore that they owed their lives to fasting. They went on to give specific instances of various diseases from which they had suffered and in most cases were given up for dead by the conventional healing profession and by undertaking a fast they recovered. This included many people with heart conditions, many with arthritis and quite a few with cancer as well as practically all other known diseases.

It wasn't too hard for me to accept the fact that a person with a heart condition benefitted through fasting, or a person with an arthritic condition, but when people with cancer told me they benefitted or got rid of the cancer, this was too much for me to believe or accept. And I must admit that it took a lot of convincing and investigating to make me even consider the fact that cancer could be driven off by a fast.

If you examine the fasting situation, you will quickly learn that most of the fasting institutions throughout America avoid cancer patients. Yet many people who had cancer told me that they benefitted and as they claim, cured cancer by fasting, and I wondered then why the fasting experts refused to take cancer patients. But investigation and questioning turned up the reason and it was most logical. I learned that the medical profession didn't interfere or bother very much at all if these fasting institutions treated people with practically any known condition as long as they didn't treat people who had cancer.

When a cancer patient died at one of these fasting institutions, there was literally hell to pay and all the legal and law enforcement machinery that could be moved by the medical profession immediately stepped into action . . . and many of the fasting healers found themselves up against the law and whisked off to jail. The result was that these fasting institutions refused to accept cancer patients. You see, it was all right as long as they handled these patients, providing they didn't die. But when they died, then the trouble began and they wouldn't take that risk. Today I note that they will accept cancer patients . . . evidently the medical profession has had its teeth and claws dulled or pulled.

For a layman to accept that fasting can be of benefit is sometimes extremely difficult. We have been taught from the cradle that we must eat at least three meals a day and the missing of even one meal is considered an event in many households. Most mothers in America today just about have a fit when one of their children — especially when they are young — misses a meal. They think it is a major catastrophe.

But don't feel too bad . . . I thought it was a major catastrophe, too, up until 15 or so years ago. Talk to 99 people out of 100 and they'll tell you that if they miss a meal they get a headache. In fact, they have a headache if they don't have their meal on time. Don't laugh . . . this is absolutely true!

It wasn't more than a year ago that a very good friend of mine, a man who had been taught the principles of nutrition and health, told me that if he doesn't have his lunch on time he gets a severe headache. I tapped him on the shoulder and looked him square in the eye and I said, "What did you say?" He actually blushed then. "Well," he said, "what I said is absolutely true but now I realize how stupid it is and I know positively that it is purely mind over matter." He revealed to me a little later that since he had taken that view, missing his meal or being an hour or two late didn't cause any more headaches.

I have fasted for a day on many occasions, for two days on quite a few occasions, for three days on a few occasions, for five days once and for 21 days once, and I can assure you that on none of these occasions did I get a headache from missing a meal. I do admit, though, that having a headache would often start me onto a fast. But as I haven't had a headache for 15 years, then obviously I don't have to fast because of headaches.

Now I'd like to tell you about a little experience I had a few years ago. In July, 1968, I took a trip and was away from my home and business for about 30 days. Before the day set for my departure, part of a filling broke off or fell off one of my teeth on the right hand side. I called my dentist and he could not take me for the next few days and by then I had to be off, so I thought I would survive with the piece of filling missing and away I went. Because of the missing piece of filling I did no heavy chewing on the right hand side and the left hand side took the complete burden. After I had been away for three weeks, I was in Los Angeles at the time, I recall biting down fairly hard on a piece of tough food. This can be understood if you realize that I eat much of my food raw and my diet is made up of a lot of grains, seeds and nuts. So when I clamped down I must have jammed a bit of a filling somewhere — at least that's the way it felt — and this caused me quite a bit of pain. The pain continued . . . at first just sort of subdued, but I felt it, and that night I couldn't sleep. In the morning the tooth still ached and I decided to fast.

I knew that I was flying back the next day so I didn't bother to contact a dentist in the Los Angeles area. But on the plane the ache became worse and while I am not a teetotaller, I seldom drink liquor . . . in fact, I seldom drink any alcoholic beverage . . . but I did take one of the wee bottles that they serve you on the plane. This didn't bring too much relief so I took another bottle and this sort of subdued the pain.

As soon as I reached home I called my dentist — it was Saturday morning — and he couldn't take me but he made another appointment for me with another dentist. He examined the tooth and I told him the story and then I informed him that I didn't take drugs of any kind nor did I want a pain killer of any kind. His reply was, "I can't touch that tooth unless you let me inject a pain killer. That tooth is so sensitive that the minute my drill touches it you'll hit the ceiling."

So reluctantly I agreed to take a needle and then he and his assistant went to work and when he had the old filling completely removed, he said to me, "With that swollen jaw and the inflammation you have there I don't think I should put a filling back in that tooth. I believe I should go down and kill that nerve. I think I'll put in a temporary filling and then we'll see what happens."

My reply was, "What's the difference between a temporary filling and a permanent filling? You'll have to drill either one out again if anything goes wrong so I suggest you clean it all up nice and put in a permanent filling and we'll play it by ear after that." This he did.

I got back home and when the pain killer wore off the same old pain was back again.

In any event, I recall clearly that I had fasted Thursday, Friday and this was Saturday . . . and at midnight on Saturday the pain disappeared completely. But my jaw was still swollen. I had promised to attend a convention on Monday but I decided I couldn't very well go with this swollen jaw so I delayed. I waited until Tuesday and by then my jaw was almost back to normal.

Then a very dear friend of mine who is a dental specialist called me and I told him my troubles. He demanded that I come and see him immediately. I said, "No, I'll wait. I'm on a fast!"

He said, "That tooth will not heal and the trouble will not go away. It's got to be opened and you have to get into that nerve.

296

You've got to let that stuff out of there, otherwise it will blow the top of your head off."

I said, "Beloved friend, I have more faith in the human body. I feel that I have removed the cause and now nature can be allowed to work and I'm going to fast until it does."

He pleaded with me to listen to him and have the work done and he would do it without charge. But I insisted that nature knew her business and I would wait. However, I promised to drop in the following day because it was on the way to the convention.

Well, I dropped in the next day — I was still fasting — and I still refused to allow him to pull out that filling. I told him that if he wanted to do something for me he could fill that other tooth that had caused the trouble in the first place, which he promptly did and he made a mighty nice job of it, too. But he still insisted that I would have trouble unless I listened to him about getting that other tooth fixed up right.

I went on to the convention and I still fasted until the sixth day. By then my jaw felt normal, my health was perfect, but I resolved to exercise a bit of care and caution on that tooth which was the source of my trouble.

Well, 3 years have gone by and that tooth has never bothered me. And I believe that the fast did the trick. It's quite simple and understandable how it did it. The moment I stopped eating I stopped irritating the tooth. But most and best of all I permitted the body to go ahead and perform its proper repair functions without the burden of having to worry about handling a normal intake of food. Furthermore, I did no chewing, which no doubt would have caused irritation.

I went on my 21 day fast because of a prostate condition . . . a very severe case of retention of the urine. They wanted to operate at once and I was catheterized a couple of times and then they put an indwelling catheter in me. I decided to go on a fast at a proper fasting institution and on the seventh day I removed the indwelling catheter and for a few days after I passed small quantities of blood. Thereafter the situation cleared up and I returned home with a perfect functioning urinary organ and bladder . . . but against the advice of the practising fasting doctor who wanted me to stay a few more days. Subsequently I learned that he was right because my condition came back at a later date and I had to have surgery. But when I left his institution and while I was there I had no problem whatsoever with my urine, as mentioned.

Now this has been my actual experience with fasting.

When I travel I try to eat as close to my beliefs and convictions as humanly possible, but sometimes it is difficult if not impossible. During the past six years I have had no trouble on my travels but prior to that when I would run into difficulty I would immediately abstain from food . . . all food except water. And as you can well imagine, the people I was with and those whom I visited pleaded with me to take some food . . . to take at least a cup of tea or a bit of juice. I refused coldly and definitely. I said, "No, I will eat nothing, but I'll drink water." And I found this one of the strongest weapons to bring the body back to health.

In my opinion the reason that fasting is so successful in most cases of sickness is because the eating or the taking of food is the cause of the trouble. It's not just food . . . it's the kind of food that you eat. I cannot visualize good wholesome natural food causing anyone trouble unless taken in excess. But nobody eats plain, decent and wholesome food anymore . . . most of us eat crap and corruption of the worst order. So when you stop eating, of course, almost a miracle takes place. You're not putting the poison and the corruption into your system so in a few days you show a marked improvement.

Probably the most important thing that I have to warn you about — if you intend to fast — is to fast only under proper supervision. Fasting alone is dangerous and can actually be the cause of your death. So if you are going to fast, fast under supervision and besides that, read thoroughly on the subject and be totally and

298

completely informed.

Of course, I know many people — dozens — who have undergone fasts on their own with great success. I also know some who have undergone fasts with poor success and some got into trouble. If you know what you are doing and if you are completely informed on the subject, you probably can fast on your own with great success. But I do not advise this.

I am acquainted with two people — one fasted 14 days and the other fasted 17 days without supervision — and both of them remained on their jobs. One drove a truck — a big oil truck — and he fasted 14 days while doing his job. The other fasted 17 days and put in a good hard day's work in a factory. I was acquainted with both of these men and I warned them and warned them. I also told them that if word got to the authorities that they were fasting, they would probably have a warrant issued for their arrest and they would wind up in a hospital by force . . . and perhaps in a mental institution.

I know three people to whom this actually happened so don't be smart and go on a fast and brag about it to anybody, because this could happen to you.

Now here I would like to give you a fasting story by Edward H. Dewey, M.D.:

"I was called one day to one of the families of the poorest of the poor, where I found a sick case that for once in my life set me to thinking. The patient was a sallow, overgrown girl in early maturity, with a history of several months of digestive and other troubles. I found a very sick patient, so sick that for a period of three weeks not even one drink of water was retained, not one dose of medicine, and it was not until several more days that water could be borne. When finally water could be retained my patient seemed brighter in mind, the complexion was clearer, and she seemed actually stronger. As for the tongue, which at first was heavily coated, the improvement was striking; while the breath, utterly foul at first, was strikingly less offensive. In every way the patient was very much better.

"I was so surprised at this that I determined at once to let the good work go on on Nature's own terms, and so it did until about the thirty-fifth day, when there was a call, not for the undertaker, but for food, a call that marked the close of the disease. The pulse and temperature had become normal, and there was a tongue as clean as the tongue of a nursing infant.

"Up to this time this was the most severely sick case I ever had that recovered, and yet with not apparently more wasting of the body than with other cases of as protracted sickness in which more or less food was given and retained. And all this with only water for thirst until hunger came and a complete cure!

"Such ignoring of medical faith and practice, of the accumulated wisdom and experience of all medical history, I had never seen before. Had the patient been able to take both food and medicine, and I had prohibited, and by chance death had occurred, I would have been held guilty of actually putting the patient to death — death from starvation. Feed, feed the sick whether or not, say all the doctors, say all the books, to support strength or to keep life in the body, and yet Nature was absurd enough to ignore all human practice evolved from experience, and in her own way to support vital power while curing the disease.

"I could recall a great many cases in which because of intense aversion to food patients had been sick for many days, and even weeks, with not enough nourishment taken to account for the support of vital power; but the fact did not raise a question with me.

"The effect of this case upon my mind was so profound that I began to apply the same methods in Nature to other patients, and with the same general results. The body, of course, would waste during the time of sickness; but so did the bodies of sick that were fed. As for medicines, they were utterly ignored except where pain was to be relieved.

300

"One of the most common complaints of the sick is that they have 'lost their appetite.' They seem to imagine that this is a terrible affliction. Quite the reverse is true, however. In the majority of cases Nature takes away the appetite because a fast is needed. They do not know that the greatest blessing to them would be to 'lose their appetite' long enough to find their hunger. Loss of appetite is simply an indication that the system is overcharged with pathogenic matter and that Nature is trying to stop the eating long enough to give these clogging, benumbing or irritating accumulations a chance to escape from the system, or it may be that the digestive organs are too weak to take care of large quantities of food. However, the laity for ages has been encouraged by the medical profession in the idea that to lose the appetite and miss a few meals is a great calamity; that this must be prevented by taking powerful stimulants in the form of appetizers and tonics. These serve to create a false and artificial appetite and cause the sufferer to stuff the weak stomach with more food, while that taken in previous meals is fermenting and putrefying, filling the system with noxious poisons.

"Many people are learning the trick of curing their colds, headaches, nervous spells and other acute troubles by missing a few meals or taking a short fast. It is the quickest, simplest and most efficient method of relieving the overloaded, food poisoned system. We would be surprised if we knew little food is actually required to keep the human organism in good condition. The majority of people are food poisoned — even those who believe they are eating moderately.

"Cornaro, the great Italian Nature Cure apostle, who lived in Venice in the Eighteenth Century, proved these facts which humanity at large has not digested and taken advantage of even at this late day. At forty he was dying from chronic diseases resulting from overeating, drinking and riotous living generally. Being gifted by nature with some intelligence and will power, he essayed the cure himself by reversing his habits of living, i.e. by reducing the daily allowance of food and drink to a minimum.

"For nearly forty years his daily allowance of solid food was

301

not more than twelve ounces. Then he yielded to the urging of his relatives and friends, who believed that he was starving himself, and took a few ounces more of food than his former quota. The result was that he immediately began to feel most miserable, both physically and mentally, and his former good health and energy did not return until he reduced his daily allowance to the old, accustomed twelve ounces.

"After the age of eighty he wrote several books on matters of health, and particularly his own experiences. His most pretentious work, which is even now in print and widely read, he finished when he was over one hundred years old. The history of this man and his experiences with moderate living and fasting should be taught in every school in the land.

"The Physiology of Fasting. Fasting is undoubtedly one of the most potent and incidentally the cheapest of all natural remedies. The reason why it is not more universally applied is that the laity at large, as well as the medical profession, are under the impression that the interruption of eating even for a brief period will greatly reduce the vitality of the individual.

"This popular fallacy is caused by the belief that food and drink are the only sources of strength. In other parts of these writings I have shown that this is not so — that the life force which is the real source of our vitality or strength is entirely independent of our material bodies (physical and spiritual) and of food, drink, medicines, tonics and stimulants; that this life force flows into us from the source of all life, intelligence and creative force in the universe; from that which we variously call God, Nature, Universal intelligence, the Oversoul, the Will to Live and by many other names. If people fully realized this fact they would not be in such great fear of missing a few meals or of undergoing a more or less prolonged fast.

"Fasting as a remedy is fully in harmony with our philosophy of the causes of disease. If disease is created through abnormal composition of blood and lymph and through accumulation of morbid matter in the system, it stands to reason that fasting will help to eliminate from the system waste matter and morbid accumulations. The most difficult feature about fasting is the breaking of the eating habit. Therefore the first three or four days of fasting are always the hardest. They are usually accompanied by craving for food, nervous disturbances, mental depression, headaches, sleeplessness, etc. We must remember that eating is the oldest and most firmly established of all habits. Therefore, it is not easily broken.

"After the habit is broken, which usually requires two or three days, fasting becomes easier day by day. One reason for this is that about the third or fourth day the mucous membrane of the intestines begin to eliminate morbid matter. The processes of assimilation have come to a standstill. The membranous linings of the stomach and intestines, which ordinarily act as sponges for the absorption of food materials, are now throwing off effete matter from the system. The sponge is being squeezed. This is indicated by the fetid breath and coated tongue which reflect the foul condition of the digestive organs. These are not fit to digest or assimilate food; therefore hunger ceases.

"The system now has to draw for food upon its reserve stores. The waste and morbid materials are stirred up and eliminated first.

"When we consider that the digestive canal from mouth to anus is about twenty-six feet long and lined all through with eliminating cellular and glandular structures, then we can better appreciate the purifying effect of a protracted fast. One need not fear the weakening effects of fasting, since of late years it has been proved in thousands of cases that fasts of even forty, fifty and sixty days' duration have no perceptible weakening effect upon the system unless the patient be greatly weakened and emaciated by disease at the beginning of the fast.

"One of our patients recently finished a forty-nine day fast. At the end of it he felt actually stronger than he did at the beginning. Up to the last day he took long walks. At the same time the chronic troubles which were caused by drug poisoning and surgical operations were greatly alleviated.

"The foregoing explains why short fasts of from one to three days' duration have not a decided curative effect. It takes that much time to start the eliminative processes in the linings of the intestines. As soon as food is taken these processes are interrupted and reversed. I would consider seven days a short curative fast.

"Why Fasting is Necessary. Aversion to eating during acute diseases, whether they represent healing crisis or disease crisis, is perfectly natural, because the entire organism, including the mucous membranes of stomach and intestines, is engaged in the work of elimination, not assimilation. Nausea, slimy and fetid discharges, constipation alternating with diarrhea, etc., indicate the the organs of digestion are throwing off disease matter, and that they are not in a condition to take up and assimilate food.

"Ordinarily, the digestive tract acts like a sponge which absorbs the elements of nutrition; but in acute diseases the process is reversed, the sponge is being squeezed and gives off large quantities of morbid matter. The processes of digestion and assimilation are at a standstill. In fact the entire organism is in a condition of prostration, weakness and inactivity. The vital energies are concentrated on the cleansing and healing processes. Accordingly, there is no demand for food.

"This is verified by the fact that a person fasting for a certain period, say, four weeks, during the course of a serious acute illness, will not lose nearly as much in weight as the same person fasting four weeks in days of healthful activity.

"It is for the foregoing reasons that nourishment taken during acute disease . . .

(a) is not properly digested, assimilated, and transmuted into healthy blood and tissues; instead, it ferments and decays, filling the system with waste matter and noxious gases;

(b) interferes seriously with the elimination of morbid matter through stomach and intestines by forcing these organs to take up the work of digestion and assimilation;

(c) diverts the vital forces from their combat against the disease conditions and draws upon them to remove the worse than useless food ballast from the organism.

"This explains why taking food during feverish diseases is usually followed by a rise in temperature and by aggravation of the other disease symptoms. As long as there are signs of inflammatory, febrile conditions and no appetite, do not be afraid to withhold food entirely, if necessary, for as long as five, six or seven weeks.

"I have treated several virulent cases of typhoid and malaria which lasted for six weeks before the acute febrile symptoms subsided. During this time the patients did not receive any food whatsoever, not even a drop of milk. I continued the fasting during the seventh week in order to allow time for the building up of the intestinal membranes which had sloughed as a result of the inflammatory processes. Towards the end of the seventh week the patients developed natural hunger. Then the feeding commenced and they made perfect recovery, gaining more in flesh within a few months than they had lost during the illness.

"In cases of gastritis, appendicitis, peritonitis, dysentery or typhoid fever, abstinence from food is absolutely imperative."

So here you have a fairly basic understanding of fasting. Use it wisely.

CHAPTER

48

BEFORE IT IS TOO LATE

I want to tell you about a very very interesting story that I
read last night. It was in a health magazine. I should say that with
care because it was a medical health magazine. I should differenciate
between medical health and natural health because there is a
difference. The medical profession wouldn't want my kind of health
to be mixed up with theirs for the world and for six worlds I
wouldn't want my kind of health mixed up with the medical health.

I take my oath that what I am recounting is actually true
only I tell it in my fashion and the story appeared in the year 1972.

This man and his wife lived to retirement age — sixty — and
they bought themselves a boat and they went down to live in Florida
to enjoy the remaining years of their lives. As all smart, alert medical
trusting Americans do he went to his doctor for his annual physical

check-up and the doctor found a bit of blood in his urine and this of course started some testing and some exploration and I presume a biopsy with the result that the diagnosis was bladder cancer. The doctor was very reasuring and hopeful and he said "There is no problem here at all. We can just put in a plastic bladder and you'll be as fit as a fiddle. You'll never even know the difference".

Our medically oriented man accepted this . . . what else at the time could he do? He didn't know where else to turn anyway and besides he had complete confidence in his doctor as he had been a hospital administrator all his life and he believed wholely in the great and noble practice of medicine and surgery. It so happened that beds were not available at the time so he had to wait a couple of weeks. In the meantime they did a little more checking up and they found that he had a little bit of diabetes too. Of course the doctor assured him that diabetes today is nothing. It's just a matter of taking a few pills and just a bit of care in the diet and everything will be hunky doodle.

So while they had to do a little bit of fixing before they could take him in for surgery on account of the diabetes a little more exploration was done and lo and behold, they came up with the new finding that he also had something wrong with his rectum and this necessitated an urgent operation which would leave him with a colotomy. But the surgery couldn't be done because his original urologist had to consult with the procotologist so that they could sort of work together as a team and one would remove one and the other would remove the other. By that time a month or maybe more had gone by and they took him in and eventually they fixed him all up with the plastic bladder, the insulin drugs and the great and noble piece of surgery known as a colotomy.

This man and his wife faced up to it boldly and in spite of all of it he still keeps active and they both try to carry on as though nothing has happened. When he's all dressed up and he is not suffering from any great pains from the umpteen pills that he has to take to prevent this and to keep that off and to maintain that and to keep his diabetes under control . . . why he's just as fit as a fiddle but

308

rest assured it is not a Stradivarius.

Now during the entire article they treated this whole thing as though it was just an every day occurrence. These things happen, it can't be helped and with the great and noble medical profession they have these things working like clockwork. In fact, I think the medical profession will have it soon that men like this with all the surgery will be able to take part in football games and wrestling and then have a bout or two of sex in the evening. At least that's the way they say it.

Now let's take a look behind the scenes here a bit. I don't want to be critical and sound like a rat or a barking dog but because of the many weeks between discovery of the first condition and the surgery, plus the many months that it took to get the man back on his feet again so he could partake of all this great activity like dancing and bowling and golfing, a long time — probably three or four months elapsed. Here and now I'm willing to stand before you and say, "Had I known that man and had he asked me or consulted me and listened to me he wouldn't have had to have the surgery and have his bladder removed, he wouldn't have needed to have the colotomy and he wouldn't have needed to take any drugs or that insulin and within two or three months he could have taken part in all those pleasurable, sociable activities without feeling the hundred and one side effects of those drugs, plus death staring him in the face.

Now lest you think that I'm really balmy or out of my head and you are gasping that I am suggesting that cancer can be cured and that a colotomy can be avoided and that diabetes can be stopped I want to say to you, "Yes, it is an absolute fact that all this can happen."

Let me also say here and now that this family's diet must have bordered on the ridiculous, on the horrendous, on the unbelievable or horrible. This diet must have contained all the conventionals like good old white bread and lots of good old white sugar and lots of good old margarine and two or three cups of

309

delicious Mashacks coffee for breakfast and then mid morning tea and afternoon tea and all the nice conventional foods from the supermarket because surely they wouldn't have time to do any food preparing with all these activities going on.

So there would be T.V. dinners, and French fries, hamburger, Southern fried chicken and lots of baked goods and pastries and cookies and cakes and pies and oh yes, ice cream that they love so much. They'd have it practically with every meal. Then of course at the first sign of a little upset why naturally they would take their alka-selzers and their aspirins or even the stronger ones with Bufferin added and no doubt they would have their shots of penicillin and antibiotics.

You see, a man couldn't get into a condition of cancer of the bladder, cancer of the rectum, and diabetes by eating raw vegetables and fruits and grains. It's just impossible. In fact, the amount of these foods that he would have eaten would be comparitively infinitesimal because these conditions just cannot happen to people who eat the foods I mentioned regularly. Of course, I stand before you and say that as soon as his condition was discovered had he read one of my books . . . for example, my "Guideposts" book or perhaps this book . . . he would immediately see the reason, the common sense, the logic behind a proper diet and the lives of two people would not have been destroyed as well as the suffering they endured plus the suffering of their loved ones. Three cheers . . . the medical profession and the surgeons score again.

Right now I'm making a very clear-cut, simple announcement. If and when such a condition should arise before you surrender yourself, that is body and soul, to the medical profession or the surgeons or before you take too many harmful drugs try the 100% raw food diet. Perhaps even with the aid of a juicer so that you can get all kinds of good fresh juices in large amounts — because time is short. I suggest that you give the raw vegetables, grains and fruits a chance for that twenty or thirty day period which you'll be waiting before they get all the loose ends tied up for the surgery and the chances are by that time you won't need their services and if so, for certain you won't want them ever again.

CHAPTER

49

IN DEFENCE OF
THE AMERICAN MEDICAL ASSOCIATION

If we are to continue our society or establishment in the manner which we like it or permit it to exist as of the year 1972 then we must have more doctors, more nurses and more hospitals and we must see to it that the medical profession and all its accoutrements are maintained in good functioning condition. If we like it that way then all we need is more money.

If we agree and like what is happening in America today or happened in the past 10 or more years then we should do everything we can to see that we have more and more medical care and better facilities and better medical plans. We must be prepared to do more surgery, to do more work with the bomb or irradiation and to make more tests and continue in full swing to make the medical scheme bigger and better. We must give more authority and greater support

313

to the entire medical structure.

The way the entire thing is set up the chemical fertilizer people supply us with the agricultural chemicals that we put on our land and then other chemical companies supply us with the pesticides, bacteriacides, insecticides and fungicides that are required to keep our plants from being eaten or devoured or destroyed by insects and other pests. Then we must have three or four or more thousand different chemicals to put into our food to preserve it, to color it, to make it tempting and do other things that the food industry finds necessary to feed the burgeoning population. The medical drug industry plays a very, very important role in our present day way of life and they must be encouraged to do research and discover more and more wonder drugs to keep our people alive and to augment their lives. Then it is up to the medical profession to do its full part in this great undertaking. They must prescribe more and more drugs and do more and more surgery and use more and more radiation, X rays and the cobalt and other bombs.

This whole gigantic colossus dovetails neatly and fits into the whole picture. Today we are living in a chemically oriented society. To break the chain or a link in any part of this tremendous leviathan wouldbe to bring disaster to the whole.

That is why I maintain that we must defend and look after the American Medical Association. They must be prepared at all times to fulfill their vital part in this vast scheme of things, they must learn to do more and more heart transplants, kidney transplants and they must learn how to transplant every organ in the body. They will not only have to do this, they will have to learn how to make animal organs fit into human anatomies because soon we will be running out of organs from human beings but I'm sure that the medical profession with the aid of the drug and chemical industry will find a way to make animal organs fit the job just as Dr. Niehans in Switzerland is doing at the present time.

Lest you think that I am jesting I assure you from the bottom of my heart that I am most serious about all of this. If we are to continue living in a chemically oriented society, all of the things that I have stated are absolutely necessary for our welfare if that is the correct term. For example, if you think that you can eat food grown on chemically fertilized soil to which the food processors have added innumerable chemical additives and get along without surgery like having your gall bladder removed, or your appendix or your tonsils or your prostate, then you are making a sad mistake. Having these organs removed is all a part and parcel of the bargain. It's like the horse and buggy . . . you can't have one without the other. If you think in our present society you can get along without barbiturates, tranquilizers, insulin or penicillin, sulfa drugs or a myriad of other drugs old and new you are making a tragic error. This too, is all part of the package deal. To give you an illustration of how this thing works let me tell you a true incident that occurred a while ago.

A very good friend of mine came rushing in to see me one day all excited and worked up and said, "They've taken my oldest son to the hospital and they are going to remove his gall bladder. Now I know he needs his gall bladder and I'm not going to let them remove it. I'm right now going to the hospital and I'm going to stay right there and not permit them to remove my son's gall bladder."

I said, "Have you talked to the surgeon?" He said, "Yes, and the surgeon told me that his condition is serious and he must remove the gall bladder immediately."

So I said to my friend, "If I were you, Bob, I wouldn't interfere".

He looked up at me with amazement in his eyes and said, "Are you against me, too? I thought you didn't believe in drugs and medicine and surgery?" and he almost shrieked these things at me.

I said, "Bob, keep cool, take it easy and just listen for a minute. Your son leads a conventional way of life, he eats conventional foods,' he smokes, he drinks and his living and eating habits are in accordance with our conventional society and gall

315

bladder surgery is part of this deal. If you interfere your son is liable to die and you'll be guilty of killing him. Now if somebody told me that you had gall bladder trouble I'd be the most amazed man in the world and would say by no means permit such surgery because you would have done nothing to deserve it or earn it. You eat practically all raw vegetables, fruits and grains the same as I do, you do not drink alcoholic beverages or coffee or tea nor do you smoke and you don't eat any processed foods of any kind and most of your vegetables come from your own garden ... well, you're not conventional and the same cap won't fit you."

With this explanation my friend nodded his head and said, "I guess you're right."

"So just take it easy, resign yourself to the situation and your son will probably come out of it all right without a gall bladder and his doctor will probably advise him not to eat this food or that food and if he wouldn't have eaten them to start with he wouldn't have had to have the gall bladder surgery."

That's the way it is, folks. If you live conventionally then you must go on for the ride on the merry-go-round and get all of the benefits . . . such as they are!

CHAPTER

50

IF I GET SICK

I am quite emphatic in stating that the proper way of living and the raw food diet never fails. I'm not suggesting that you can take people on the brink of death and quickly return them to normal health. Still, it has been done, I've seen it being done and I see it in actual progress every single day. No one can promise or guarantee anyone that it can be done but I stand firm and state that the proper way of living with a knowledgable raw food diet never fails. You have no right to make me promise that it can be done . . . still I say it is happening all the time.

That there are failures with the raw food diet and proper living is granted. Even though I maintain that this form of diet is 100% fool proof, nothing is perfect and there are exceptions to all rules. I am fool enough and stubborn enough to accept challenges whenever they are posed and I'm quite willing to stake my life that the raw food system works, provided the raw food is 100% organic and provided the method is followed to 100% accuracy without if's, and's or but's. I realize this is an extremely difficult course to follow but is imminent death not difficult? Can any measure be too demanding when one is faced with imminent or extended-time death . . . and by following this means save his life?

Here I would like to cite a few true incidents that point out the dangers involved and why there are failures. I knew a case of cancer where the afflicted wanted to live so badly and was willing to follow the routine 100% and when she started her progress was remarkable, unbelievable and then slowly the progress was halted and the situation slowly deteriorated. I was shocked, dismayed, bewildered and then through the grapevine I learned that the party, due to the insistence of her husband, was taking a cancer fighting drug recommended by her physician.

In incident 2 the afflicted was following the rules quite closely and then ran into rectal troubles. This caused me a great deal of concern and embarrassment. I could not find out why. Then eventually by accident I learned that this friend of mine just loved cold, canned tomatoes and had them every day religiously. I took him into a supermarket and picked up a can of tomatoes and showed him what it said on the label . . . contains "calcium sulphate." Each can was loaded with this chemical and definitely this chemical caused or contributed to his condition.

In incident 3 a friend who followed most of the rules and had good clean living habits could not shake a condition of the colon, no matter what she did . . . but she also couldn't give up her coffee and her wine.

Incident 4 involved coffee. This is an old lady who had made remarkable progress. She was 85 years of age but the progress was halted by set-backs at various intervals. Close questioning revealed that an occasional cup of coffee was sneaked in, not believing it could have much effect . . . just an occasional cup of coffee maybe once or twice a day.

318

Incident 5 involved a woman I knew. She really gave up all her bad eating habits and was using a fresh vegetable juice regimen closely. She even gave up smoking and made fairly good progress but I wasn't satisfied. I felt the progress should have been well nigh perfect because her regimen was perfect. Then after a great deal of investigation and questioning I found out that she was still using a mineral oil which she had been using for many years to insure herself of a good easy bowel movement. She didn't recognize that the mineral oil was depriving her body of vital, essential minerals and elements.

I stand squarely before you and say that the raw food way of eating does not fail but various boobytraps cause complications and even failures. There is no way on earth of which I'm aware that we can be sure of the 100% diet being followed without outside environmental hazards. The system is fool-proof, the system does not fail but there are many unaccountable occurrences that creep in even with the greatest of care and the best laid plans. If the raw food system can work on an 85 year old body which has been in poor health for much more than 10 years, (I can only guarantee 10 years because that is as long as I've known the party but obviously the sickness was of much longer duration) and six months on a raw food diet brought results that were nothing else but phenomenal . . . that is what nature, that is what proper food, that is what proper living can do for you and for anyone.

I can truthfully state that from my actual experiences the raw food diet works almost directly in the proportion to which it is followed. Follow it 100%, you get 100% results and from there on it goes down. In these cases you sort of get back what you put into it . . . what more can anyone ask?

O.K., you accepted my thesis, you believed what I taught and told you. You accepted my arguments and you followed the way of life that I advocated. Then suddenly out of the blue . . . you are stricken. It could be something wrong with your stomach, or a heart attack. It could be retention of the urine, it could be any one of the ten thousand different things that can and do go wrong with the

319

human body. In simple terms, you are sick.

Now here I am standing beside you and say to you "If you have followed the practices and the principles that I advocate you can't get sick." But you say, "I am sick." And I repeat again, " You can't be sick if you follow the practices and principles that I advocate".

Some years ago this actually happened and the young man, a close friend of mine 9 years my junior, insisted that he was abiding by all the rules, practices and principles but he was sick. He was weak, he didn't have enough energy to work. I asked him. "Did you consult a doctor?"

He said, "Yes, much to my disgust and he could find nothing wrong with me".

So I went back to my rule book and said, "I'm sorry, there can't be anything wrong with you if you have followed and done as you told me you have. Then an idea struck me and I asked, "Is there anything different that you've been doing in the past few days or past few weeks that you don't normally do?"

He replied, "If you mean about eating, well I haven't changed my eating habits at all or my living habits."

But I said to him, "I've noticed you haven't been here every week-end lately like you used to be. What's the reason that you're here so infrequently?"

"Oh," he said, "That house that I own here in town needs painting and I've been doing the work myself, painting it indoors".

"How long has this been going on?"

"Well," he replied "I've been doing it every week-end. I start late Friday afternoon and work part of the evening and I work all day Saturday and all day Sunday. Then I go back to my business in

Toronto on Sunday night".

"Maybe it's the fumes or the gases or the odors or the emanations from the paint that's contributing to your trouble".

"I never thought of that", he said.

"How much more have you got to go?"

He mused for a moment then said, "I should have it done in another two week-ends."

"My suggestion is, chum, that you should get yourself a gas mask if you want to finish that job"... which he did and he has had no more trouble. Now don't laugh, this is an absolutely true story.

O.K., we are back to my earlier thesis. What do I do, where do I go, to whom do I turn if I do get sick? Again I reiterate ... if you follow the eating, living and drinking habits that I advocate you can't get sick. So now you are becoming annoyed and firmly state, "Let's be realistic, let's use the common sense we are supposed to have."

People do get sick in spite of this, that or anything. I am quick to answer, I'm the first to admit and grant this. To live in this polluted world of ours today, especially in America or in any industrial country it is impossible to avoid all risks. We are being infected by the air that we breathe, by the water that we drink and of course by the food that we eat, even the best organically grown food is still subject to contamination by air and water or fallout.

If anything happened to me, in spite of my protestations that I do everything right, I would immediately abstain from all food and drink and take only water. I'd certainly make sure that my water was good water, preferably from a spring that's uncontaminated. I would stay on this total fast for two days or three days but not longer than 10 days. Three to five days usually accomplishes the purpose. I warn against long fasts at all times. I admit that long fasts may be

321

necessary to a person who is exceptionally loaded down with contemptibles and such. But for these people I have no concern because I do not involve myself with them. If you are polluted go and see one of the fasting experts. I am not an expert on fasting or anything else.

Here and now I must make it clear that none of us has lived properly since birth and to make matters worse most of us only accepted the proper way of living in the past few years at the most, and maybe only in a modified way. There are very few people I have ever met who have been on a proper diet for more than 20 years. In fact, I do not know of one single person who has eaten raw food, organic food and avoided all contemptibles for 20 years. Therefore, it is possible that some of your earlier sins are catching up with you. If that is the case one couldn't possibly know where to begin to treat or to advise. Therefore, the short fast is in order. It may work. It usually does, unless the damage has been severe and then perhaps a long fast might be indicated. I do not say that it is indicated.

Following the short fast from 3 to 10 days I would advise a 100% raw vegetable, grain and fruit diet with the accent on the green vegetables and the fresh ripe fruit but the proportions must be at least three quarters raw vegetables. Let the fruitarians rave as they will about the merits of fresh fruit. I know from studies, observations and experiences that fresh vegetables are better. Now these methods that I have advocated work, especially among those who have for some time lived properly. The only means or method of treatment with which I am acquainted and which I can recommend is proper food, raw food or the total abstinence of food. If that doesn't work then nature refuses to forgive and you are paying for your past indiscretions or gluttony. I regret that I cannot offer you drugs, pills, potions, vaccines, narcotics, surgery, X rays or cobalt bombs, in which to drown your sorrow.

Among my wide acquaintanceship with people who eat and live properly none of those that I know have yet reached the 100% raw food diet, yet no serious problems have yet arisen. If it works for hundreds it should work for thousands and millions. I reiterate it

322

works but you must do it.

The big reward for leading a proper life with proper food and proper drink is that you just don't get sick, now or ever. Therefore, there is nothing left for you to do but to stay well. Now this is serious writing. It's not meant as a joke and it's not to be treated lightly. Those who eat right and live right stay healthy – those who eat conventionally get conventional diseases and die at the conventional time . . . before their time.

CHAPTER

51

WE TAKE A CLOSE LOOK AT SICKNESS

Sickness . . . what is it?

There are various terms by which one can describe sickness . . . ill health, disease, body malfunction, a morbid condition of the body resulting from disturbance of physiological functions, abnormal state of the body interfering with the functions of one of its organs or systems, departure from functions or integrity of the living organism, failure in normal physiological actions, a seriously abnormal state of the body, a physical derangement.

No doubt we could find another one hundred words and phrases to describe sickness but this is ample, I think, for our purpose.

This is all right as far as dictionary terms are concerned but I

325

am more interested at this time in finding out what sickness is all about and for the sake of this discussion we'll deal with you and me.

O.K., I'm sick . . . I don't feel so good . . . I realize something is wrong with me and I know I must do something about it. The first thing I ask myself is, "What have I done to make myself sick?" Unlike you, I don't say, "Some malevolent creature — be it a deity, enemies or as the ancients used to believe, an evil spirit — is seeking my downfall and therefore is making me sick." Believe it or not, most people believe that to this day, except they don't say it the way I have said it. They blame it on ill luck, the fates or upon everything and everybody but themselves, where the blame really belongs.

However, it's my problem this time and I say, "Tobe, old crock, what have you done to bring this condition about?"

I answer myself, saying, "I really don't know what I'm looking for but realizing I am to blame I must find out what I did".

Then I start going back step by step and in most cases I can pin down the culprit and it is practically always something I should not have done or something I should have done and didn't do.

One of the first things we must recognize if we are going to accomplish anything in this discussion of sickness is that sickness is, in the main, remedial to the body and not an attempt to do harm to the body. Here and now you must get this straightened away in your mind. Probably in the olden days they believed that it was something or somebody trying to get rid of the body or do it harm. But I think we can rest safely and securely on the premise that sickness is basically remedial . . . that is, the body is trying to do something to rid itself of the problem or the trouble and regain health.

The body has many remedial actions and functions at its disposal. The simple ones that we know of are disgorging the stomach contents through the mouth (vomit); or eliminating unwanted substances through the pores of the skin (sweating); excreting them through the bladder (urination); by means of frequent watery bowel movements (Diarrhea); or a runny nose, coughing, spitting and high temperatures (a cold). In these actions the body seeks to eliminate the materials that are causing the umbrage. Thus we see that the human body is trying to correct the condition and restore you to health again.

Then how do we look upon a condition like arthritis where parts of your bones or such calcify and you become crippled? What's curative about that? In all instances you have received frequent warnings through pain, aches and stiffness and this was clear evidence that your body cannot properly metabolize the cooked food you are eating and you should immediately switch over to a raw vegetable, grain and fruit regimen.

Take a heart attack, for example. All of a sudden you find yourself out cold or worse, in agony and unable to do anything for yourself but lie there like a mummy. What's remedial about that? No one ever gets a heart attack out of a clear blue sky. There were headaches, pounding in the head, tightening in the head, shortage of breath, loss of energy and a hundred other warnings for which you took aspirin or other medication. Besides, few first heart attacks are fatal, so a quick change to proper diet and living habits can almost without fail eliminate heart disease as a future cause of death.

Then again, what's remedial about cancer? Stomach cancer, for example? Somehow I can't conceive of a man in good health until he is 80 suddenly getting a pain and finding that he has cancer. My knowledge about the functions of the human body tells me that this just doesn't happen in this way. You probably had ulcers or colitis or some other pains and aches and warnings and malfunctions for years . . . yes, probably from five to twenty or more years . . . and you thought it was dyspepsia, stomach distress, gas or some hard to digest food you ate. So you ignored the remedial processes and didn't act until the final blow fell.

However, there is no doubt about it that the body does try to warn you of serious harm being done to it. The common cold is the best example on earth of the body's desire to help you regain your health. I had my share of colds when I was young but in the past 15 years I doubt if I've had more than a couple of colds in that period . . . and none of them has been anything but slight. But a cold can be positively recognized as remedial.

For years I have outlined what I call the prescription for a cold . . . smoking, drinking, carousing, burning the candle at both ends, bad food (and I don't mean poisoned food but mostly processed food that is lacking in proper nutrients), lack of sleep, exposure, a heavy salt intake, heavy feeding on refined carbohydrates. Today it is a positive fact that we do not catch a cold but clearly earn one and most of the aforementioned abuses are involved.

True, I have never known an experiment to be conducted along the line that I'm going to mention but I'd be willing to wager any one the sum of $1000 that more smokers have colds than non-smokers, more liquor drinkers have colds than non-liquor drinkers, more coffee drinkers have colds than non-coffee drinkers, and I could go down the line quite a bit further but I'm quite sure that you will get my point quickly.

It is known that the average individual, when he gets sick, reaches for some aspirin or some other cureall or drug. That has never been my way or attitude. I always ask myself, "What have you done wrong? What have you eaten that you shouldn't have eaten? What have you drunk that you shouldn't have drunk?"

Through my lifetime most of the colds that I suffered from were due to lack of sleep. I used to try to kid myself and make myself believe that it was because I worked so hard but I knew then and I know even better now that that was not the cause of my trouble. If I didn't get enough sleep, it was usually due to the fact that I was trying to have too much fun and wasting time whereas I should have been tending to business and then when I had my commitments to meet I overworked and worked long hours and I just didn't get enough sleep. Of course, it was due to my own errors and omissions, but I do know that lack of sleep and overindulgences have been the cause of most of my colds or minor ailments.

I am also convinced that those are the causes of most colds and minor sicknesses that afflict younger people. The older people are usually wiser and don't abuse their bodies and try to get by without sufficient sleep. Besides, they have much fewer demands made upon their time and therefore they don't lose their sleep. However, it must be recognized that when older folks get a cold or feel out of sorts it is mainly due to their poor diet and smoking, alcohol or too much coffee or tea.

If any of you are so naive as to believe that you can catch a cold, I want to positively state that you never catch a cold . . . you always deserve it. I know that I never had a cold that I didn't earn, and neither did you.

Because the cold is the world's most common ailment, it is the easiest one to pin down. Of course, it's also the condition for which there are the most drugs, medicines and cures offered. Any person who is so stupid as to seek medication for a cold does not merit consideration for being a sane, sensible human being. Any man who would medicate himself for a cold must recognize that he is actually impeding his body in the process of helping to make him well. In other words, the body has the cold to fight and now you're adding the extra burden of the harmful drugs which it has to get rid of as well.

Normally a cold has a regular course to run and as an old, old family physician told me, "A cold runs its cycle in about 14 days and if you use drugs it gets better in about 2 weeks or longer." But today colds seem to hang on and on and on. Now you may be puzzled at this but to me it's very, very simple and the reason is this. You are getting a new cold before the old one has run its course. Therefore it seems to run continuously. No, I am not fooling you, this is my simple explanation of why colds drag on so long. The body is expelling the toxic materials but you keep adding them as quickly as the body throws them out and you're too stupid to recognize what is happening.

329

Disease to me is a cause and effect procedure. Remove the cause and the disease or the effect will disappear.

One of the simplest ways to prove or disprove my simple theory is to stop eating solid food of any kind the minute you get a cold. Drink lots of natural water but never fluoridated water. Take only fresh juices made by your own hands . . . carrot, apple, turnip, celery, beet or any other fresh fruit or vegetable juice. Stay on this a few days and the condition will disappear. Of course, there is to be no smoking and no coffee or liquor drinking. If this doesn't lick your cold, bring it to me and I'll take it and wear it around my neck.

I challenge you to try my system of breaking a cold!

CHAPTER

52

WHO IS TO BLAME?

We could easily lay the blame right on the back of God, the Lord, Jehovah, the Creator and that would end it there. He's loused us up . . . we are sick, we are ailing, we are dying before our time. God is to blame. But you know and I know that that's just not true so let's deal with Dad and Mother. Well, I guess they are the ones who should be looked to.

Father isn't home enough to lay the blame on him. He's out making a buck — although the mothers are out making bucks today too — but still dad doesn't prepare the meals or put them on the table. That's mother's job . . . so mother, I guess you're it. You are the one who feeds us at the table, you are the one who does the shopping at the supermarkets. Therefore, if we are sick, if we are ailing mother is to blame. Who else? I don't think there is any question or doubt about it. The deplorable health of the people of

America, especially the children, today rests squarely on the shoulders of the mothers. Yes, I fully realize that mothers will not take this lightly. They will screech and scream and holler that I'm a despicable louse and worse and that I'm desecrating the holy name of motherhood but I'm willing to stand up and take the responsibility.

I say the mothers are to blame because they are the ones who put the food into our mouths or on the table. They are the ones who buy it and if the stuff is no good they shouldn't buy it and if they do have it and it is no good they shouldn't put it on the table. If decent food is ever to be served to our children or in our homes it will be the mothers who do it just as they are putting the horrible concoctions on the table now. They can plead innocence, they can plead ignorance, they can plead lack of guidance or any one of many excuses but that will not alter the fact nor will it cover their guilt. I'm not a judge and I'm not a jury but I attach a great deal of the blame on the mothers of America for the deplorable state of the health of the people of America today.

I have the pleasure and the privilege and sometimes the displeasure of watching what mothers put on the table. Most of the days of my life I watch what the mothers buy in the supermarkets and I'm telling you as straight as an arrow that I can't condemn them hard enough. Mothers today are the cause of the ill health and disease of the children of America. I'll repeat it a dozen times if necessary because it's true.

The government has proven itself to be responsible whether it be the Canadian or the American government. Both governments are corrupt, both governments are ridden with bribery and the information that the government agencies pass out about food and health consists of half truths, lies and downright falsification. Both governments and those processors who sell this food know the truth yet they still perpetrate this horrible outrage and the mothers accept it because it is convenient for them to accept it. There are mothers in America who feed their families properly but they are treated as outcasts because they do not go along with the conventional way of eating and feeding their families. There are some mothers in

332

America today who give birth the natural way without drugs. There are not many but there are still a few thousand on the American continent who do give birth in this way and who have given birth in this way. They have mighty healthy children to show for it and if they go to that much trouble most of them also go to the trouble of feeding their children right, starting off with breast feeding.

Most mothers today smoke, most mothers today drink alcoholic beverages besides tea and coffee and soda pop . . . all of which create sickness and prevent children from being healthy. It is just too much of a chore today for the mother to prepare decent food for her family. Why bother preparing when in the supermarkets you can buy all of the food and drink prepared and practically ready to eat? There is no doubt that the mothers will have some excuse and perhaps even a vestige of innocence in the matter. But what apology can the mother make for children who get sick and who acquire serious diseases and who are retarded and crippled when all of this is absolutely preventable? It doesn't have to happen. I cannot feel any remorse or sympathy in my heart for mothers who give birth to sick, to palsied, to retarded, crippled children when during pregnancy they smoked and drank and used drugs and didn't eat proper food to nourish their bodies and their offspring.

A child has a right to be born healthy and strong. It is a mother's duty to bring into the world only healthy offspring. It can be done if the mother has the strength and the courage and the decency to forego smoking and drinking and the use of contemptible, damnable foods that will prevent her from having a healthy normal child. Of course, today the normal child is a sick child suffering from any one or many diseases or conditions.

If a mother has a sick child, in 99% of the cases that child is sick because the mother allowed it to become sick or made it sick by the care she gave it. I fully realize that this will not endear me to the mothers of America but that doesn't worry me much. I only hope that this article will show them the error of their ways. Everything I say is proveable. In fact, no one will even bother challenging what I say because they know that what I have said is the truth even though it may hurt many mothers. Nevertheless, I hope perhaps it's still not too late, maybe their next child will be a natural healthy one.

Here is the old Mother song.

M is for the million things she gave me
O is only that she's growing old
T is for the tears she shed to save me
H is for her heart of purest gold
E is for the eyes with lovelight shining
R is for right and right she'll always be.
Put them all together, they spell MOTHER.
The word that means the WORLD TO ME.

Here is the modern version.

M is for the mucky guck she fed me.
O is only I won't live to grow old.
T is for Tit that could have saved me.
H is for the horrid food she was sold.
E is for my eyes with glasses cover'd.
R is for the raw food she didn't feed me.
Put them all together, they spell MOTHER.
The word that means Bad Health to me.

CHAPTER

53

IT COULDN'T BE NUTRITION

A friend dropped into the office to see me. Whenever he comes, which is most infrequently, we always have a chat that lasts half an hour or more.

Isn't it strange how loosely we use the word "friend"? I knew this man quite closely 45 long years ago — before I was married! I am now a grandfather with four grandchildren. For 30 years I had not seen him . . . until one day he dropped in at the nursery. He'd been receiving my Growing Flowers catalog and had read my name in the newspapers so he dropped in.

I had recognized him instantly in spite of those elapsed 30 years and we enjoyed our reminiscing about those good old days. He kept coming back about once a year. I would like to see more of him because he's a very fine man. He was when I first knew him and he is every bit as good today . . . handsome, understanding, intelligent and good humored — as you know, a wonderful combination in any individual.

Somehow we got to the subject of health, which is one of my pet interests, and in the course of the discussion I mentioned to him that it was my humble belief that nutrition was the cause and control of practically all diseases known to mankind.

"Don't be ridiculous!" he told me. "Food isn't that important in the life of mankind."

"You are dead wrong, friend," I responded. "From what I have seen, studied, learned and felt, food can directly or indirectly cause practically every disease known to mankind and correcting the diet can cure it."

"Poppycock!" he retorted vehemently.

"Inform yourself," I said to him. "Study and learn and you will find that what I say is absolutely true."

"Listen to me," he blurted out, as though he had had enough of this nonsense. "I'm going to give you a case right here and now to prove how ridiculous your theories are about nutrition and disease."

"Go ahead, friend. Shoot!" I commanded daringly.

"Let's be seated," he suggested . . . and we did.

"Just a short time ago my older brother developed a most serious and strange malady of the eyes. He went to one of the leading eye specialists in Toronto and he was told that he had an unusual disease of the eyes. My brother then told the doctor that our mother was also suffering from an eye derangement. She was taken to the same doctor and both were discovered to have the same disease. This disease, because it affected both mother and son, was so unusual that after considerable investigation, study and treatment the

336

doctor wrote a teatise on these two cases which was published in the Medical Association Journal and appears in the records. The eye specialist claimed it was a genuine clinical phenomenon.

"Now I am not sure — I did not make a record of the name he attached to the condition — but I believe it was 'paralytic strabismus'."

He stopped, as though to invite my remarks, but I said, "You're not finished. Go on. I'm listening."

"While individual cases of this malady are found in different parts of the world, never before have two cases been found in one family. It consists of a derangement of the eyes which causes them to focus and see only straight ahead. They can see neither above, below nor to the right or left . . . just as though they were wearing blinkers. The doctors have yet found no positive method or means of curing this trouble."

Here my friend stopped and looked straight at me contemptuously. "Now", he said, "show me where that's got anything to do with nutrition!" Then he snorted, "Pugh! What a theory! Boy, are you nuts!"

I sat for a moment thinking. His derision didn't bother me or phase me one iota. I'm so used to that in discussing problems with my friends that it's just like water off a duck's back. In fact, it sometimes tickles me a little bit or maybe actually pleases me.

Then I said, "You're married and don't live at home. How long since you lived with your brother and mother?"

"About 10 years," he said.

"Is your brother married?"

"No, he is a bachelor and lives with Mother and Dad."

"Tell me," I asked, "when you were home, do you recall anything about your brother's eating habits? Was there anything strange or unusual about them?"

"Naw, he just ate like everybody else, I guess."

"Come, come," I said, "Think a little closer and deeper. Wasn't there anything unusual that you noticed through the years of living with him — something that he liked or disliked or wouldn't touch or had to have?"

He stopped for a moment and by the look on his screwed up face I knew that something was going on within his head.

"By jove!" he snapped, "Come to think of it, Wes did have a lot of crazy notions about food. Holy smokes, now I remember that his likes and dislikes were most fixed."

"O.K. chum," I added, "Stop thinking about him for a moment. Tell me something else. How were your mother's eating habits?"

"Ah, I didn't pay much attention to what mother ate. In fact, I couldn't very well. But wait — now I remember. She used to encourage him in many of his prejudices and peculiarities about his food because she was like that herself. She said that she was glad someone in the family took after her."

He got up off his chair somewhat agitated, rubbed his forehead and began walking towards the front door. I heard him mumble, "Why in hell didn't that smart eye specialist think of that?"

That's the last I've seen of him He hasn't been back since. However the year isn't up yet.

CHAPTER

54

HEART ATTACKS ARE FOR CHUMPS

Any man who dies from a heart attack or any other cardiovascular or heart disease is a nutritional ignoramous. He could also be an informed man who has deliberately taken the calculated risk.

If you fear a heart attack I can tell you how to avoid one with 90% accuracy. I say this with the full realization and understanding of what I am saying, whether it be contrary to the government or to the medical association or to any group of scientists on earth. I still maintain that a heart attack is the easiest condition on earth to prevent and no man need have a heart attack, let alone die from one.

To begin with, the good old Bible tells you in no uncertain words how you can prevent a heart attack. In fact, if you followed that simple injunction of the Bible, in two places, you never could have a heart attack.

I have long maintained that you could take the average human heart and you could work or run or jump or exercise until you fell to your knees or were prostrate because of sheer exhaustion, yet your heart would never konk out on you.

As a matter of fact, up until 50 years ago men seldom ever had heart attacks. I'll tell you a few of the things we use now that bring on heart attacks: pasteurized milk, pasteurized butter, pasteurized cheese or any other pasteurized dairy products. Pasteurization is a cause of heart disease throughout the world today. In countries where pasteurization is not followed you will find very few cases of heart attacks, if any. Of course, wherever they heat or boil milk or dairy products, then heart attacks will be common again. But wherever milk or dairy products are used without pasteurization and without heating and without treating, they will not cause heart trouble.

The answer here is very simple and there is no mystery about it. Even a six year old could understand it. It is because the factor found in milk that prevents heart problems is destroyed in the heating process. That's why, when mothers feed their babies, they feed direct from the breast and the same goes for every other animal that exists on earth. None of them boil or heat the product before feeding it to their offspring.

The heat liable factor is lecithin. It is what would prevent the accumulation of cholesterol in your arteries or your blood and heat destroys its effectiveness and this permits the cholesterol to form and it is a cause of your trouble. Of course, your doctor will not agree with me but that's nothing . . . I probably don't agree with his antics either.

The body makes cholesterol but, let me tell you this, the kind of cholesterol that your body makes will not clog up your arteries and the body only makes cholesterol when it is needed, because cholesterol is definitely required by the human body.

Therefore, if you would avoid trouble with your heart, just avoid or cut drastically down on all forms of animal fat. This includes milk, cheese, cheese products, cream and all forms of dairy products, as well as meats containing a fair amount of fat or much fat, although all meat contains some fat and don't kid yourself that it doesn't, even the lean meats with the fat trimmed off. Organ meats also contain a lot of cholesterol, as do eggs. Now raw eggs will do you no harm but cooked eggs will cause or contribute to your trouble.

I contend that it is virtually impossible for a man who consumes no animal fats or margarine whatsoever to have a heart attack. I am fully aware of the fact that the medical profession advises the use of margarine but margarine is hydrogenated and hydrogenated fats are worse, much worse, than any animal fats and they will do you more harm than any of the animal fats. Again I say, I make this statement clear and to the point despite anything that the medical profession can say to the contrary. Yes, I am fully aware that most doctors advise the use of margarine and they also use it themselves. Well, I don't mind them using it themselves but they shouldn't advise their patients to use it. If they want to kill themselves that's their business but they shouldn't kill anybody else. And if you think I'm kidding, just examine the statistical records and you will learn that doctors are more prone to heart attacks than any segment of our society. Therefore, do not use margarine, any brand, any kind or any name. There is no good margarine.

Lest you run off with the idea that there are no other factors that affect your heart, I want to state that that would be giving you the wrong impression. Smoking will definitely harm your heart and so will a diet that is lacking in proper nutrients . . . natural oils, specifically alpha-tocopherol, or Vitamin E. Your heart can also be harmed by the use of white sugar. It is clearly demonstrated that white sugar can cause heart trouble.

But the danger of a heart attack, as it appears in our society

341

today, is mainly due to the heavy intake of animal fats in our diet, especially milk products that have been pasteurized.

CHAPTER

55

STRESS, HEART ATTACKS AND FARMERS

Some authorities would make us believe that stress is an important contributor to heart attacks. In fact, a famed Canadian specialist was one of the first to state that stress was the cause of, or the main contributor to, heart disease. Of course, that was 15 years ago. I notice that this respected high authority has learned the error of his ways and he does not stress the stress factor as much now.

On frequent occasions when someone I knew as a business man dropped dead of a heart attack the old story was thrown in that hard work killed him, that the stress of modern living and modern business and the pace of our existence in this modern age killed him. Through the years I've known virtually hundreds of men who dropped dead or died of a heart attack or heart disease and to be honest with you I don't recall one that worked very hard or was affected by stress. I would definitely state that most heart attack

343

victims neither work hard nor are they involved with stress factors. Hard work positively and emphatically does not cause heart attacks . . . in fact, to the contrary I maintain that those who do work hard physically and mentally seldom have heart attacks. It is those in sedentary occupations and who have the cushiest jobs and the ones with the least responsibility who die of heart attacks. Yes, frequently they are heavy drinkers and smokers.

For many years whenever someone I knew or was acquainted with had a heart attack I immediately investigated as closely as possible the individual's living habits and I can assure you that my research and findings seldom if ever indicated that the individual had a stressful life or did a lot of hard work. Farmers, for example, are living proof that hard work is not a factor or a cause of heart trouble. I contend that farmers are our healthiest and longest lived citizens and I give herewith what I believe to be the logical reasons.

(1) They work hard.

(2) They work long hours.

(3) Their work is invariably physical and involves a great deal of activity.

(4) Most farmers use, or did use, unpasteurized milk, butter and cream.

(5) The farmers usually eat fresher and better vegetables and fruits.

(6) The farmers seldom eat meat with diethylstilbestrol. If they have cattle they usually keep one animal around for butchering themselves and that animal is seldom if ever fed diethylstilbestrol which the other animals get.

(7) Farmers usually use chickens — and eggs from such chickens — that run on the range and are not cooped up like the chickens that other people buy and use.

344

(8) They breathe better, fresher and less polluted air.

(9) In most cases they drink unchlorinated and unfluorinated water.

(10) They generally go to bed early and get up early. They have their necessary quota of sleep.

(11) Their vegetables and fruits have the least of sprays. No doubt most of their vegetables have no sprays at all but the fruit that they sell is usually plastered.

(12) In my day and I think even to the present day farmers tend to can their own fruits and vegetables and do not as a rule buy the chemically treated, commercially canned goods.

(13) Their waste water and materials don't go into the sewer but back to the land.

(14) They would normally answer nature's call promptly and thus get rid of body wastes without delay.

(15) They say the farmer's work, like the housewife's work, is never done. Most farmers work six and seven days a week. If they have animals and they have chores to do then it means at least partial work for the whole seven days.

All of these factors tend to make the farmer live a more wholesome and a better life which adds years, good years to his life.

CHAPTER

56

SUGAR AND YOUR HEART

I regard good carbohydrates as the most important and vital food for man, over and above protein and fat. Not everyone will agree with me but that doesn't mean anything to me. However, sugar, in whatever form you want to consider it, is a mighty, mighty important food or so-called food, depending on how you look at it.

Now strange to relate, sugar isn't a very old commodity ... that is, it was in 1785 that the first reference was made to sugar cane as we know it. It was known in the middle ages as the Indian honey bearing reed. It was introduced in the 15th and 16th centuries by Spanish and Portuguese explorers, throughout the old and new worlds. It is, however, comparatively new to the world. But we know that man has always had a sweet tooth. Of course the Bible tells us that they used honey in those days. But somehow I have the feeling that the bees just wouldn't be able to make enough honey for the world if we didn't have other sources of sweetening.

Did you know that dates make good sugar sweetening ... among the best? All you have to do is dry them and grind them up and you've got a really good quality sugar. Of course it will always have a slight taste of dates.

I'm sure there are other forms of sugar but how they were used in the old days I would not know. The well known licorice plant has a high content of sugar and is used in syrups and medicines because of its sweet, unusual flavor. However, I am trying to convey that at the present time sugar is a very, very essential and important commodity in the diet of man.

There are two kinds of sugar in commerce generally. One is the sugar that we know best ... cane sugar. The other is beet sugar. Whether you believe it or not, when the two sugars come out of the refinery as a finished product there is no living man who can tell the difference between beet sugar and cane sugar. The only people who can tell the difference between cane sugar and beet sugar are some people who happen to be allergic to beets. Cane sugar doesn't do anything to them but beet sugar ... wow! It can almost kill them. Now this is not a fable – this is a fact – and any allergist can vouch for what I have said here.

Cane is harvested by cutting down the plant stalks. These are then pressed several times to extract the juice. The juice is concentrated by evaporation into dark sticky sugar. Much of this is sold locally.

Refined sugar, less nourishing as food, is obtained by precipitating out the non-sugar components ... leaving almost pure sucrose. This is the main commercial product.

By-products obtained from sugar cane include molasses, rum, alcohol, fuel, livestock feed and from the stalk residues, paper and wallboard.

Then there are the various kinds of refined or semi-refined sugars like raw sugar, brown sugar, yellow sugar, turbinado and clean-raw as well as white sugar, loaf sugar, icing sugar and fruit sugar. All of these come from the sugar cane plant, Saccharum officinarum, a member of the Grass family, with much similarity to our Sorghum and Corn plants.

I think we generally understand that white sugar is the least nutritious of all the sugars and sweeteners in existence but this does not include any coal tar derivatives like saccharin and the cyclamates which are not sugars . . . still plain white sugar is the most popular. The reason for its popularity is quite simple . . . it can be used in thousands of ways in sweetening to perfection without imparting any foreign flavor or flavor of its own. That is why it is so beloved by all of the food processors who use it.

However, white sugar, the most beloved of all the sugars, is still the most harmful of all so-called natural forms of sweetening. Saccharin and cyclamates are much worse but they are not sugars. Actually, I hate to attach the word "harmful" to something of which I am so fond but right now I am being very truthful. I want to tell you, folks, that sugar is a harmful substance. If you work backwards, the least refined of the sugars is the least harmful and the most refined is the most harmful.

Sugar is implicated in a number of ailments to which man is prone. The leading one is dental caries. It is positively established and accepted that it does destroy the teeth of mankind. And if you want any proof of this, go to England and Scotland and look at the people. Look at the kind of sugar and the amount of sugar they use and then look at their teeth.

Of course sugar is also a prime suspect in diabetes. Now you won't find very many diabetics who don't like sugar or sugar products, but that's not really very conclusive proof because everybody likes sugar. Anyway, sugar is implicated in many conditions.

349

At this moment I would like to mention something that is comparatively new — at least within the last ten years — and that is that sugar is seriously considered a factor in heart disease. Now I have read and read and re-read and inquired concerning the possibility of sugar being a factor in heart disease and I haven't been able to reach any positive conclusions. Dr. John Yudkin of London, who has been working on this angle for a number of years, claims with positive assurance and clinical evidence that sugar is a factor in heart disease. The more sugar you use, the more danger or risk you take of having heart disease.

Now this Dr. Yudkin has sort of gone out on a limb and stated most emphatically that sugar is more dangerous and a greater contributor to heart disease than fats. That's a rather strong statement. As yet I have reservations about accepting sugar as a contributor to heart disease as Dr. Yudkin claims but on the other hand, there are now researchers in Czechoslavakia who claim that they have substantiated Dr. Yudkin's findings and that sugar is definitely linked to heart disease.

Soviet investigators claim that excess carbohydrates are not only involved in diabetes but also in hardening of the arteries. This all adds up to substantially support Dr. Yudkin.

There are three groups of sugars (a) monosaccharides (b) disaccharides (c) trisaccharides.

The monosaccharides are the simplest sugars and include fructose and glucose. The disaccharides are formed by the union of two monosaccharides with the loss of one molecule of water. Disaccharides include lactose, maltose and sucrose. The trisaccharides are of little consequence to our needs and studies.

Dr. K. S. Petrovsky, a Russian researcher, claims that excess sugar, especially the refined saccharose, not only leads to fat deposits but disturbs the basic metabolic processes of the body, lowers the activity of essential microbes in the digestive system, decreases the body's synthesis of certain vitamins (including B-12), and raises the quantity of cholesterin in the blood. Yes, Dr. Petrovsky stresses that refined table sugar (used at the table or in prepared foods and drinks) is a major source of excess cholesterin . . . the factor blamed by many scientists for hardening of the arteries and resultant heart disease.

He further claims that the refined sugar remains in the blood stream for prolonged periods, which generally had not been the accepted concept. He goes on to state that we should use honey and recommends it strongly. Honey is very sweet and has a strong sweetening effect on other foods yet it contains a very small quantity of saccharose and much sugar in the form of fructose.

Dr. Petrovsky believes that one of the biggest benefits from eating sugars in fruits and vegetables comes with the so-called roughage (cellulose) they supply. Soviet research indicates that such food roughage definitely helps to lower the cholesterol level in the body. Besides that, the pectin factors in fruits are markedly beneficial to the digestive system.

So there you have it for what it's worth, folks. It looks as though, if you want to avoid heart trouble, along with other things you'd best avoid white sugar. Be smart . . . switch completely over to unpasteurized honey. Switch — avoid a heart attack, avoid diabetes and stay alive.

CHAPTER 57

NEW VIEW ON HEART DISEASE

I claim that I was one of the first people in America to recognize the harm and the danger of a heavy animal fat diet and its effects on the heart. Thirty-five years ago I warned of the danger. Yes, dating back to 1937 I warned that a heavy diet of animal fats contributed to heart disease.

This may surprise some people because I am not a healer of any sort nor am I a scientist but I am an observer and I am an inveterate, avid reader. Also, I am an inquirer.

Nothing yet has made me change my mind about the effect of animal fats on the heart. But in the past 25 years other factors have arisen and the heart disease cause situation is rather clouded or muddled. For instance, today we definitely do know that smoking contributes to heart disease. We also know that heavy coffee drinking

353

contributes to heart disease. Alcohol today is recognized as a contributor to heart disease. Then when you realize that drinking coffee and alcohol and smoking are indulged in by 99% of the population you can see what a crazy mixed-up situation it becomes.

Then, as mentioned earlier, along come some researchers who maintain most vociferously and emphatically that white sugar is a contributing factor to heart disease. It must be admitted that the animal fat theory is definitely not the only factor. It may be the most important, it may be the biggest contributor but it certainly is not the only cause.

The latest figures available, statistical figures up to 1970, reveal that 54% of all deaths in the United States were caused by heart disease. So if more than half of the deaths in the whole nation are due to heart disease then you can readily understand that more than one factor is involved. For some considerable time it was believed that stress was a factor. However, I'm quite certain that most of the authorities have been wisened up and realize that stress is not a factor, at least it's a very cogent factor.

It has also been recognized that the treatment of heart patients has been unwise, if not downright disastrous. Putting a heart patient into a wheelchair or confining him to bed and eliminating all effort and movement is no way to cure or improve a heart patient. I think the thing that a heart patient needs more than anything else on earth is a means of working off that build-up of cholesterol if cholesterol happens to be the factor.

There is a factor in heart disease that has never been given any consideration by scientists or the medical profession and I consider it a very, very important consideration. The example that I have cited is an ordinary garden hose. Let us assume that the ordinary garden hose is made to withstand pressure of 80 pounds per inch. If the pressure goes above the 80 pounds there is a strong likelihood that you are apt to burst the hose. And I'm sure most of you have seen or heard of a hose bursting because of pressure being too great. A hose can be manufactured to withstand any given amount of pressure, 100 pounds or more so when the hose bursts it is due either to too much pressure or the walls of the hose are too weak to withstand the given pressure.

Now the same principle applies to your arteries. Your arteries are normally built to withstand a pressure of say 120 over 80 but if that pressure is increased to 220 and in some cases it goes up even higher than that, then the arteries are subject to bursting — in medical science they call it a myocardial infarction. Therefore, if your blood pressure is high, either bring it down or strengthen your arterial walls so they can withstand that pressure. I suggest of course that you bring down your blood pressure. On the other hand if you have weak arterial walls or have allowed your arterial walls to deteriorate then even the nominal 120 pounds pressure could cause a rupture.

Rutin, a substance found in Buckwheat is definitely known to strengthen arterial walls. It is also found in abundance in Hungarian red peppers and lemon juice. Szent-Gyorgyi extracted it from these peppers and called it Vitamin P.

It is claimed that people who eat foods containing buckwheat as they do in many European countries have a very low incidence of hemorrhoids, varicose veins and heart disease all of which are due to either too much pressure or weakened arterial walls.

Rutin is a crystalline glucoside of quercetin which is closely related to hesperidin. It is mainly derived from buckwheat, especially the whole plant. It is known to be found in at least thirty eight specific plants of the vegetable kingdom.

Taber says it is used "to restore increased capillary fragility to normal, preventing vascular accidents in patients with hypertensions in various hemorrhagic conditions in which permeability, or capillary fragility is involved."

Here is a note of caution. If you are under the impression that by cutting down on the animal fat intake and substituting margarine for butter you are doing yourself a favor, I want to warn you definitely that the margarine can be as harmful or even more harmful to your heart and to a cholesterol build-up than butter. Margarine is not the unsaturated fat that you have been taught to believe it is. Margarine is, in practically all cases, hydrogenated and in the process of hydrogenation the unsaturated fats have been turned into plastic and they are much more harmful and deadly than the saturated fat. Besides, some saturated fats are essential for your health and well being. Please do not be deluded into believing that margarine is a food or that it is beneficial or that it is safe for your heart because these things are definitely not true . . . margarine is a killer. I cannot stress this too strongly.

CHAPTER
58

SURE REMEDY FOR BACKACHE

There's not much point in discussing or describing the pains and symptoms concerning backache. If you have suffered, or are suffering from backache I don't have to tell you what it is. And if you haven't suffered from backache then you won't know what I'm talking about.

Some people describe it as a sudden jolt, a sharp stab, twisting paralyzing agony, and the late President John F. Kennedy described it as "something like having a toothache."

They claim authoratatively that one out of 3 adult Americans is tormented by such pain every day of the year. With so many Americans suffering the agony of backache it is obvious that the healing professions reap a harvest.

Yet from my close investigations, studies, and experience, there is not one single thing they can do to help you. The medical men can give you drugs to partially drown your misery but neither medical men, orthopedic surgeons, or chiropractors, can move you one iota closer to a remedy. They can give you temporary relief and that is the best they can do.

The medical journals tell us that the principal victims of backache are those in their middle years and then they say, when muscle tone begins to weaken and the joints stiffen backache is the result. Still backache is no respector of age.

They claim that it afflicts those who bend too much or who slouch too much, or who sit too much, or reach too much. Medical men offer you their panacea, their cure-all, their magic aspirin as a means of relief. They also suggest bed rest. But they also admit that a sneeze can trigger another attack.

Of late the medical profession has started a new method of attack. They are performing surgery. The American Academy of Orthopedic Surgeons estimates that 2.5 million backs are permanently impaired and furthermore, each year back injuries to workers of America cost industry practically $1 billion.

Here are some further reasons that the medical profession gives for back troubles. They blame the muscles which keep you erect by supporting your spine. In the upright position gravity constantly pulls downward on the vertebrae of your S-shaped spine.

They go on to tell you that topmost are the 7 cervical vertebrae which control head, neck and upper back movements. Then they continue by saying there are 12 dorsal vertebrae to which the ribs are connected. Then below are the 5 lumbar vertebrae, which are most vulnerable to stress because they support the weight of the upper half of the body.

Here in the lumbo-sacral joint (sacroiliac) at the base of the spine is where most severe back pain originates.

One renowned orthopedic surgeon goes on to state "The most common cause is a combination of poor posture and obesity. The burden is just too much for the supporting abdominal muscles and too much strain is thrown on the spine." He suggests that bending over without bending your knees is another way to trigger backache.

Many housewives get a terrific jolt in the back just from leaning over to dust the table, he tells us. So do a lot of young mothers who bend to pick up a child over and over again. The strain may be too much for their muscles. It is a matter of leverage. Unless the knees are bent in a squatting position, the back has to do all the bending with your vulnerable sacroiliac acting as a fulcrum.

Another famous doctor tells us that after a 5 year study of 93 mothers aged 18 to 23, who had persistent back pain following child-birth, a typical mother experienced pain not only when she lifted the baby but when she carried heavy objects or performed routine household chores.

There was also pain after sexual intercourse. Examinations disclosed that these mothers had poorly developed abdominal muscles as a result of physical inactivity since childhood. They had never ridden a bicycle, they rarely danced, swam, bowled, skated, golfed, or engaged in any regular exercise through school years or since marriage.

Another famous doctor tells us 90% of all back pain comes from stress at one or more of 4 pain sensitive areas in the musculoskeletal system. These four areas are known as facets, the nerve roots, the dura mater, and the posterior longitudinal ligament.

Then he goes on — when the spine is overstrained one of these vertebrae can be dislodged. The resultant pain is agonizing. This is the familiar "crick in the back," or "subluxation".

The highly sensitive nerve roots are in proximity to the flat little discs of fiber and cartilage that separate adjacent vertebrae. The discs contain a spongy, gelatin-like substance that helps them to act

359

as shock absorbers. But heavy lifting, bending or jumping, may crack the protective covering. Thereby the spongy substance oozes out and presses on a nearby nerve root, causing sharp pain that radiates down one leg. This refers to the classic symptom of a slipped or herniated disc. Sciatica occurs when the sciatic nerve is affected.

Other renowned surgeons and physicians go on to tell us "for a person to have one leg from a quarter inch to an inch longer than the other is not unusual."

President Kennedy used to have a special woman physician to look after his back. And this physician pointed out to him that his trouble was due to the fact that he spent many hours walking along the sand when he was vacationing in Florida and was putting a strain on his back by the sloped surface of the beach. Corrective shoes were prescribed for the President.

Women after menopause frequently develop microscopic fractures that do not show up on X rays and osteoporosis or fragile bones. These conditions are linked to hormonal imbalance and the menopausal woman may need minerals as well as estrogen to obtain relief.

Further, we learn from the medical men that 9 out of 10 backaches respond to simple treatments including such home remedies as aspirin, hot baths and bed rest. Medical therapy may range from local injections of analgesics to immobilization of the spine by the use of pelvic traction, along with exercise both in and out of traction. Sometimes a leather brace is prescribed for men or a special corset for women as a temporary support for strained muslces.

Then they go on to tell us that "medicine has worked many miracles but it has not yet come up with one for an ailing back."

Please forgive me for taking you through this maze of references to backs and back disorders but I had a very special motive in taking you through all of this. And the lesson learned will thus stay with you for the rest of your days.

I suffered with back trouble for more than 40 years of my life and I know, better than anyone else, just how serious backaches can be, but I also found the solution and it's a solution that the poor medical men, who have worked miracles, have been unable to find. What's more — they never will find it, nor will they recommend my method, which is 95%, at least, effective, because they don't want to lose that much business.

My method will not even be recommended by chiropractors for exactly the same reason.

Now I'm sure that the thought racing through your mind at the present moment is this — how could one individual layman, who is not trained in medicine or in chiropractic or in healing, find a solution that has plagued mankind since time immemorial and is plaguing millions of people daily throughout the world?

Well I can't answer that question for you. But the fact is that I have found a solution and it is so simple that mankind has passed over it because of its simplicity. I tell the whole story in detail in my book on the subject but I'll tell you here and now all you need to know. So be prepared for a shock. Here is the denoument.

As soon as backache strikes, eliminate wheat from your diet, whether it be in the form of cakes, bread, biscuits, crackers, pizza, or any one of a 100 other forms in which wheat is found. This means noodles, spaghetti, and macaroni as well.

To be absolutely safe, go on to a raw vegetable diet for 5 days and your back troubles will clear up like magic. I give you my word of honour that this will work in better than 95% of all the cases of backache.

Yes, I realize that you are wondering how this can be true. But true it is nevertheless. I recall a nephew of mine who was suffering the agonizing pain of backache and I told him to lay off wheat and he looked at me in utter disbelief and said to me, "Uncle, my spine feels as though it were made out of jelly. How can bread or

361

wheat have anything to do with that?" Well, I could explain that, too.

It's a long story, but the fact still remains that that jellylike spine will regain its normal rigidity in less than 5 days if you lay off any form of wheat.

Through the years I have received hundreds of letters from people who have told me that this method has worked, that it has given them comfort for the first time in many long years. I've had friends and other people who have followed my advice come to me to thank me personally. I also want to tell you this that I have never known my suggestion to fail, if it is followed.

So if you are suffering from backache, no matter how skeptical you are, no matter whether you distrust me or disbelieve me, just try it and be relieved.

I admit that I found it very difficult to remove bread from my diet, especially the good dark homemade bread. I occasionally indulge and I find that as soon as I start to eat any quantity of bread my legs begin to stiffen and if I maintain bread eating my back troubles begin.

More than 12 years have passed since I discovered the cause of my trouble and I've never had any serious backache since that day. But if I go on a bread eating binge, in a few days I get a few warning shots of pain and I immediately desist.

Don't pass up this remedy for your backache because it is too simple.

CHAPTER
59

ARTHRITIS

If you have any form of Arthritis read this chapter carefully in its entirety. You are presented with two approaches ... that of The Arthritis Foundation and the approach of John H. Tobe.

First I will quote from a bulletin put out by The Arthritis Foundation entitled "The Truth About Diet And Arthritis".

The truth about diet and arthritis may surprise you. It is simply this: There is NO special diet for arthritis. No specific food has anything to do with causing it and no specific diet will cure it.

Well-meaning friends may tell you otherwise. Food fanatics and peddlers of "health and nature" foods and self-styled "experts" who write books praising their miracle "discoveries" about food and arthritis are more interested in their personal profit than they are in

363

your health. Don't let them convince you.

The fact is, the possibility that some dietary factor either causes or can help control arthritis has been thoroughly and scientifically investigated and disproved. The only exceptions are in gout and when adjustments in a normal diet need to be made for an arthritis patient with an individual problem, such as overweight. These are explained below.

The proper diet for an arthritis patient is a normal, well-balanced nourishing diet. Good nutrition is essential for good health whether you have arthritis or not; and it is even more important that you eat well-rounded, adequate meals regularly when your body must resist and fight off the ravages of a disease like arthritis.

There are many sources of reliable information on good nutrition. **If in doubt, call upon your local chapter of The Arthritis Foundation.**

Weight — Overweight. People with arthritis tend not to move around very much and may become overweight. This can put a burden on arthritic joints, increasing the inflammation and the pain. If you need a reducing diet, your doctor can advise you.

Underweight. Arthritis sometimes can make you rundown and underweight, leading to fatigue and lowered resistance. You may need extra nourishment, more high calorie foods. Let your doctor tell you what to do.

Gout: Gout is a special kind of arthritis, caused by an inherited defect in body chemistry, not by "high living." However, overeating and overindulgence in alcohol can trigger attacks in some patients who already have gout. Doctors recommend not drinking beer and not eating such foods as kidney, liver and sweetbreads. With new drugs, gout can be well controlled today.

NUTRITION NONSENSE

A great deal that you hear and see advertised about special food products for arthritis is outright quackery. It is fantastically profitable for the sellers. For you, the arthritis sufferer, it leads to false hope and wasting of your money. So don't be lured into treating yourself. Arthritis experts do have an answer for you.

Arthritis pain now can be controlled and crippling prevented by prompt and proper treatment. See a qualified physician.

Here is another pamphlet issued by the same Arthritis Foundation entitled "The Truth About Aspirin For Arthritis".

SHOULD YOU SEE A DOCTOR, AND IF SO, WHY?

"Yes, because only he can answer these important questions: Do you actually have arthritis? If you do, which kind is it? (There are many forms.) Should you take aspirin for it? (Maybe you are one of the few people who can't tolerate it.) How much should you take? (Maybe you can't take as much as someone else without having side effects.) What else should you do for your arthritis besides taking aspirin? (To control arthritis and prevent disability, medication is only part of a total treatment program which needs to be prescribed and supervised by a qualified doctor.)

WHAT ASPIRIN CAN DO FOR ARTHRITIS

Aspirin is a truly remarkable drug. It was originally developed years ago specifically for rheumatoid arthritis — the kind which makes people sickest and causes the most pain and crippling. Aspirin relieves pain — but it does much more than that. It also reduces inflammation — and inflammation is what does all the damage in joints and what causes the swelling and stiffness and pain. When taken properly, aspirin helps arthritis victims feel better, move around better, function better, do treatment exercises better. It doesn't just relieve the symptoms, it treats them.

HOW MUCH, HOW OFTEN? — YOUR ASPIRIN PROGRAM

You are an individual, not quite like anyone else. Your arthritis is not quite like anyone else's arthritis. How much aspirin you need for your disease, and how much you can tolerate, is for a qualified physician to decide. You make a serious mistake when you act as your own doctor and try to figure out your own dosage schedule.

For severe rheumatoid arthritis, the doctor usually prescribes as much aspirin per day as the individual patient can tolerate. You should have your aspirin-taking program . . . to be kept up day in and day out even when you are feeling better. If you skip taking it on schedule when your pain subsides — the way you would when a headache has gone away — you lose the full anti-inflammatory effect. Steady dosage is what keeps inflammation under control. So keep in touch with your doctor; if your program of medication, rest and exercises should be changed, let him be the one to decide, not you.

SIDE EFFECTS

Overdoses of aspirin cause ringing in the ears and slight deafness. These symptoms go away when the dosage is reduced. And some people can't or shouldn't take aspirin at all because it upsets their stomachs or because they are allergic to it or because they have certain conditions — like peptic ulcers, for example — which might be made worse. If you can't take aspirin, there are several other drugs effective in arthritis which your doctor can prescribe instead.

Just remember that aspirin is safe for most people, but for the rare few it can be bad. Don't let advertisements tell you how to treat yourself with aspirin. Play it safe. Find out about you and your arthritis from a qualified doctor.

WHAT BRAND?

If your aspirin program calls for ten or more five-grain tablets a day, the cost can really add up. If you don't want to spend more than you have to, you should know that highly advertised brands *(especially those with added ingredients) are the most expensive. Plain aspirin is what helps your arthritis. Many unadvertised brands of plain aspirin do the job just as well and cost far less.*

The least expensive way to buy plain aspirin effective for arthritis is in bottles of 1,000 tablets. Ask your doctor for advice.

Have you seen ads or commercials for buffered aspirin, liquid aspirin, coated aspirin and time-release aspirin? Maybe one is just right for you, but don't let advertising tempt you into trial-and-error self-medication. Again your doctor is the one to decide.

ASPIRIN ADVERTISING

Aspirin is big, big business. Millions of dollars are poured into aspirin advertising each year. More and more of it is being aimed at arthritis sufferers because they are big aspirin buyers.

The Arthritis Foundation says that aspirin itself is good for arthritis but a lot of aspirin-for-arthritis advertising is bad.

There you have the whole story as told by the Arthritis Foundation. Now listen to what I have to say.

It is claimed by reliable sources that in America 17 million people suffer pain, the anguish and the woes of arthritis. It has long been established by the medical profession and the Arthritis Foundation that there is no cure or help for arthritis except aspirin.

In reply I ask, "How can people tell such horrible lies? How can an organization like the Arthritis Foundation condemn 17 million people to a life of agony when it is absolutely unnecessary?"

Please believe me, you don't have to continue suffering if you have arthritis. No, I admit there is no cure for arthritis anymore than there is a cure for cancer or a cure for heart disease or a cure for diabetes, Yet, I seriously claim that each and every one of these

367

diseases can be conquered and your body can be rid of it.

Perhaps I am just playing with semantics. Perhaps I should be saying to you directly and clearly that cancer, arthritis, diabetes and heart disease can be cured. That they are being cured and that they have been cured. Undoubtedly, there are tens of thousands who can swear and attest to the fact. Still I stand forthrightly and say there is no cure.

To me the word cure means taking a drug or a medicine, a concoction, or a pill, and presto . . . the affliction disappears like magic. I say there are no cures. I say again, that these conditions can be corrected in spite of what the American Medical Association and the Arthritis Society tell you.

The process of causing arthritis to disappear is a simple one . . . in fact, to cause practically any disease known to man to disappear the same method is used. Because here we are dealing with the lives of 17 million people and their suffering we must omit the play on semantics and get down to cases.

There is no arthritic who lives in America today who cannot materially help himself to ease and remove the pain and improve his condition by a beneficial change of diet to raw vegetables, grains and fruits. This change of diet can remedy arthritis and does not fail.

From what I read and from what I am told, arthritic sufferers undergo greater pain and agony than those who suffer from any other disease. One of the few or many things that I cannot stand is to see human beings suffering. And it's even worse in this instance because they don't need to suffer. Still the medical profession maintains that diet has no effect on the disease. At least they have been telling themselves and the world this since the profession started back in Hippocrates time.

I heard it when I was a young boy and I hear it today, although their voices have been somewhat softened. To be truthful I must admit that some doctors today even recognize that some

368

diseases are involved with nutrition.

About 10 years ago Dr. Jarvis wrote a book called Folk-Medicine, which has sold, I believe, more than 20 editions and if I'm not mistaken it is still selling by the hundreds of thousands in paperback form.

In this he told how thousands got rid of their arthritis by the simple expedient of a mixture of cider vinegar and honey. Even though the medical profession didn't like it, even though the government tried to intervene and impede the sale of the book, they could not stop it.

Many nasty things are said by the medical profession of Dr. Jarvis but he was a reputable physician, a member in good standing of all the associations and they were powerless in their attempt to discredit him. I'm not standing before you to defend Dr. Jarvis or his cider vinegar and honey. But obviously, it was most effective.

And I give the simple reason why it was effective. Because in most of the cases where Dr. Jarvis used it, it was unpasteurized cider vinegar and it was unpasteurized honey and it was effective because it was probably the only raw unprocessed food that these people ingested.

William S. Clark, M.D. national president of the Arthritis Foundation says "As far as is known today, no single food or combination of foods causes arthritis, nor can any food or combination of foods cure it." Dr. Clark goes on to state this medical statement will shock many sufferers, those, for example who believe that eating meat causes an acid that triggers arthritis. Or that drinking special hard teas, or eating honey and vinegar, will cure them.

Now, if you know anyone who has arthritis, tell him that a raw food diet will be of great help to him and will in due course, if the disease has not advanced too far, probably clear up the condition. He doesn't need to see a doctor. He doesn't need to consult any healer. He doesn't have to consult the Arthritis Foundation. All he

369

has to do is go on a raw food diet, including regular daily quantities of fresh vegetable and fruit juices.

While normally I do not advocate the use of juices, where depletion has taken place over a period of many years, concentrated quantities of these deficiencies can be utilized with excellent results and that is where the fresh vegetable and fruit juices play an important role.

It will take some weeks before even slight progress is made. But progress will take place and after a few months the improvement will be clearly noticed and from there on you get better, you have less pain, you are able to make better use of your limbs, slowly but surely. As you continue your diet the improvement goes on and on and on.

The medical profession has taken other retrograde steps by announcing surgery for arthritis. Oh yes, they also recommend the gold treatment. It's gold in more ways than one. I understand each gold treatment gains a physician $100.

I don't have to say that gold injections harm a patient but a raw food diet is much better. It costs less and there is absolutely no risk involved. The only thing that can happen is that a person who follows the diet will get well.

So don't believe the American Medical Association, your individual doctor or the Arthritis Foundation when they tell you that no food can cause or cure arthritis because they are telling you a deliberate lie.

Of course you want to know why the medical association and the Arthritis Foundation take this stand. Well, it's the same story that exists in a thousand and one other instances. The golden calf is here involved. The doctor gets paid for his services even though he brings you no good and often does you harm. The Arthritis Foundation has everything in the world to gain by seeing that there is no cure ever found for arthritis because the moment a cure is found, they will be snuffed out of existence.

Now I'm not making any insinuations, not making any charges. I'm relating the story as I see it. I have with my own eyes watched and noticed and observed through the years hundreds of people show improvement and get well after a serious bout with arthritis because they changed to a raw food diet.

Do you believe the Arthritis Foundation when they say arthritis cannot be cured?

You can see that this organization sells more aspirins than all the advertising the aspirin people can do for themselves. They would make you believe that arthritis is caused by a deficiency of aspirin in your body so you are supposed to add aspirin to your diet to correct that condition. They tell you "Aspirin is truly a remarkable drug". I'm telling you that it is a positive poison and causes and contributes to many diseases including deafness, stomach hemorrhage, ulcers and many other conditions. Yet they tell you, "Just remember, that aspirin is safe for most people". They recommend that you go to your doctor to find out how to use aspirin. Can you think of anything more ridiculous than that statement? Pay a doctor or a medical specialist a fat fee to prescribe aspirin . . . a poison!

We note also, "The Arthritis Foundation says that aspirin itself is good for arthritis". They tell you also that a proper diet for an arthritis patient is a normal, well-balanced, nourishing diet but nowhere do they tell you what a normal, well-balanced, nourishing diet is. Reason? They don't know what it is and therefore they can't tell you. They only know how to perpetrate themselves in a well paying enterprise besides gaining support and probably financial assistance from the drug corporations.

Note also, "Nutritional Nonsense: A great deal that you hear and see advertised about special food products for arthritis is outright quackery. It is fantastically profitable for the sellers." But they do not tell you that their foundation is far more fantastically profitable because they give you nothing for the money you give them and they probably get paid from the chemical or drug companies as well.

The best way to prove once and for all whether or not they speak the truth or I speak the truth is for an arthritic sufferer to test the 100% raw food diet.

I do not have any product to sell . . . only truth to tell.

CHAPTER

60

DIABETICS ARE MADE NOT BORN

There are a lot of diabetics throughout the world but I guess most of them are in America.

From records that I have seen and been able to get, it would appear that diabetes affects more Americans, at least people living in the Northern Hemisphere, than any other part of the world. I've given considerable thought and analysis to diabetes and diabetics. Actually, I am more interested in the diabetics than in the disease or condition itself.

I have had a goodly number of my family, relatives and friends who were affected and stricken with the disease, and thus I have felt that it bears some study. For some years now I have stoutly maintained that when a boy or man before marriage became a diabetic, he was made a diabetic by his mother. I repeat that he

373

didn't become a diabetic by accident but was made a diabetic by his mother. Then, if a man became a diabetic after marriage he therefore became a diabetic because his wife made him into one.

You will probably censure me for being so harsh on mothers and wives, but I will stand my ground and maintain that what I say is true . . . and proof and research will bear me out.

But now I've come up with something different on diabetics. I contend that a diabetic is a human-being of a certain specific state of mind. In other words, there are people who become diabetics and there are those who would never become diabetics, not because of their physical build-up, but because of their character and mentality.

For example, I know two brothers. By the treatment afforded them by their wives both of them should have or could have become diabetics. The true story is that one became a diabetic and the other did not and I doubt if he ever will be one. I contend that this is solely because of the different mental make-up of the two brothers.

I am trying to explain or illustrate that an individual by the things he rejects or accepts mentally, does or does not become a diabetic.

Here I stretch my neck way, way out. I contend that diabetes, like all other diseases but just a little more so, is a disease of ignorance. Please hold your fire a moment. This ignorance is not necessarily on the part of the person who becomes a diabetic but upon those responsible for his upbringing and feeding. I can't think of any disease in the world that I can label an ignorant disease more than diabetes and I'll pin it down in this clear-cut manner. People who think that health is found in eating much rich, cooked, seasoned, highly refined food and have the responsibility of preparing it for their families are the ones to whom I refer.

Here I want to state that a person can become a diabetic himself or herself, even without the aid of his father or mother or wife or husband, but again it is the make-up of their character that permits this.

Two children may have the same mother and be given the same food, yet one becomes a diabetic and the other remains normal and healthy. How does this come about? Well, I'll tell you. One probably had a revulsion for some of the food being given or forced upon him, while the other one either liked it or accepted it. You know only too well that there are those of us who can sit down with a pound box of candy and eat every one of them without feeling a twinge of remorse or over-indulgence, yet another will eat one, two and perhaps three and then call it quits, because he feels he has had enough of that good, luscious, delicious, rich food.

From my actual observations, discussions and searchings, I have come up with the conviction that diabetics as a rule would rank probably a little higher on the I.Q. level than non-diabetics. You may wonder again why I would call diabetes a disease of ignorance when the I.Q. of those afflicted was higher than the average. I would even go further and say that diabetics, before they became diabetics, were probably the most energetic people with more drive, push and ambition than the average.

What I am trying to say is that there is a sort of diabetic character or make-up. Then I could go on record as stating that a diabetic lacks self control or perhaps a better word would be self denial. He may have complete control over his temper or emotions, but he lacks it when an extra drink is offered him or an extra serving of a delicious, appetizing food.

The people who say, "Oh, to hell with it all, I have enough worry and trouble and concern, and I work hard enough, I can afford to have this little extra of something I like". I suggest . . . those are the folks who are destined to become diabetics.

The man or the woman who can't say "I won't eat this, I won't eat that; I'll have half as much of this or half as much of that or none of this and lots of that," and mean every word of it, is apt to wind up a diabetic.

That does not necessarily mean that diabetics lack strong will or will power. This would only affect them or bother them when it came to their own sweet selves. It might not at all affect them in their relationship and dealings with others.

I would like at this time to challenge the concept that diabetes is hereditary. The only connection that diabetes might have with heredity is the fact that food habits, food likes and dislikes may be passed along from parent to children and also among the members of one's family. But that is purely environmental and has nothing whatsoever to do with heredity.

Men or women who would normally become diabetics can be prevented from doing so by a strong partner — husband or wife — who by a rigid regime of food control can prevent one who might normally become a diabetic from being one; or by the one partner exercising a firm guiding hand, a combination of control, sagacity, kindness and reason. I was a witness to such an experiment and can attest that a diabetes-prone person can be saved or spared by a partner, guided with kindness and reason.

This might not work out if the husband who is susceptible has a good share of his meals out or is a traveller. Then, of course, he could give free rein to his choice and his weaknesses, whereas if he were home his wife could control his diet and prevent his becoming a diabetic.

From what I have seen, and I have seen many, I know that diabetics are difficult to control in their dietary habits.

I do not have any records to indicate or prove the point I wish to make at this time . . . that is that diabetics are noted for their refusal or inability to take instructions and follow a safe regime. I understand that many of the diabetic specialists put their patients into the hospital where they can be under supervision and that is the only way that their diet can be controlled. Any person who has had experience along these lines would quickly recognize whether I speak the truth or not.

I have run down the list of all the diabetics that I have known more or less closely or intimately and I would say that this rule holds extremely close to the truth. There is not much sense in giving a diabetic a set of rules because he just won't follow them. He will follow those he wants to follow and that he can follow and which he finds convenient to follow, and the rest he completely ignores.

The common suspicion, or acceptance that diabetics are stout people who like rich foods is not necessarily true, but they usually follow along one of these lines . . . that is they like rich food, they like good food, they like cooked foods; they prefer enormous and often frequent servings. Another weakness is they have very marked preferences for certain foods and eat enormous quantities of these in proportion to all other foods, completely throwing their metabolism out of kilter. In this regard the individual may not even be a big eater. But let's say he likes bananas. Well, he will eat bananas to the exclusion of most other foods, and yet not have a big meal or consume much food.

People of the executive type seem prone to diabetes and the explanation given is that they assume so much responsibility that they feel they are entitled to allow themselves to indulge in a little bit of excess now and then or with a fair degree of regularity.

It probably may seem strange to anyone reading this treatise on diabetics that nowhere have I mentioned the cause, effects or symptoms of the disease, and to me that is quite irrelevant. I am dealing with the situation from the aspect of the individual and the individual's characteristics. Nor do I attempt to set myself up as an authority and point out the certain specific foods that cause diabetes, nor will I go on record as saying that over-indulgence in sugar, white bread, large quantities of salt and much rich foods are the sole cause of diabetes. Yet many diabetics I have known were great eaters or habitually ate fair or large quantities of these so-called foods.

While according to my beliefs and convictions, food and its misuse are the cause of diabetes, yet I make no attempt to pinpoint

377

the foods in question.

CHAPTER

61

MUSCULAR DYSTROPHY

Would you like to get muscular dystrophy? Of course not. But I think I have learned how you can get it in case you do want to get it. I'll discuss a fairly simple and direct method of acquiring this disease. Of course you realize that muscular dystrophy is not to be sneezed at.

Now I have mentioned on frequent occasions that I am not a healer of any kind and that I know nothing whatsoever about pathology. But this condition or disease usually comes under the heading of muscular atrophies, dystrophies and related disorders. Dystrophy is usually reserved for hereditary myopathies, characterized by progressive weakness. So probably you could get all of those three or more conditions if you follow the rules that I am going to give you here. So if you know of any young people who want to get the disease, pass this information along to them.

(1) Use cookware, pots and pans, that are made of aluminum. Pressure cookers made of aluminum will also do the trick.

(2) Be sure to drink lots of cola drinks and pop of all kinds, especially the ones with the artificial flavorings and artificial sweeteners.

(3) Eat lots of cheap chain-store ice cream ... is there any other kind?

(4) Eat mainly processed, cooked and preserved meats and cold cuts.

(5) Be sure to get your polio shots and be sure you are vaccinated. Get all the shots and inoculations that you can get. This is of great help in getting these diseases.

(6) Eat TV dinners regularly or as often as you can.

(7) Try to have your biscuits, cakes, buns and other baked goods made from quick mixes.

(8) Use largely frozen foods.

(9) Be careful to avoid fresh fruits and vegetables and always select the canned and preserved items.

(10) If by chance you do eat nuts, make sure they have been chemically treated and coated with the various chemical coatings. Be sure they have been kept exposed in those heated and lighted display cases.

(11) Be sure to eat lots of that attractive looking candy that is displayed and sold everywhere, containing loads of glucose, white sugar, coloring matter and artificial flavoring.

(12) Avoid exercise. Never run if you can walk. Never walk if you can remain still. Never stand if you can sit. Never sit if you can

lie down. And never get up if you can sleep.

Follow these instructions and then take all of the drugs that are recommended and it won't be too long before you will have a good chance of getting one of the dystrophies.

If anyone wants to rid himself of Muscular Dystrophy the simplest and most direct means is by following a raw food diet. I realize that what I say is hard to believe but it is still true . . . a well balanced raw food diet is the safest, surest way to overcome muscular dystrophy.

As of this writing, in Germany Dr. Jos. Evers, a qualified medical doctor in good standing, is helping hundreds of sufferers rid themselves of this dread wasting disease. Furthermore, he has been helping muscular dystrophy sufferers for many years.

CHAPTER

62

THE COMMON COLD

If I were to suggest that the common cold was a benefactor of mankind the idea would be ridiculed or thought preposterous but perhaps there is more truth in that statement than the average individual realizes. If you were about to walk into a trap unknowingly and someone shouted a warning which prevented you from being harmed or destroyed would you consider that warning a harm or benefit?

I am suggesting that the common cold is the body's reaction or warning to a wide build-up of abuses or neglects and the body is telling you to do something about it before serious harm results. In fact, a cold is the body's reaction to the onslaught of harmful factors and the body is struggling in every way possible to shake off the evils that seek to destroy it.

Within the past year there has been a great deal of publicity given to the Nobel prize winning scientist, Linus Pauling, and his stumping for vitamin C as a cure for the common cold. In fairness it must be stated that the beneficial effects of large doses of vitamin C to prevent or stop a cold have been known for at least 25 years and many people whom I know have been using vitamin C in large doses to successfully knock out a cold for many years but it is not as simple as it sounds. I admit that extra large doses of vitamin C will definitely knock out the cold symptoms. Now I did not say it will knock out the cold, I said it will knock out the cold symptoms but it may also be the means of creating something more serious in the future.

Warning signals are not sounded merely as a warning nor are they something to be avoided, they are actually sounded as advice and counsel for you to do something about it of a more permanent nature. However, most of us use the warning to sidestep the issue and think no more about it, whereas the intelligent person will do something about it so that the warning button will not have to be sounded so frequently or in vain.

I will not deny that the use of vitamin C does present various benefits, especially if vitamin C is used in its natural form and the reason that it is beneficial is because most people in America today do not get sufficient vitamin C in their diet and even those who do get it in sufficient quantities lose it through smoking, drinking and the consumption of drugs and devitalized food. Therefore, it is now realized that most people in America receive inadequate quantities of vitamin C in their diet.

I have studied the cold situation for many years and have reached the conclusion that when one has a cold it is usually due to one, many or all of the following . . . an inadequate intake of natural vitamin C in food; lack of sufficient sleep; overwork or overexertion; smoking; over-indulgence in drinking — be it alcohol in any form, tea, coffee or other beverages including soft drinks; lack of fresh, nutritious vegetables, grains and fruits; a drastic change in body temperature without protective clothing; too much salt in food

384

causing an overloading in the body; too much processed and fried food; or too many drugs. It is a positive fact that the common cold can be prevented by avoiding or correcting the conditions mentioned above.

The safest and sanest way to clear up a cold is to remove the causative factors and to add the essentials for our way of life and permit natural, normal bodily functions to take over. People who follow the way of life I advocate do not have colds or if it does happen it is indeed a rare occasion. For example, I have had only two colds in more than ten years.

I would also like to stress that the cold should be regarded as a warning and as a friend so that effective preventive measures can be taken to prevent more serious breakdowns or harm in the future.

CHAPTER

63

LET'S TALK ABOUT CONSTIPATION

It has long been held by the authorities and practitioners that taking laxatives for constipation creates more problems than it sets out to cure.

There is danger without a shadow of doubt in the use of laxatives. On the other hand, I also am acquainted with people fairly close to me who have been taking various laxatives for more than 50 years and are still in comparative good health. Among these people are some who have never had a normal bowel movement without the aid of a laxative since they were children. The laxatives that these people have taken run from the most common old fashioned type like senna leaves, castor oil, epsom salts, chocolate Exlax, prunes, figs, Milk of Magnesia, enemas and colonics to the common or various mixtures of herbal laxatives, pills and otherwise.

I know two men who are now in their mid 80's — one almost 90 — who have taken enemas regularly for at least 50 years. Now I am not telling you all this to convince you that enemas or laxatives are satisfactory or all right, I'm merely reciting facts about constipation.

I believe it was Sir William Arbuthnot Lane who was supposed to have said, "The principle cause of cancer is constipation or impaired elimination." It is claimed he also stated that never in any case of cancer did he find that constipation was not involved. Obviously Sir William Arbuthnot Lane felt that constipation was either one of the causes or the contributors to cancer.

Yet above I've cited cases known personally to me who have had constipation all of their adult lives and still were in comparative good health in their 70's, 80's and beyond. Let it be clearly understood that I am not minimizing or treating constipation lightly. I think it is unnecessary, I think it can be prevented, avoided and that remedial steps should be taken in every single instance.

In America and in the western world in general the taking of laxatives is like the taking of aspirin. Practically everybody does it just as though they were breathing. It's no more of a problem or a task than breathing is. As another writer put it, "The simple logic of the situation is that the bowel normally reacts to the presence of either an excessive bulk of waste content or some form of irritation — often due to putrefaction."

As for the frequency of bowel movements, in an article by Dr. Abraham Marcus in the Observer back in 1961 he noted that in primitive peoples a bowel movement after every meal is quite common. Then it is also quite often found that with some people a movement once in two, three or even four days may be compatible with good health. Basically, a great deal depends upon how great an excess of food is eaten and whether or not the over abundance of food is prone to putrefaction. Then of course the health or condition or the tone of the intestines and their muscular ability are factors.

It is clearly understandable that if one measured his intake of food rather carefully and selected the kind and the variety to meet the demands of the day that the excretion and the frequency of movement and the volume would not be very great but if one was given to gross over eating and the ingesting of large volumes of cooked and over-cooked foods, especially of the protein variety, that one would have more copious, more frequent and more bulky bowel movements.

It is also easy to understand that the bowel in good physical or muscular tone would respond more readily to a bowel movement than one that was flabby and weak and over-distended. It is definitely easy to understand that having big, bulky, regular bowel movements every day or twice a day is not specifically a sign of good health. One would gather and understand that if we took a purgative or a potent laxative and had a complete emptying of the bowel today that we could not expect a normal or even a copious movement tomorrow but yet that is precisely what some people expect. Of course, if they don't get the bowel movement the following day they immediately feel they have to resort to a pill or a laxative or an enema and of course in this way they get a bowel movement ahead of time and this interrupted or unseemly situation continues day after day and that's how people get into the laxative habit. In other words, trying to produce tomorrow's or the day after's bowel movement today.

It is claimed to be a scientific fact that the absorption of toxic materials into the blood stream is usually greatly increased by the administration of an enema. The reason is given in this way. "With relatively dry bowel contents, there is little or no transport of materials through the bowel wall and into the vessels which line it. There may be stasis — a lack of forward movement — but there is no danger and the tissues are not irritated. But add water, and immediately there is a rapid absorption through the walls: with the inflow of water there is also an invasion by soluble toxic material. True, this may induce an even more vigorous evacuation, by producing an acute inflammation of the bowels, but the body as a whole has been seriously burdened with additional toxins. Bowel

389

emptying will occur, but without any real advantage to the patient: what had been a quiescent mass has been transformed into an extra task for the kidneys and the other blood-cleansing organs."

There is little or no doubt that refined foods and especially refined carbohydrates are the basic cause of or a contributor to constipation. Where foods are eaten whole, and of course contain the normal bulk, constipation would seldom if ever be a problem. I find constipation a consideration where people are very, very selective in what they eat and who select only the choice and tasteful morsels. This, combined with eating refined foods, would definitely contribute to constipation.

There appears to be some disagreement among the experts as to whether drinking adequate water or mixing adequate water with one's meal poses a hazard or a benefit. My own personal experience has been that drinking with meals or having foods that are watery rather than dry contributes to better bowel movement. I have found that a dry stool is usually a difficult one so I prefer to have my food on the wet or soggy side.

I must definitely disagree with the experts who do not recommend water taken in sufficient quantities. They seem to think that it is in error because the water can be absorbed through the intestinal walls. I'm sorry but I cannot accept that thesis. There are many people who regularly consume various quantities of foods that would improve bowel movements such as figs and prunes. Raw potatoes are claimed to be somewhat laxative. In this case I suggest rotating these and other foods that tend to promote evacuation so that they will not tend to make the bowel lazy or become ineffective.

From all the evidence it appears that where proper food is taken with adequate bulk and with adequate quantities of it raw there is little danger of ever having constipation. Upon changing to a proper or natural diet one must be patient and allow time for the system to regulate itself. Given raw, natural food it will do so and will function properly and normally. Confidence in the ability of nature to handle the situation is essential and also most rewarding.

CHAPTER

64

BALDNESS — IS IT PREVENTABLE?

Actually every known condition that affects or impairs health has some form of remedy. There is a logical answer to virtually all physical impairments. Even cancer, heart disease and the difficult Parkinson's Disease and Multiple Sclerosis can be healed or remedied but as yet I've never been able to discover even the slightest remedy or hope for baldness.

For the record, personally I began to lose my hair at 17. By that I mean I was losing more hair than was growing back. I did not become bald until my 40's but I knew back when I was 17 years old that the chances were that I would become bald. I knew this because I'd recognized that there was a strong hereditary factor in baldness and all of the men on my mother's side of the family were bald but all of the men on my father's side retained a good head of hair throughout their lives. So it was clear to me that I took after my

393

mother's side and felt that I would be bald.

Don't misunderstand . . . I strove in every way that I could think of or any way that I could learn about to prevent this from happening and the different means and methods that I tried would fill a good sized book. And don't for a moment think that I didn't try some that are considered good, logical ways which included massage, change of diet, drugs, natural substances such as lanolin, bear oil and goose grease. I could go on and recite a host of other things that I did and used but I just want to clearly make you understand that I did do everything that any human being could do to prevent the loss of my hair. Yes, I consulted physicians and tonsorial specialists. In my youth I had a beautiful head of wavy, dark brown hair and I hated to lose it but lose it I did. That is, up in the centre . . . around the sides or the fringe I have plenty.

I found that practically all barbers are hair experts. They recommend various tonics which they have available and ready for application at so much a treatment, but in most cases they are themselves bald or balding.

Back in my youth it was always the men who suffered from falling hair and worried about it but today evidently it appears almost as frequently among women and with them it's a much more serious affair than with men as you can readily understand. As a matter of fact, it is estimated that in 1970 women spent more than 750 million dollars buying wigs and other hairpieces to bolster or camouflage their receding scalplines. After a rather detailed survey of the situation it is revealed that aging, heredity and hormones are factors in baldness but as to the exact cause of baldness there appears to be no definite conclusion and as for any reliable cure or preventative, no such thing exists or even promises hope. Various drugs, pregnancy or a serious illness involving a high fever will cause temporary baldness and when the siege of the disease is over the hair grows back — in most cases as good as it was before.

It is strange but massage is involved in practically every hair treatment offered by the so-called experts and hair stylists and

394

beauty specialists yet there is not one shred of scientific evidence to indicate that massage contributes one iota of benefit in restoring or growing hair and as for seeking help from the legitimate medical profession as compared to the other kind of operators there is not one shred of difference. Neither can do a thing for you and I'm not sure which one will take most of your money faster or which can do you more harm.

I found some consolation in the fact that scientists claimed that all sexually virile men were bald. Well, I'll admit that I was sexually virile and even in my youth indulged in sexual relations frequently or should I say as frequently as my female companions would permit.

During all that time that I was seeking to correct my condition or find a means of stopping it I was reading on the subject and studying and trying to gain knowledge. I did come across some very valuable information but I learned this late in life when the damage had been done. I believe if I had known then what I know now I could have prevented my baldness. Of course, some may say that it was a hereditary condition and could not be helped but I do not believe that. I believe, heredity or no, I could have definitely helped my condition. However, I do admit that hereditary factors are a major predisposing factor.

I've since learned that two very important factors are involved in baldness. One is the use of salt, especially the excessive use of salt and I was a most excessive user. The second factor is a deficiency of good natural fat or oils. The finest oils on earth, in my opinion, are the oils derived from seeds, or roots such as carrots, beets, parsnips, turnips etc. A seed contains these oils in greater abundance and in a more pleasant and readily available manner. I had my share of seeds but I've learned that cooking or treating seeds destroys the important vitamin factors so essential for maintenance and growth of hair.

The connection that I discovered was that both sex and hair require the same nutritive factor and obviously I didn't have enough for both so the sex glands got the nod. The experts claim that,

"Inadequate intake of protein enriched foods like fish, milk and eggs deprive the hair of the vital amino acids so important for growth and lustre." My answer to this is 'baloney, bunk, bosh', because those were the specific foods that I ate and used in abundance during that part of my life and my hair fell out without abatement. There are more experts on hair and more experts on dermatology — who would do a lot of spouting but who in my opinion know nothing — than there are in any other field. Some advise using a stiff brush and others say to use a soft brush. Some say to brush gently, some say to brush vigorously. From all of the counsel and advice of the experts I say just one word "nonsense". There are only two factors that I have found involved and that is an excessive use of refined table salt and a deficiency in essential oils such as are found in seeds and in raw root vegetables.

I will agree, however, that the frequent washing of the hair ... especially with the use of soaps and shampoos ... will do serious damage to the hair. I won't say it will cause baldness but I will definitely state it will affect the hair in a harmful manner. No head of hair can remain long in good physical condition when subjected to the treatment with soaps and shampoos or other hair treatments and the punishment that women's hair gets in the hairdresser's shop is nothing short of cruel and tragic.

Today another very vital factor has entered the field and that is the use of diethylstilbestrol in our meat. It definitely does cause hair to fall out. Some experts might here point out that the use of DES will also cause excessive hair growth. This is granted, but it is usually unwanted hair in unwanted places. This is important. It has been found that because of the birth control pills women's hair sometimes falls out. This is due to the same factor as in meat ... that is diethylstilbestrol is the factor involved. However, once you stop using the pill or the DES in the meat the condition usually corrects itself.

Now it is my positive conviction that the factors involved in baldness are: 1. Diet 2. Salt 3. Incorrect methods of washing or shampooing. You'll note that I omitted in this instance the oil factor . . . the proper oils are included in diet. One's diet should consist of sufficient quantities of these fresh, whole, uncooked and untreated grains that contain adequate or more than adequate quantities of the essential oils. I believe that a teaspoonful or two a day of any living seed, be it flax, wheat, barley, rye, sesame, sunflower or pumpkin, will give the body sufficient oil that could prevent falling hair and baldness but this must be started in childhood or youth and not after the damage is done in middle or old age.

Some authorities believe that a deficiency in Vitamin A causes the hair to become dry and brittle. A test done on animals indicates that a diet low in vitamin E is reported to cause the fur to remain infantile and unusually white in the young while in the adult it becomes coarse, sparse and discoloured. In another experiment two teams of researchers report that dryness and scurfiness of the fore and hind paws is the earliest and most constant symptom of the deficiency, occurring while the animals are still growing, after only 10 days or a few weeks on the deficient diet. The condition of the paws returns to normal within 3 to 5 weeks when linoleic or arachidonic acid is given.

CHAPTER

65

CANCER AND THE ANTI-CHOLESTEROL DIET

Recent studies and conclusions seem to show a distinct and clear-cut relationship between cancer and a low cholesterol diet. This will come as quite a shock to many people because the tendency has been among the more erudite to cut down drastically on animal fats of all sorts to prevent a heart attack.

However, to make up for the loss of these tasty, enjoyable foods, other foods have to be substituted and evidently these other foods, or the lack of the nutrients found in the cholesterol foods in some strange, unusual, or poorly understood manner, seems to be involved with cancer.

My investigations indicate that when people seek to avoid animal fats they eat a whole array of processed foods and other foods containing unsaturated fats, specifically margarine and perhaps lean meat, which is low in fat but high in diethylstilbestrol.

If lean meat, which is the basis of a high protein diet is adopted in an attempt to eliminate the animal fats like butter, cheese, milk, cream, ice cream and fat meats, then you are getting a big dose of diethylstilbestrol from the large quantity of lean meat.

Do not ignore the implications of the heavy intake of diethylstilbestrol, because diethylstilbestrol has long been known to be a prime cause of cancer. There is a great amount of positive, unquestionable, scientific, statistical proof that diethylstilbestrol causes various forms of cancer.

There is no argument, there is no doubt, there is no question involved. Diethylstilbestrol does cause cancer and as meat, whether it be beef or chicken, contains large amounts of diethylstilbestrol, this in itself could be the cause of cancer . . . and probably is one of the main causes.

Personally I am somewhat reluctant to lay the whole blame on the lean meat and the heavy content of diethylstilbestrol. We must not ignore the change-over from dairy products and fat meat to lean meat and a wide range and variety of processed foods — foods that have been manufactured, packed, concocted, treated, fancied up and flavoured for taste appeal, as substitutes for the animal fats and the dairy products.

So, therefore, the evidence is that you may help your heart by going on an anti-cholesterol diet but you greatly increase the risk of cancer if you follow the diet recommended by many cardiologists . . . that is, a diet low in saturated fats, meat and dairy fats and high in poly-unsaturated fats, which are the liquid vegetable oils.

Two Los Angeles medical doctors reported an unexpectedly high incidence of deaths from cancer among elderly men and women who were on the traditional cardiologist's heart diet. This was revealed at the recent annual meeting of the American Heart

Association held in Atlantic City. Drs. M. Lee Pearce and Seymour Dayton of the University of California, said that in an 8-year study of 846 elderly men they found that among those on a low saturated fat/high unsaturated fat diet the death rate from cancer was double that of a control group that ate the typical American diet high in butter fats and meat fats.

In another report, Dr. Kenneth Carrol of the University of Western Ontario linked a high-fat diet to breast cancer in laboratory animals. Animals treated with a cancer-causing agent, he said were found to be more susceptible to the disease if their diet was high in fats, and particularly unsaturated fats.

Neither of the studies was considered conclusive by the assembled scientists. In reference to the Los Angeles study, Dr. Gardiner C. McMillan of the National Heart and Lung Institute pointed out that many other studies of patients on a poly-unsaturated fat diet have yielded no evidence that such a diet increases cancer risk.

On the question of whether the 'heart' diet actually plays any role at all in the prevention of heart disease, the assembled scientists were still hung up in debate and disagreements, as they have been for years. A suggested 'definitive' study would involve 50,000 men over a 5-year period and cost $50 million.

The great and most important consideration that is ignored by the entire medico-scientific fraternity is the role that hydrogenated fats play in this vital affair.

Here I am going out on a limb . . . one that looks precarious to conventional scientists, medical men and nutritionists, but I feel it is a sinewy, wiry limb that can take the full impact of my suspicions and allegations.

I unhesitatingly state, based on my studies, that hydrogenated oil is the cancer-causing agent in the unsaturated fat anti-cholesterol diet. Allow me to point out that Margarine, Peanut Butter and a

401

thousand other processed food products are actually loaded with hydrogenated oils. Couple this with the diethylstilbestrol-treated lean meat diet and you have the greatest union of cancer-causing agents ever used in foods throughout the whole world.

I am warning all that diethylstilbestrol and hydrogenated oil do cause cancer, and today they play a major role in all the food we eat. Cancer is sweeping America like a prairie fire.

CHAPTER

66

CANCER IS EPIDEMIC

I have been a calamity howler for 30 or more years so I guess everybody has taken me for granted. I have pointed out the dangers in chemical fertilizers and the dangers in chemical sprays and dusts. I have pointed out the dangers in the chemicals in our food and the dangers in the fragmentation of our foods and also the danger in the oils we use in foods.

I maintain that chemistry is destroying our soil organisms. It's making them sick and sick soil organisms make sick soil. Sick soil makes sick plants. Sick plants make sick animals and sick plants and sick animals make sick human beings.

All right, we would die soon enough from this but then to add another blow the chemicals in our food and the drugs in our medicines are doing the job much faster.

America, they say, is still the best fed and the healthiest nation in the world, according to our government and according to government spokesmen and the American Medical Association and hosts of nutritionists and scientists.

Listen to me, friend. Today cancer in America has already reached epidemic proportions. The statistics do not show this for many reasons. Perhaps the doctor wants to be kind to the family and he says pneumonia or this, that or the other caused the death instead of cancer on the death certificate. There may be other reasons why they don't put cancer on the death certificate and one of the reasons might be because they claim that they can cure cancer with the cobalt bomb and surgery and if everybody were dying of cancer it would look as though their boasts were baloney . . . which they really are.

Now I'm not afraid of them shooting me or putting me in jail for what I am going to say, so I am repeating to you that cancer in America has reached epidemic proportions. First of all, the statistics that we have available as of now, November, 1972, are statistics that are at least two and one half years old . . . and I say, even older.

Women everywhere are having lumps removed from their breasts. They're having surgery performed just like a common everyday occurrence.

O.K., let them jail me, let them hang me or let them do what they will . . . but I am still telling you the truth and no matter what happens to me, the truth will out and my statements will be verified.

You may ask how I know and why I am predicting such a thing. Well, I'll tell you, my friend, I have eyes and I have ears. I see and observe, I read and I study. Thousands, and I repeat, thousands of letters cross my desk in the course of a few weeks and thousands are crying out to me, "Help me, I've got cancer!" Or it may be, "My wife's got cancer," "my sister's got cancer," "my brother's got cancer," or "my child has cancer." So what am I supposed to do? Say that there isn't any cancer?

Besides this, I get telephone calls from California, from Florida, from Texas, from Iowa, from Ohio and from New York, telling me, "My brother (my sister, my uncle or my aunt) has cancer. Can you help?"

Well, the truth of the matter is that I am not a doctor or a healer. I have never professed to be a doctor or a healer. Yet thousands of people are coming to me with cancer. Why don't they go to the doctors? Why don't they go to the hospitals? Well, most of them have been there and the horrible, dissected, mutilated remains are crying out for help. Then, of course, there are a small minority who refuse to take the medical and hospital treatments. And let me tell you this, they are lucky. At least their bodies haven't been torn, butchered, dismembered and poisoned or their cancer metastasized.

I can speak freely because I do not believe in a cancer cure, nor do I offer one. I am telling you absolutely and positively that there is no cancer cure and I'm equally positive that surgery and the cobalt bomb are not the answer to cancer. I seriously maintain that synthetic drugs, surgery, the bomb and radiation, without exception do only harm and never, never benefit the human organism. Yes, I realize that the medical profession claims that they save lives by these means but I say these lives would have been saved better without. Besides, drugs, surgery and radiation kill more than survive the ordeal. Of course, the medics say that early detection will prevent or cure cancer. And that, my friend, is the biggest lie ever told. The earlier it is diagnosed the earlier you will die. The sooner you start taking treatments the sooner you will die. The sooner you have surgery performed the sooner you will die. And the sooner you have the bomb applied to you the sooner you will die.

However, that does not mean that people who get cancer are without hope or help. To the contrary, there is more reason to have hope and help and alleviation from cancer than ever before in the history of mankind. So take heart, those of you who are afflicted and those of you who fear affliction, cancer can be conquered and the individual himself or the afflicted one is the best person to do the conquering.

405

I have a few suggestions for those who would rid themselves of the affliction. Now please remember, I said and I maintain that cancer cannot be cured but it can be conquered.

The medical profession tells you that any day researchers will produce a breakthrough. Well, Hippocrates promised a breakthrough more than 2,000 years ago and there were many other healers who promised breakthroughs 3,000, 4,000, 5,000 years ago and yes, as many years ago as mankind has existed. But there won't be any breakthroughs because the only person who can conquer a disease is the individual himself and he can do it by removing the cause.

I strongly and emphatically maintain that cancer can be prevented. That is the easiest way to beat cancer. Do unto your body that which is necessary and cancer will not be a threat to you ever.

The best way that I can tell you what I know about cancer is to answer a question that I have been asked on many occasions and that is, "What would you do if you got cancer?"

I'll tell you what I would do. In the first place I would put my affairs in order and assume that I had but a few months or a few years in which to live. Remember, I am 66 years of age and I'm telling you what I would do if I got cancer. Then I would immediately go on a 100% raw food diet, consisting mainly of fresh organically grown leafy green vegetables, adequate quantities of root vegetables, grains, fruits and nuts in that order.

The most important are the green leafy vegetables and the second are the root, stalk, stem and flower vegetables. Then come the grains, such as, wheat, barley, rye, oats, rice, millet, flax, sesame, buckwheat and other seeds. Then come the fruits, preferably fruits native to your own area. And then last but not least, nuts . . . preferably those native to your own area. I would not make a fetish of any one of these but I would eat them all regularly and in as broad a variety as humanly possible. None would be heated, processed, cooked or treated in any manner, shape or form and I would crack the nut shells with my own hands.

Wherever possible I would have a garden and organically grow every single item that I could, and on these I would rely. I would make sure that my soil was in good tilth and as far away from contamination as possible. I would use no commercial fertilizers and no dusts, sprays or other pesticides.

If humanly possible — and I think in my case it would be possible — I would make an environmental change. If I lived in the north I would go to the south. If I lived in the south I would go to the north. If I lived in the east I would go to the west and if I lived in the west I would go to the east. I contend that the single greatest factor in the conquering of cancer is an environmental change. The reason I stress the environmental change is because of that one simple stroke . . . you eliminate most of the causes of cancer in the individual case.

This would take a fair amount of elaboration and I cannot undertake it in this book. But I expect to do so in a forthcoming book dealing expressly with cancer in all its vast array.

When the environmental change has been made, the next most important factor is to have a plot of ground and grow your own food just as I have suggested previously. If you have succeeded in making both of these changes . . . making the environmental change and growing a lot of your own food . . . you have made a big enough step to conquer cancer right there and then.

I'd make sure my drinking water was not tampered with and came from a spring or a good well. I would keep away from television, especially colored television, and if I did view it at all it would be for a short period and from a distance of at least 10 or 12 feet . . . never closer.

Permit no aluminum utensils in your home. Do not use an electric heating pad. Do not use fluorescent lighting. Do not permit yourself to be X rayed. Do not take drugs of any kind . . . not even a single aspirin.

407

Eat no fragmented, processed, treated food or food not prepared by your own hands. Make sure you get a good share of wholesome air and sunlight but be sure not to overdo the sunlight. Keep active. Walk and exercise as much as humanly possible. Keep active, active, active . . . mentally and physically. Keep busy, as busy as possible.

Under no circumstances drink milk, tea or coffee or any other processed or manufactured beverage. You can allow yourself wholesome herb teas prepared by your hand.

Make sure that your bowels move regularly and freely. This should give you no problem on a strict raw food diet but if there is a problem, use an enema with only lukewarm water and nothing else.

Do not use tooth paste or tooth powder. Do not use soap. Do not use deodorants or cosmetics. Do not use shampoos. If a male do not shave but permit yourself to grow a beard and keep it neatly trimmed. If you use glasses, try to do without them especially when you are outside. Let the sun and the air get to your eyes.

Do not allow moth balls or the substance from which they are made into your home. Use no chemical sprays or fly catchers or insect destroyers in your home or on your grounds. Do not use an air-wick or any other chemical means of destroying odors in your home.

Eat no baker's bread — it's cooked anyway. But you can make and use raw breads. There are many recipes available. Never eat ice cream unless you make it yourself . . . even then, milk products are not recommended.

I presume you do not smoke. Smoking in any form is deadly. No liquor, but homemade wine is permissible and so is homemade beer.

I strongly advise the eating of large amounts of raw vegetables. If you find a juicing machine will help you consume more of these, then a juicing machine is permissible. A blending machine would be better but blended foods don't taste as good as the fresh juices.

It is your responsibility to make sure that the food you do buy is untreated. Never buy sulphured fruits. If you are buying your vegetables — especially your green leafy ones — it is of great importance that they not be sprayed because leafy vegetables today can contain a tremendous amount of harmful toxic sprays.

I would not submit to a biopsy, X rays, the cobalt bomb or surgery. If you must die, then die with dignity. You will live as long or longer without treatment as with treatment. This is as sure as the sun rises and sets. But by following the suggestions that I have given you, you will probably live your normal span of life in comparative good health and your cancer will disappear.

Now I don't say that you shouldn't go to a doctor. If you feel you should, then by all means go . . . go as regularly as you like. I wouldn't go because I feel I could help myself a lot better without his attention than with it.

Don't be afraid to leave your family, because if you take all the treatments as most people do you probably won't live long anyway. In this way, if you have to leave your family it will only be temporary, they can visit you if they want to and you'll probably be alive and around and well to visit with. The other way your stay on this planet will be short and you'll part from your family permanently.

Don't allow yourself to be frightened. Conquer fear. The advice I've given you is the best, the most sensible and the sanest way to conquer cancer. Millions have died and are dying with all the best treatments that all the best healers in the world can give them. You can do more for yourself than any man on earth can do for you, including the medical profession and all other healers.

I can sincerely tell you that hundreds of people of my

acquaintance through the years have conquered cancer. Yes, and you can take encouragement from the work of a Danish woman doctor who developed cancer in both breasts and refused to have them removed. In her stirring little book she tells of how she conquered cancer and lived to be in her mid-eighties. Yes, she lived 30-odd years after cancer was diagnosed . . . and she did it by means of a raw food diet. And she tells of how when she went off her diet the lumps in her breast quickly reappeared. But as long as she remained true to her diet there was no sign of the lumps. The book is available if you want it. It's an inspiration and can give you great hope and courage.

I am fully aware of the fact that it will take a person of great courage and ability to follow the procedures that I have indicated. It will take perseverance and determination and it will be hard. But on the other hand, what choice do you have? Is it easier to die like a lamb being led to slaughter?

Here is an opportunity for you to fight for your life and you can drive cancer from your door. Here is a case, a true case, where no one can help you . . . you must go it alone. But it has been done, it is being done and you can do it, too.

I am fully aware that there are thousands, tens of thousands, of people and organizations who are offering cures for cancer. Don't be misguided or misled. Don't be fooled. I realize that a person who has cancer is desperate and will grasp like a drowning man at any straw and pay lots of money. I understand your predicament and probably with a lack of knowledge I would do the same.

But no method on earth or no method ever devised is as logical, as sensible, as practical and as truthful as the method that I have just outlined for you. The medical profession and the cancer fund organizations warn you against quacks. I tell you that the greatest, the most dangerous and the most insidious quacks are the medical trust and the cancer fund organizations. They are just dragging a red herring across the trail.

The set of rules that I have laid down for you can work and

will work, because in following this guidance you are removing the causes of cancer and when the causes are removed the body will, if not interfered with, heal itself.

By every means possible give your body the opportunity to drive off the cancer ... which it will do. Let me also state that I know people who followed these principles and were brought back to normal health but then they became careless — they felt that they had conquered the condition — and they went back to their previous way of life and the cancer quickly returned. I warn you that this is what usually happens.

The course that I am mapping out for you here is the course that you will have to follow strictly for the rest of your life and you can make it a long life. But you cannot deviate.

Cancer is an irreversible pathology. You can make it go away or disappear or earn a remission but you cannot go back to your old ways of living without having it come back just as it came before.

So there you have it, you know what I would do if I got cancer!

CHAPTER

67

SURGERY AND CANCER

Some time back I read an article in one of the medical magazines where a researcher linked frequent surgery and cancer. The essence of the article was that each advent of surgery performed on the human body took you one step closer to cancer. The researcher evidently studied all the cases of cancer that he could get records for and then checked up and tried to find out whether or not the person who had cancer had had any surgery performed on his body. He found the more surgery the individual had the greater was the risk of cancer. From the article I felt that the researcher had established his case and that there was a positive link between surgery and cancer.

It so happens that a handful of people with whom I had close association over a period of many years died of cancer and in every case these people had had surgery performed — a tonsilectomy, a prostatectomy, an appendectomy, a hysterectomy or gall bladder surgery. It is also coincidental that in four out of five of these cases with which I was acquainted four happened to be women. So I did a bit of investigating and here is what I have learned.

We'll start with tonsils. According to the medical description the tonsils function and act as a filter to protect the body from invasion of bacteria and aid in the formation of white cells. Their most recognized function is the formation of lymphocytes.

The Vermiform appendix is a small tube about 3 to 4 inches long and 1/4 inch thick which is about the size of a goose quill which opens into the caecum or large intestine and is closed at the other end. Its inflammation is called appendicitis. The Columbia Encyclopedia states that the appendix has no function and is considered a vestigial remnant of some previous organ or structure that was unnecessary in man in his evolutionary progress. Infection of an accumulation and hardening of waste matter in the appendix may give rise to appendicitis symptoms.

The gall bladder is a pear shaped sac on the under-surface of the right lobe of the liver holding bile from the liver until discharged through the cystic duct. It is 3 to 4 inches long and 1 inch is its greatest diameter. Its capacity is 50 to 75 cc concentrated bile, equivalent to 1 1/2 pints of liver bile. For those who are afflicted with or have gall bladder trouble it is suggested that they avoid chocolate, fats, ice cream and all foods containing fats, condiments, strong coffee, salt and strong flavored vegetables and all fried foods.

A prostatectomy is an excision of part or all of the prostate gland. The most usual form of prostate surgery involves an incision into the bladder. This type of surgery is usually performed when the enlarged prostate causes retention of the urine or serious bladder discomfort. Often kidney disorders are created as well.

A hysterectomy is known as the removal of the uterus either through the abdominal wall or through the vagina. It is usually removed because of the presence of tumors both benign and malignant. However, many hysterectomies are performed without any

414

signs of disease or infection and many women approve of the hysterectomy and have it done as a means of preventing conception.

Now let's discuss the tonsils from a layman's viewpoint. They are two ovid masses composed of lymphoid tissue situated on either side of the throat between the pillars of the fauces. The true function of the tonsils is to act as a filter against disease organisms. For some strange reason medical men usually advise removal when the tonsils become diseased or chronically enlarged and this condition usually prevails in childhood and in early life. Some medical men believe that the enlargement or the frequent inflammation of the tonsils poses a threat to health.

It is my belief, based on studies, that when the tonsils are enlarged and inflamed it is due to these organs fighting the battle for the health and the life of the individual. So much improper food and toxic substances are being ingested that the tonsils become enlarged and inflamed because of continually fighting the battle of survival. Then along come the medical men and take these fighters out with surgery and tell you that now you won't have any trouble. Of course, usually you wind up with many other more serious and more harmful conditions.

Through my lifetime when I heard or knew of such circumstances I said to the child or the parent, "Stop eating conventional foods, especially anything containing milk, drink lots of water and eat fruit" and lo and behold, almost invariably in a few days the condition would correct itself. Chronic enlarged tonsils definitely indicate a continued intake of foods or matter or toxic substances that is causing the trouble. This matter was brought into sharp focus to me about a month ago.

A man came to visit me from the west and in the course of our conversation he related this little story and I'm very happy that I remember it. He was the principal of a school and he was a little bit of a nut like me. That is, he was health-minded. There was one child in the school who was continually suffering from a malady and the teacher had great difficulty with the child because the child could

415

not breathe properly and the child was continually uncomfortable and making all the other students uncomfortable as well.

The teacher kept reporting this to the principal and eventually he called the child's parents and said to them that they had to do one thing or the other . . . take the child out of school or have the matter attended to by their physician, once and for all. The physician advised surgery and the parents refused surgery but the principal refused to allow the child to come back in that condition. So in a discussion with the parents the principal said "I can't force you to have surgery but you must do something". And the parents said to the principal "What would you do if the child was yours?" He said, "I'd take the child home and make her drink a lot of water and give her only fruit to eat for a week".

So the parents did just that and at the end of the week the child was at school and the condition had completely cleared up. In this case he told me it happened to be a very heavy dairy diet that caused the trouble.

It is my belief that the removal of tonsils is actually a criminal act because the individual suffers many other conditions for the rest of his life. I do not say that it is never advisable to remove tonsils but I do advise every individual to hold on to them if humanly possible.

Now about appendicitis. Back 50 years ago they removed most appendices and tonsils at the drop of a hat. I knew a very fine old physician, Dr. Stutt . . . he was quite old then, highly respected and in great demand but he was a very frank, outspoken individual. I was going to high school at the time and this physician used to come into a drug store where we used to gather occasionally for a soda. Now I remember his remark about the appendix.

He said, "When a doctor suggests or advises the removal of the appendix he is admitting he doesn't know what is wrong with the sufferer because it is never the appendix that is actually to blame for the condition or the symptoms. But as the medical men recognize no particular use for the appendix they will take it out so it can't rupture and cause peritonitis . . . and besides there is usually a fee of a few hundred dollars involved."

I do not deny that the appendix becomes inflamed but it is due to the action of other organs. That is why when there is ever the slightest sign of trouble they yank out the appendix but this doctor stressed that the appendix, being an inactive organ, could never be the actual cause of the trouble. People who eat proper food never have trouble with their appendix. For that matter they don't have trouble with any other organ.

When a person has trouble with his gall bladder — and I have known literally hundreds of people who have had gall bladder trouble and had gall bladders removed through my lifetime — always they were the fried food eaters and those who violated every decent known rule of proper diet. I have no great sympathy for people who have gall bladder trouble except that they have perhaps received poor nutritional guidance or were improperly directed by their parents.

Let me tell you a little bit about the gall bladder and the gall. The gall or better known bile, is a bitter alkaline fluid of a yellow, brown or green color which is secreted by the liver. It is composed chiefly of water, bile salts, acids, bile pigments, cholesterol, lecithin and inorganic salts. The bile pigments are derived from the decomposition of the worn out red corpuscles. Bile or gall is stored temporarily in the gall bladder and through the cystic and common ducts it is secreted into the small intestine where it aids in digestion. Bile emulsifies fats so that they can pass through the mucous membrane of the intestines. It prevents a decomposition of food while it remains in the intestine and it stimulates the muscles of the intestines and therefore the movement of their contents. The flow of bile is impeded by inflammation, by gall stones or other abnormality and digestive disturbances and jaundice are frequent results.

Now I give you this so that you'll understand that when the doctor tells you that the gall bladder is not important and removing it won't affect you he is not telling you the truth or the whole truth

417

and he is looking for the few hundred dollars that are involved in performing the surgery and of course there is something in it for the physician too. Once the patient has his gall bladder out the chances are he'll have many more other complaints and this is just plain good business.

I have known many people who have had all four of these operations performed . . . tonsils, appendix, gall bladder, and uterus or prostate. In the case of a male it runs like this . . . tonsils, appendix, gall bladder and prostate. With the woman it runs . . . tonsils, appendix, gall bladder and uterus.

Now there are many people who are 70 or 80 years of age and maybe older who have had all of these four organs removed but so far I haven't come across any. If you know of any please let me know.

About 25 or 50 years ago cancer and heart disease did not pose the great danger that they pose today and 50 years ago heart disease wasn't even known in America and there were much fewer cases of cancer. Well, in those days the doctor was hard pressed to make a buck or a living. I personally knew many doctors who existed only because they could write prescriptions for liquor. In those days in Ontario you couldn't buy liquor unless you had a prescription from a doctor. The doctor could write a specific amount of prescriptions for liquor every month. So the doctors actually made a living from the liquor prescriptions they wrote and the only way they could make an extra buck or two was by yanking out someone's tonsils, adenoids or appendix. But the gall bladder and the hysterectomy and the prostate operations weren't so prevalent in those days.

Therefore I contend that hundreds of thousands of people in America have had their organs removed needlessly . . . well I shouldn't say needlessly, needlessly for the patient but necessarily for the doctor for his income . . . and many thousands, tens of thousands or more died premature deaths because of the removal of these organs. As to the link with cancer I did not grasp this until it was pointed out to me in the article I mentioned earlier and I feel certain that this researcher established his case. No one will ever convince me that the body contains unnecessary organs, including the appendix.

I maintain the appendix performs a function, only we in our ignorance have not as yet discovered that function and the removal of any organ lowers the entire functional ability of the human body and the more organs that are removed the greater the functional impairment.

CHAPTER
68

WHY A CANCER CURE WILL NEVER BE FOUND

I don't know if others have said it before me but I know I have been making this statement for a quarter of a century. I don't think there is any mystery about why a cure for cancer will never be found. I think it's really very, very clear. Here it is, right on target. I suggest that cancer is the best paying disease in the world and millions of people make billions of dollars out of it so therefore the chance of a cure is astronomically remote.

A new book on cancer and cancer research by Pat McGrady, science editor of the American Cancer Society, titled "The Savage Cell," gives some very valuable information and in the book he states that the American Research Program is set up (and controlled) so that most of the money goes, inevitably, to only those "researchers" who explore fashionable, acceptable, "safe" and usually dead-end avenues of research. In my language this means that if you are a researcher and you are going to do research on cancer where there is practically no hope of finding a cure then you will be given a research grant.

Now I'd like to cite an example. They wouldn't give me a grant to do cancer research because my work with natural raw food would no doubt turn up some very valuable evidence that might lead to cancer being obliterated. Well, these people who control the cancer funds never, never would want that to happen because that would put an end to their supply of money . . . in truth I wish their grant could put them out of business.

Don't laugh this off because it isn't a laughing matter. If you stop and analyze it carefully you will see that I speak absolute truth and good common sense. Now at this point I want to mention that the medical profession regards any treatment that they give to a cancer patient that enables the patient to drag along for five years, either during or with or after the treatment, as curing the individual and they chalk up a cure in the official cancer cure score book. Now this is a positive statement that I am making. So therefore, the medical profession can boldly state that every year they cure tens of thousands of patients by means of their medicine, their drugs, their surgery and their cobalt bombs, X rays and radiation. In this most ridiculous counting system they run up a fairly high score claiming that they cure anywhere from 30 to 60% of various kinds of cancer. Now if the cancer patient who is cured dies one day after the fifth year from cancer that doesn't count, he was still cured of cancer.

About 20 years ago it was estimated that it would cost you a minimum of $7,000 to die of cancer. Today, the cost is much higher. I would judge that you can't die of cancer today for less than $10,000. Of course, with those who can afford it and where the disease drags over a longer period the cost can run $20,000, $25,000, $50,000 and more. So when you multiply that by millions of cancer patients yearly you can quickly see that we are talking about money — big money, real money, cash money and with such goings on who, in their right business mind who makes a living from cancer, would be crazy enough to bring forth a cure even if one really could be

422

found?

But why talk about cures? Just tell me, exactly how many cures has the medical profession come up with since the first medical doctor came into existence? I'm acquainted with many diseases and as I look through my medical dictionary I find literally hundreds of different diseases but I don't find many cures. Here I'm racking my brain right now like mad to see if I can come up with a known cure for a certain disease. I'm thinking of malaria and quinine but quinine is not a cure . . . it will in most cases hold the disease in check. I'm thinking of pneumonia and they use penicillin and other antibiotics to knock it out but what happens is that almost invariably the same patient comes up with another condition so all that the penicillin and the antibiotics did was drive the disease out into another guise.

For years the medical profession claimed cures for tuberculosis, for syphilis, for gonorrhoea, for smallpox, diphtheria . . . oh, and many more but really, were they cures? Of course not. You can count all of the cures brought forth by medical man and medical scientists on the fingers of your hands and have enough fingers left over to write or pitch a baseball. Come on, you're a bright fellow, you think up the different cures, genuine cures that the medical profession has discovered. I really can't come up with any. Of course, they're expecting a big break through any day with a cure for cancer but medical science has been waiting and expecting an imminent breakthrough since the time of Hippocrates . . . And that's how many thousand years?

In this mad search for a cure for cancer I'm reminded of a man of fame and fortune who travelled around the world and after spending a lifetime in futility he came back home dejected to spend his last days and he found what he had been seeking all over the world for years right in his own back yard.

The control, the answer, the end or call it the cure for cancer has been here all along, right at home and no money is required to dig it up or discover it. All one need do is to remove the cause and the condition will disappear on its own accord. This has been proven

423

repeatedly and is being proven every single day. Then why haven't the researchers discovered it? Reason enough . . . they've never looked for it. They were looking for ways to spend money, they were looking for ways to fill in time, they were looking for miracles, they were looking for complicated, deeply buried secrets and they couldn't see the answer walking all around them, right there in the open.

Of course, when a case of cancer that has been cleared up is brought to their attention they invariably say, "Oh it wasn't cancer." "But it was diagnosed as cancer. You diagnosed it." "Yeah, but we made a mistake. It wasn't cancer". And often when they're in a real box they will say, "Well, a spontaneous remission occurred which is a shear accident or act of God".

You see they have an answer, at least some sort of an answer for every time that a cancer victim recovers without their help. In this way they can keep on searching and searching and searching . . . I was going to say forever, but no, as long as money will hold out.

Now a certain group tells us that Amygdalin, Nitriloside or Vitamin B17 is a positive cure for cancer. This wonder drug Laetrile or whatever name they call it is found in the kernels of apricot seeds but it's also found in most if not all seeds so why take vitamin B17 when all you need to do is eat a handful of live seeds every day and prevent cancer or cause it to disappear or obtain a spontaneous remission in this manner? The answer to cancer is clear and simple and it works for everyone who follows the rules scrupulously . . . a wholesome way of life and proper nutrition through balanced raw foods.

CHAPTER

69

YOUR BRAIN NEEDS FEEDING AND EXERCISE TOO

"Use it or lose it" is still as applicable today as it was 2,000 years ago in "Matthew" about the talents. Those who made good use of their talents were rewarded and he who failed to make use of them was chastised and demoted. So it is with people who make use of whatever intelligence they have. I think in general people are given equal amounts of brain power but some make more of it than others. The more you use your brain power, the more work you give it, the more useful it becomes.

It is not the amount or the weight of the brain or brain power that you have, it is more what you do with it. This does not mean you have to be a scientist, an engineer or a banker . . . the most intelligent and enlightened men that I have known were businessmen and working men, not necessarily men of great learning.

425

We are told that the body is fed by the bloodstream.

Now let's ask ourselves some very straight-forward, candid questions. What kind of blood can liquor, coffee, hamburgs, French fries, white bread, white sugar, cokes and other soft drinks, cigarettes, fried pork, fried pancakes, calorie-less cereals and other such foods produce? They not only cannot produce decent blood, they can do irreparable harm. You can't have good blood without good food. On top of all this most of these so-called foods are loaded with harmful, toxic chemicals. Now isn't it shear madness to try and feed your bloodstream with a concoction made from the list that I have just given you?

Now let's take what nature has provided . . . fresh vegetables, viable seeds and grains, fresh wholesome fruits and nuts or even fresh milk without chemical treatments and without pasteurization, fresh eggs laid by chickens who were not penned up in a cubicle or even meat from healthy animals. These foods can make good blood that in turn will properly nourish every organ of the body, especially the brain.

I do not believe there is one normal intelligent human being who doesn't realize that the refined pap that is supplied by most of our restaurants and food establishments cannot properly nourish the body and the brain. You cannot encumber the body with the thousands of chemical additives in food which wind up in the body and expect your bloodstream or your body to function properly.

Most people, especially young people who have not yet informed themselves about food, still like to believe that ice cream is made from cream and fruit and sugar . . . it's not. It's made mainly from synthetics that have little or no food value and from chemicals which the body cannot utilize and which in turn make the body sick. You must realize that the hamburger you eat is not made of meat — good wholesome meat — it is only a fragment of the hamburger. The rest is protein made from processor's wastes . . . garbage in other words, plus chemicals and salt and sugar and fat. Most do not realize that practically all of our processed foods are adulterated, coloured,

426

homogenized, hydrogenated, preserved, disrupted, corrupted and rendered unfit for decent human use.

The body cannot be any better than the food which nourishes it and this also applies to your brain. It can't be any better than the kind of food that enters your body. You still can't make a silk purse out of a sow's ear. You can't make a healthy body and a well functioning brain out of chemical additives and processor's wastes. You need food — decent, wholesome, fresh, natural food; not chemical or synthetic compositions.

CHAPTER 70

MENTAL HEALTH, DRUGS AND FOOD

In my discussions and arguments with friend and foe I'm frequently confronted with the individual who says, "O.K., I can see where food can be a factor regarding the health of an individual, say as far as diabetes is concerned or even arthritis or heart disease but don't try and convince me that food has an effect on a person's mental health".

Please believe me that this kind of an argument has been thrown at me frequently and it actually means that many people will buy my bill of goods that food is important for physical health but most people just won't accept it as being a factor in mental health. They seem to have the idea that people just go nuts. In fact, most people won't even accept the fact that food and nutrition have any effect on a nervous condition.

I have postulated, since first I gleened that nutrition was a factor, that mental health is just as much affected or even more so than physical health. To me it is inconceivable that anyone could separate mental from physical as far as health is concerned. The brain governs every action, every movement, every thought. So how can people separate it when one discusses health of the body in general?

The medical profession has been foremost in fostering the principle that nutrition is not a factor in mental health. In fact, they won't even accept the fact that it is an important cog in physical health because the doctors, at least most of them, still believe that the American diet is the best in the world and is absolutely adequate and they can see no harm in French fries and cokes or a cigarette and coffee and they recommend packaged cereals for children. So there is not much point in arguing with the great and mighty medical profession on these grounds.

However, the famed Linus Pauling has become involved, I think he's in trouble also with the medical profession and even with certain segments of the scientific fraternity. Evidently, both the scientists and the medical men resent the fact that Linus Pauling has stuck his nose into their business. After all, Pauling is quite a boy. He has been awarded two Nobel prizes and that's probably irked the scientists enough without having Pauling becoming an authority in the field of nutrition and health.

Evidently, all this started many years ago when Linus Pauling wrote a research paper supporting the theory that niacin and ascorbic acid were useful in the treatment of schizophrenia. Of course everyone knows today that Pauling stood flat-footed and claimed that vitamin C will knock out a cold and he recommended massive doses. But even before Pauling made this great announcement it was known by many that massive doses of vitamin C would knock out a cold. I've known it for at least 5 years but I never recommended it for the simple reason that I don't believe in vitamin supplements when the food is available.

In any event, the medical boys have got their big guns trained on Pauling and if he can be laid low they are going to lay him low . . . they are going to try darn hard. They contend that he has at last ventured beyond his established competence and they further claim that his conclusions are totally unsupported and that he cannot prove them by controlled, clinical studies.

Now in Pauling's paper on schizophrenia he was evidently doing some sustained bio-chemical research in what he refers to as the "molecular environment" of the mind. He claims that he was able to perceive direct connections between chemical imbalance in the brain and irrational and erratic behavior, generally diagnosed as schizophrenia. Pauling went further and he found evidence to support the findings of medical researchers who had discovered that massive doses of vitamins with the emphasis on the B vitamins plus ascorbic acid enhanced the body's ability to repair its "orthomolecular" deficiencies and to provide for restored chemical balance in the brain.

Here Pauling went on and emphasized that mental disease is frequently the result of a low concentration in the brain of thiamin, nicotinamide, pyridoxine, cyanocobalamin, biotin and ascorbic acid. He stressed the need, especially of niacin and ascorbic acid. Pauling outlined all of these things in his paper which appeared in the Science magazine of April 19, 1968 which is published by the American Association for the Advancement of Science. Fortunately for Dr. Pauling, he is supported by some of the world's best researchers which evidently his medical attackers do not bother to investigate.

All you have to do is look in Bicknell and Prescott's "Vitamins And Medicine" and you will find most of the references that Dr. Pauling has given or similar ones. Actually, Pauling didn't have to do the research, all he had to do was look up Bicknell and Prescott's "Vitamins And Medicine" and presented there was the sum and substance of the whole story. There definitely is a relationship between chemical imbalance and mental disease. Poor nutrition or poor dietary habits are clearly identified frequently as the cause of mental symptoms.

In clearly stating that nutrition is a vital, an important factor in mental disease it does not rule out that there can be or that there are other significant factors such as emotional pressures and genetic factors. However, it is important to know that one can prevent or even clear up mental conditions by a proper diet and when I say a proper diet I don't mean a government proper diet or a medical proper diet but a diet composed mainly of raw vegetables, grains and fruits as clearly outlined in this and other books . . . a diet that the conventional authorities do not advise or recommend.

Of course the medical profession rejects any suggestion that anything but drugs or shock treatments or other medical and surgical practices can have any value in the treatment of mental diseases. It is clearly established today, to any human being of normal intelligence who cares to look and investigate, that the medical profession causes or contributes to more mental disease than any other factor in our present society. Now I'm not changing my tone and deviating from my story that mental disease is caused by malnutrition but I'm sort of adding a corollary in stating that a great number of mental conditions are created by doctors and the drugs and treatments they give. These are known as iatrogenic diseases. I go further and state that the very drugs and medicines that doctors prescribe for mental conditions create graver, deeper and more incurable mental conditions.

My experiences and studies clearly indicate that practically all mental and psychological conditions readily respond to a raw food diet and proper living habits and conditions.

CHAPTER

71

CAN YOU PROVE YOU'RE NOT CRAZY?

Take it easy, just don't laugh yourself sick at the above heading because one of these days you may just have to try to prove it to prevent yourself from being put in the bug house. Yes, what's more you'll find it's mighty, mighty difficult to prove that you're not mad.

Sad to relate, tens of thousands of people in America have been put away while they protested and proclaimed loudly that they were innocent and sane. Let me warn you, your protestations have no merit, value or deterring effects upon those who are bent on putting you away. If a couple of doctors think you ought to be put away the chances are very strong that you will be put away. Does this worry you? Does this frighten you? If it doesn't, it should.

Actually, in the past few years I have met with or

433

corresponded with at least 10 people who have been committed, who are not now locked up but who claim that they were as sane when they were committed as they are today and I found them logical, reasonable and sane. "Why were they committed?" you may ask. Who knows, no doubt there are many reasons and underlying factors and I'll give you an example with which I am very well acquainted and for which there is documented proof.

This man went on a fast for health reasons. He had read various books which made him feel that fasting was the answer to his health problem. He stayed on the fast for 30 days and then abruptly broke it off and then a few weeks later he felt that he should have continued and he started on another fast. He then called a doctor acquaintance of his and asked for a bit of advice. A few days later he was taken into custody and committed. The story of how he eventually got out is a book in itself but the point is that the man was as sane then as he is now — a reasonable, intelligent, capable individual, a scientist of stature — yet he was committed. And had it not been for the efforts of relatives and a few friends he would still be there.

Remember, when a complaint is lodged against you there is usually no jury, no lawyer, no witnesses . . . just the judge and if he believes the complainer, usually a doctor or healer, you are confined and you have no appeal and you may be there for the rest of your life. Frightening isn't it? And it's all true, too.

No, this does not take place in Russia or China or Bulgaria . . . it takes place frequently in the United States of America and in Canada. The crime with which you are charged is mental illness. Granted, this does not often happen but it does happen. If you have children, a family and friends, it is not too likely to happen to you because you have someone who will fight for you in the event such a thing occurs but if you are lonely with few friends and few or no blood relatives and especially if you have some money that somebody would like to get ahold of, it could very well happen, especially if you are an individualist like me and have ideas of your own and give them licence. The truth is that it takes only one doctor to do the trick. He can usually get another doctor to support him but he doesn't even need that . . . a supporting layman, or an individual is sufficient.

There is no formula for insanity or mental illness or whatever you want to call it. In each province of the Dominion and in each state of the Union there are different laws that govern mental illness or insanity. There are many acts and deeds that are regularly done and committed by normal human beings like you and me which could easily be construed or misconstrued as mental illness or insanity. I am sure that you know many instances in your lifetime where a nice, decent, normal individual, man or woman, because of some provocation or incident went off into a streak of anger which could readily have been interpreted as insanity. When you get upset, annoyed, troubled or provoked it's justifiable but if someone else should do it it is easy to believe or suggest that it is insanity, be it of a mild or virulent nature.

If you are wealthy and if you are comparatively young you can afford to indulge in tantrums and in idiosyncrasies but if you are old and if you are poor I would advise you not to try these shenanigans or give vent to your idiosyncracies because you may readily find yourself in an institution or standing before a judge to be committed.

I have actually witnessed two cases of committment where I knew the person was not insane — disturbed perhaps, but not insane. They were committed by their own family in their blindness or ignorance. In one case the husband had his wife committed. I saw the reason while the rest of the family did not. He had an affair with his housekeeper and his wife objected so he planned it and arranged it and his wife was committed, so don't tell me it can't happen because it does happen. I also know of a case where the father was committed by his sons because they wanted to take over his estate and succeeded in so doing. The man was no more insane than you or I but he did have strong likes and dislikes and many idiosyncrasies which when he was younger were indulged in by his friends and relatives but when he became older the selfsame expressions and acts

435

were sufficient to convince the judge that he should be committed.

There are today in the United States well over a million mental patients confined in institutions. More than 70% of this million are from the low income or poverty group. The same 70% are over 65 years of age. Now the startling thing about all of these million people being committed is the fact that more than 65% of them were committed involuntarily.

I recall the case of a woman who was involuntarily committed. The complaint against her by her neighbours was that she had all the lights in her home on all night and that she ran about in her home without any clothes and that they could hear her screaming and shouting and singing at the top of her voice while carrying on voodoo or other insane antics, incantations and dancing. Also, that she had her radio or record player blaring at all hours of the night. After she had been committed for some time she was brought before a judge for a hearing because in the institution her behaviour was exemplary. The judge was a reasonable man, which is not always the case, and he gave her a chance to explain the situation and here is what she told the judge.

She was the youngest of 10 children and it had fallen to her lot to look after her parents who were strict Methodists. They did not permit singing or dancing, they went to bed when night fell and arose at daybreak. They permitted no noise, nor did they allow music or a radio and of course never any alcoholic beverages.

She explained that eventually when her parents died and her obligations to them had ended she decided to indulge in some of the things that she had never enjoyed or been permitted to enjoy. So she bought this house, moved into it and she slept when she wanted to sleep, got up when she wanted to get up, sang when she wanted to sing, danced if she felt in the mood, played the radio or the music machine whenever she felt inclined to do so and had an occasional cocktail. She minded her own business but the neighbours thought it was strange and unusual. The judge ordered her release.

It must be admitted that many of the older and poorer people who are committed to these institutions are committed for no other reason that they have nowhere else to go. Today another insidious aspect has crept into this mental situation. In practically every instance when an enforced patient is brought before the judge he or she is usually heavily dosed with tranquilizers or other drugs. In this condition they are not fully capable of defending themselves or relating their story plausibly and reasonably and what chance do they stand against a medical doctor or individuals who are intent upon having them committed?

Just how you can avoid being committed or having this happen to you I do not know. The best advice that I can give you is to have a few friends if there are no blood relatives around to protect you as you grow old.

I want to tell you three stories. To the best of my knowledge and belief they are true. They were told to me directly by the individuals themselves. I will not give their names, but if anyone definitely wants the names for any legitimate purpose, I will supply them.

Case No. 1. The first one we'll call Watson.

This man had a wife and three children. They had a farm and were fairly successful. They ate conventional food but they did practise organic gardening and believed, to a degree, in the natural way of life.

The wife began to have some trouble in her breasts and she felt some lumps and thought she'd best go to the doctor. The doctor felt there was some cause to be alarmed and had the woman put in the hospital. After tests and examinations it was recommended that she have her breasts removed. And because of the advancement of the condition they felt that surgery should be done immediately.

The wife demurred and said she would like to talk to her husband before she made any definite decision. So the husband was sent for and he came and her condition had now developed to the stage where she had a private nurse. So they had a lengthy discussion and they decided that because of their way of life and belief in natural foods, and also because of their convictions, they did not wish to have surgery performed.

The next day the husband informed the surgeons of their decision. The doctor told Mr. Watson the following — "The private nurse in your wife's room and the other nurses observed your actions. Unless you consent to having the surgery performed on your wife, we will have you committed to an institution."

Then the surgeons spoke to the wife and told her that if she did not consent to the surgery her husband would be committed to an institution and that as she was unable to look after the children, being in the hospital, the children would be put in the care of the Children's Aid Society. He gave them 24 hours to make up their minds.

They consented to the surgery and within two years the woman died.

Case No. 2.

A well known scientist whom we'll call Johnson was working with the highest scientific bodies in the U.S.A. He decided he had had enough of the rat race and retired to a farm in the New England states. He was not a raw fooder. He was not a hygienist, but he did have his own ideas concerning food and fasting.

On the farm he purchased, he built a shelter which was supposed to guard him even against an atomic bomb attack, which he considered a likelihood in the not too distant future.

He decided to undergo a long fast. After he had been on the fast for about 15 days, he called a local doctor for a bit of counsel. Then a few days later while still on the fast he called another doctor in the area for further advice. Now you and I well know that medical

438

doctors know nothing about fasting and they are positively opposed to it.

Within 48 hours a State Trooper drove into his farm driveway. He knocked at the door and he asked Mr. Johnson if he could come in and talk to him. Mr. Johnson invited him in and they had a chat.

The State Trooper asked Mr. Johnson some questions and after the questions he asked Mr. Johnson if he would accompany him to their office. Mr. Johnson consented and instead of driving him to an office he took him to a mental institution and there he was committed.

He remained there for some months. In fact, he lost track of time. They forced him to accept medication, which included tranquilizers and he realized the chances were he would never, never leave the institution.

One day he was called down because some visitor was there to see him. When he went to the visitor's room there was his sister with a lawyer and a preacher . . . and of course the doctors of the institution. A heated argument began and the lawyer and the preacher demanded that he be taken to a Judge. The doctors refused, but eventually because of the lawyer's insistence and quoting of the law, he was taken before a Judge for a hearing.

All during this time, he was kept under tranquilizers. At the hearing the two doctors from the institution testifed that he was a sick man and it was not safe to allow him out of the institution, that he was dangerous, both to himself and to others.

Mrs. Johnson was called upon and because of the treatment with the tranquilizers she told them she didn't care where they left him, that he was all right in an institution. But his sister and the lawyer and the preacher insisted that he be allowed his freedom, realizing that he had been kept under sedation of some kind.

439

The Judge was hard-pressed about making a decision. Here was a man who didn't know enough to ask for his own freedom and didn't care. Here were two qualified doctors who said that he should not be permitted out. It so happened by a dint of fate that the Judge and the preacher knew each other. And only because of this did the Judge grant this man his freedom.

Case No. 3.

There was a provocative, talkative, health nut in California. He was bold, he was aggressive and permitted himself to be involved in various unorthodox movements. In any event, on one occasion he was arrested and committed to an institution.

There he was forced to take medication which included a wide variety of drugs and when he objected he was severely beaten and manhandled and as a result he was crippled for life.

Now I have not gone into details on any of these stories. And if any official or individual desires to investigate any one of the three from the ground up, I will furnish the names and addresses, for while the woman died of cancer, her husband is still alive and both of the other men are still alive.

The lesson to be learned from these three stories and I assure you there are many more with which I am acquainted, is that if you are going to go on a little fast, for example, or if you intend to live as a raw fooder, or as a hygienist, or you intend to go on any extended fast or purification program, you keep your mouth shut. Live as you like. Eat as you like. Fast if you want to. But don't make too much noise about it.

There was another man I knew . . . in fact, I still know him, he is still around. He drove an oil truck and he decided to go on a fast and he dropped in to see me. At that time he had been on the fast for 3 days during which he drank nothing but water. When he told me what he was doing I was aghast. I said, "Fasting may be all right. The fast may do you good, but in heaven's name, don't tell anyone what you are doing because, sure as you're born, within the next day or two the word will get around and the police will pick you off the street, with your truck, and ground your truck and take you to the bughouse. Now be sensible, man. Either you go off your fast, or keep your mouth shut".

He decided to keep his mouth shut and I swear and attest to you that he fasted for 14 days and worked every single day and worked hard. I didn't believe this could be done. In fact, I thought it would be dangerous, especially if you have to work — and driving that huge truck was not easy work.

But he did it. He lost more than 20 pounds while he was doing it and he claims when he finished he felt better than he ever had in his whole life.

But had the word gone out about what he was doing, he would likely have been picked up and his family would have had a mighty hard time getting him out of the looney house. And yet the man was as sane as sane can be.

I hope that I have made my point clear. And remember, I'm not justifying anything, nor taking sides one way or another. I'm just casually handing out some advice to you, that if you are going to do some of these offbeat things, don't make too much noise about it.

CHAPTER

72

ABOUT DRUGS

If there is a monster — a hideous, dangerous, deadly, death-dealing monster — on the face of the earth today, it is drugs. I am sorry, ladies and gentlemen, but I do not have one single kind word to say about drugs.

Oh, yes, I am very, very familiar with the medical adage and have heard many M.D.'s state, for example, that aspirin is our best and our most useful drug and the medical profession could hardly get along without it. Well, to me aspirin is nothing but a poison that can do naught but harm — serious or less serious, depending on the amount used — but harm it does do everyone who uses it. Every single aspirin that is taken by any individual does a degree of harm. But aspirin, while it is one of the most insidious or hardest to recognize harmful drugs, is still by no means the most harmful.

A well known doctor of high repute and rank made the bold and clear-cut statement to me that he was taught in medical school — one of the first things he was taught — that there is no such thing as a harmless drug. Therefore, it is obvious and clear that the medical profession knows the harm or the deadliness in drugs. When I say this I mean that some doctors know this or many doctors know it or that some doctors remember it . . . because an awful pile of doctors do not accept this last statement that I made; that is, that there is no such thing as a harmless drug, in spite of the fact that that is what is stated in medical school.

The doctors who recognize that drugs are harmful boldly state that while they recognize the harm, the danger and the side effects of drugs, still when a patient who is suffering comes to them it is their duty to relieve that suffering and they do it in the best manner that they know . . . and some drugs are the best method that they know. Well, who can argue with that kind of logic? Who could act otherwise? Who can deny a suffering person relief that only drugs can bring?

I recall many years ago a nephew of mine gave me this argument and I replied, "Why don't you tell the patient the truth, that his trouble is caused, for example, by his way of eating and if he would change his way of eating he wouldn't need to take the drug and he wouldn't have the pain or the trouble?"

He said, "Uncle, I tried that, please believe me, and in most cases I lost the patronage of that patient and in some cases the patient stood up and said to me, 'I didn't come to you to get a lecture about what I should eat or what I should do or how I should live. I came to you to get medication to relieve my condition. Will you give it to me or will I go somewhere else?' "

My nephew claimed that because of this general, widespread attitude he changed his tactics and he metes out to his patients the kind of treatment that they expect, request or demand.

For years I blamed the medical men for the boom in the drug

business but I have learned to change my mind about this. The drug men have millions if not billions of dollars to spend on promotion in a thousand different ways. In fact, they use every way known. So they orient the individual to take drugs, to need drugs, to desire drugs and to demand them.

I see this every day of my life . . . among my employees, among my friends, my relatives and my associates. They have been conditioned through the mass media of the newspapers, magazines, radio and television that drugs are the things they need. The lack of aspirin gives them a headache. The lack of a tranquilizer makes them restless. The lack of laxatives makes them constipated. The lack of a diuretic fills them with urine. The lack of murine makes their eyes sore and itchy. And this goes on and on and on.

I maintain that every drug in the world causes various side effects. It is agreed that some of the side effects are slight and some are very noticeable, but they increase in severity to the extent that some are absolutely deadly. In many instances − in fact, in most instances − the drugs create a worse condition or a more serious condition and a longer lasting condition than the disease or sickness they were supposed to cure. In fact, I am acquainted with innumerable cases of people who have for years suffered with a condition brought about by the drug that they used for some other condition. These are known as iatrogenic diseases and various authorities give various figures and they claim that anywhere up to 30% of all the diseases treated in the hospitals are caused by medically prescribed drugs.

Just for a moment I would like to deal with one drug, cortisone. It has been heralded as the miracle drug of the ages. It brings relief to suffering people when no other drug or treatment would be of help and it is still a very widely used drug. Yet in spite of the full knowledge that it brings serious harm − in fact, in most cases they know it will do more harm than the relief it brings − doctors still use it and I presume patients request it or expect it. Cortisone is positively known to cause or bring about conditions that can never be cured . . . cataract is one of them. Yet so many people

445

take cortisone for comparatively simple conditions. But people just don't want to suffer. They want to get rid of the condition that is bothering them today and never mind the condition that may strike them tomorrow. Today is when they want relief . . . instantly. You know this is the day of "instants". Everybody wants everything instant.

As I see it, the tragic thing about drugs is that they are in every case given to sick people. Now everyone knows that a person who is ill, ailing or suffering needs understanding, needs guidance, needs help, but by giving him a drug you are doing just the opposite. Remember, he is sick . . . his body is in a weakened and broken down condition. He needs good food, he needs a gentle hand, he needs guidance and leadership, and not poisons. We have been taught and we know not to rub salt into an open wound, so why would we inject poisonous, harmful, deadly drugs into the body of a sick and ailing or suffering man? Yet the sicker the man is, the closer he is to death's door and the more he is suffering, the more potent is the drug that is administered.

Tell me, folks, tell me, please . . . does that make sense? Even to a moron or a half-wit, does it make sense? It's worse than flogging a sick man! It's worse than kicking a man when he is down! It's as bad as burying a man alive. That's what I think about drugs!

Believe me, I am fully aware of the tremendous advantages of drugs in surgery as well as in hundreds of different conditions, for example, anti-hemorrhagic drugs so necessary in surgery. However, I advocate the kind of living that will eliminate 99% of all surgical operations. What I said about drugs still stands.

CHAPTER 73

CYCLAMATES, SACCHARIN AND MONOSODIUM GLUTAMATE

I have won a great and glorious victory. I have lived to see the cyclamates labeled for what they are . . . a cause of cancer and many other diseases . . . and they have been ordered removed from the supermarket shelves. Saccharin is admittedly considered suspect as a cause of cancer. And at the same time I achieved another great victory. Monosodium glutamate was removed from children's foods and perhaps from some other foods as well.

I am kicking up my heels and dancing with glee
I am jubilant for I have won a great victory.

But in this sweet hour the taste in my mouth grows sour because I see already that my triumph is turning out to be a Pyrrhic victory. The heat of the battle has not even died down and I see the enemy forces have already been recruited. I suspect that they allowed us to win this so-called victory, so that we might let down our guard and be battered into submission forever. No I am not fooling, I mean every word.

Already the new evil forces are on the market. For example, there are (1) ammoniated glycyrrhizin, (2) "Wonder Sweet" modified saccharin, (3) a dipeptide sweetener known as Aspartyl phenylalanine methyl ester, (4) a sugar substitute that uses glycine, one of the amino acids generically referred to as amino acetic acid.

So we were victorious and we licked the cyclamates . . . but now we have five greater and stronger enemies to contend with. Oh, what a great victory we won! Remember these forces have billions to spend and they know how and where to spend it to do the most good . . . for their cause. They never allow us to win a great victory until they have an even greater defeat in store for us. Don't underestimate them, they are all powerful.

And now to the MSG and our other great victory. Already they have at least three substitutes to take the place of the one that has fallen. Again I fear that the three substitutes are all much more harmful, much more deadly than the one that we have vanquished.

They are called by the soothing simple sounding names of Hydrolized vegetable protein, Disodium Inosinate, Disodium Guanylate — all of which contain supposed flavor-enhancing qualities in strengths greater than M.S.G.

The increase in strength ranges from two to three times as great as the "original toxic substance".

I have read of no animal tests made to establish the safety of these products but no doubt some were made by the chemical manufacturers but sufficient time has not elapsed to establish any great certainty one way or another. However, a most interesting sidelight comes into focus on this occasion. I suggest that the chemical boys were not caught by surprise for these relief substitutes had been warming up in the bull pen for some time, awaiting the nod to be called to the mound when ageing old MSG was knocked out of the box.

This was exactly the case with sodium cyclamates.

How long will the chemical boys continue to traffic in human health and life as though they were but pawns in a gigantic game of chess?

Again I say, oh, what great victories we've won!

CHAPTER

74

THE HARM OF FOOD PROCESSING

According to the latest figures obtainable it is learned there are at least 3,000 different additives that are allowed in food. Some authorities claim that there are closer to 4,000 different food additives used today by the food processing industry. Of course the chemicals used vary tremendously in name and in chemical structure but there is one thing that they all have in common and that is that all of them, 100%, are harmful to the animal anatomy and they do absolutely nothing to improve the nutritional quality or the health-giving properties of the food itself. This is a positive, direct, unequivocal statement and therefore I feel it is vital and important to repeat it. Not one of those up to 4,000 chemical food additives brings any benefits or adds any nutritional value to the food in which it is used.

You have the right to ask, "If they don't improve the food,

what are they used for?" Ah, that's a most disturbing question. Those food additives perform many functions, some of them even believed or claimed to be useful. One of these is, they retard biological deterioration. Everyone knows of the scheme of nature . . . a seed sprouts and grows, bears its flower and later fruits and then goes back from whence it came to complete the cycle. Food chemicals are used in many different ways to retard, to slow down, to prevent or to stop this normal biological cycle. It is granted that the chemicals do retard spoilage and thus permit food to be stored or to be shipped long distances and to be kept virtually from one season to another. In the olden days many natural ways and means were resorted to, to perform the same function. Every farmer, for example, had his root celler and later a cold storage room or plant.

Chemical food additives are used for many other reasons — for coloring, or as it is referred to for cosmetic purposes to prevent signs of deterioration, to make people think it is fresh when it is really stale — and I could go on endlessly but the point that I am intent upon making is that none of these food additives benefits the health and well being of the human body, be it the newborn infant, the child, the adolescent or the adult. Healthwise, you get absolutely nothing. In fact, as I have constantly pointed out, you receive varying degrees of injury and harm.

Apart from the chemical additives there are other ways in which food processing does serious harm to our food supply. For example our fruits and vegetables are washed in harmful detergents, they are blanched, they are irradiated, they are frozen, they are candied and many are dehydrated. In every one of these processes some serious or casual losses occur. Of course in the process many or most of the water soluable vitamins are lost, depending on the kind of produce, and a great deal of the vitamin C is lost in the process.

Fruits, for example, are usually sulphured and this process has long been regarded with grave suspicion. Normally, if you were to dry peaches or apricots or even apples in the sun you would find that the fruit would become dark. In fact, so dark as to render it

452

unattractive to the average individual's eyes but the sulphuring process does much for industry. First, it prevents the loss of most of the natural juices. This of course increases weight. A thoroughly sun dried apricot, for example, weighs just one seventh of its original weight. In other words, it takes seven pounds of fresh apricots to make one pound of dried apricots by the sun method but by the sulphuring process I doubt if they lose more than half their weight. Then the sulphuring permits the fruit to emerge a sort of golden colour which is attractive to the eye but the damage to the vitamins, specifically the thiamin and vitamin C is deplorable.

I might also add that in the sulphuring process fruit is often washed and cut and various forms of heat, various forms of solvents, detergents and other chemicals are used.

The freezing process is generally regarded as safe and it is assumed that only a small nutritional loss is incurred but usually the fruits or the vegetables are washed or blanched or dipped before undergoing the freezing and further losses are inflicted. Just exactly how much loss occurs to food in freezing has not been positively established but even if the loss is negligible in the freezing much harm appears to result in the thawing process. Then if we go one step further and we cook the defrosted, frozen food the loss now becomes tragic. It is also unfortunate that so many people regard freezing as harmless and they practically assume that frozen food is as good as fresh food. Nothing could be farther from the truth.

Of all the harm that the food processing industry does to food — and ultimately to our bodies — none is greater than the harm they do to cereals and grains. My own experience and investigations have taught me that grains and seeds, for example wheat, barley, oats, rye, corn, buckwheat, sesame, flax, millet and rice are excellent foods in themselves and capable of giving almost complete nutrition to the human body. However, in their natural form they are considered not palatable or attractive enough to induce buyers to eat them. So, the processor goes to work and removes or as he calls it refines away various components with the result that he presents to the public a food that is probably more palatable and attractive because they usually add sugar, glucose or other sweetening agents, but it's practically devoid of any nutritive content. The many processes and the milling usually alter the nutritional value of the food by removing various parts of the grains' nutritional factors. This, of course, means the removal of vitamins and minerals and even the good part of the protein and part of the carbohydrate values. Actually, in the refining and the processing the heart and the soul of the food is removed.

Besides this, various processes are performed like the bleaching of flour with various chemical treatments. Chlorine is usually used in this process and various minerals are lost or rendered unassimilable . . . for example, copper, iron, zinc, manganese, potassium, cobalt and others are removed or lost. The rice is polished, the barley is pearled and all along the line the various wholesome grains are devitalized. Of course the millers and the processors will tell you that all this is taken care of by their enrichment program. They actually, as I said before, remove the heart and soul of the living organism and replace it with a few fragments of synthetic chemicals and pretend that all is well and that the needs of the human body are taken care of.

Food processing has grown in America to become a tremendous vital industry in our economy but no industry does more harm to the health of the American people.

CHAPTER

75

DO THEY KNOW WHAT THEY DO?

I'm sure all of you are acquainted with the famous saying "Father, forgive them, for they know not what they do". I feel sure that all of us within our hearts can forgive an error, especially an error in judgement or even an error due to ignorance.

Today in America we have a sick, sick nation. I claim sicker than any nation on earth including India, Pakistan or you name the nation. The incidence of sickness and disease in America is higher than in any country in the world. If you don't believe me or wish to take issue with me on the subject, before you do, I suggest that you get a copy of the official statistical abstract of the United States. Get the 1972 issue or the latest one you can and then look under the vital statistics and see the number of sick people. Make inquiries concerning the number of people suffering from the leading causes of death; heart disease and cancer. And while you're at it look up the number of people suffering from arthritis, emphysema, diabetes, rheumatoid arthritis and go all the way down the list until you reach the number of retarded children or children and individuals in institutions of various kinds throughout our vast America. You will find the numbers so high they will stagger you.

If you want further information call your local Cancer Society or your Heart Society or your Diabetic Society or Muscular Dystrophy Group and ask them the number of people sick and ailing with their specific disease. Until you investigate you'll not realize that I speak the gospel truth.

Now if you believe me then the next question that should come into your mind is, "Why are all these people sick?" We have the best supply of food of any nation in the world, we have the best variety of food of any nation of the world. We have the best transportation system which will enable us to get the food from every corner of the country into the other corner. We have the highest standards of hygiene and cleanliness . . . all of this should add up to health and long life and freedom from disease. Now add a little more — keep your pencil handy — the number of doctors in America, the number of nurses, the number of hospitals and the hospital beds, the number of institutions for the sick and ailing. Then take a look at the number of drug corporations and the number of drugs that they make and the quantities of each drug they make . . . my friend you'll come up with some staggering figures. O.K., we're back to our original question. With all the facilities for health why are we all so sick?

The number one enemy in my sincere opinion is processed food. Number two enemy is the chemical additives in our food. Number three, the chemical fertilizers and sprays and dusts supplied to our soils and crops. Number four, drugs. Number five, beverages. Every bit of food that you consume apart from the fruits or berries and vegetables that you grow in your own garden has been treated with chemicals. In order to increase shelf-life various chemicals are added. In order to make the canned goods stand up well chemicals are added. In order to retain the color, the firmness, the quality, the appearance or 101 other purposes chemicals are added. All of this makes us sick. Oh yes, I realize that you are going to tell me that the Food and Drug and various other arms of the government protect us and make sure that no harmful chemicals can be used in food. Sure, that's quite all right if that's what you want to believe. Belief is one thing, fact is another.

Every single chemical used in food processing can and does cause serious harm to the human anatomy.

The next question is, does the Food and Drug, does the Department of Agriculture, do the processors, do the distillers and the brewers, the manufacturers of tobacco and the chemical corporations and the fertilizer manufacturers realize or know the harm they are doing? I maintain that every employee in these corporations from the sweeper of the floors to the secretary or the technicians or the president knows exactly what he's doing. No man can be alive and educated and breathing in North America today without realizing positively that chemicals do harm — serious harm, devastating harm. I've talked through the years to hundreds of people who are employed or are in management of these corporations. In each case my conversation leads me to believe without a shadow of doubt that they realize full well the harm in the products that they sell and the same applies to doctors who administer drugs and surgery. They know the harm they do but a Cadillac and a $100,000. home and all the nice things that money can buy are great blinkers. Bribery has been used, I presume, since the world began and for a thousand dollars or a hundred thousand dollars or a million dollars a man can fail to see that which is staring him right in the face. For the promise of a better paying job with more money and security like the chemical corporations offer to various or certain Food and Drug employees, it is easy to understand why they wouldn't recognize their own best friend. Obviously the stakes are high and that is why so many employees who were once with the Food and Drug are now employed by the chemical corporations.

Furthermore, for a number of years people like myself have challenged all of these organizations to a debate in public concerning

457

the harm or the merit of their products but they never accept the challenge, they never will. The same applies to the people who are fighting for fluoridation. They will never at any time meet people like me who oppose fluoridation. In fact, the fluoride people warn them not to get into arguments or debates because they can't substantiate their claims.

This all adds up to what I'm trying to say . . . that these people all know the harm they do, the damage they do and the criminality they perform. But then you bring in the fact that they, too, have children and loved ones. However, by the same token I suggest that cigarette manufacturers smoke and probably their wives and children smoke and I presume that the distillers' wives and children use liquor and that the wives and children of the employees of the Coca Cola company or the beverage companies use their products as well. But again I admit that I cannot always explain the workings in men's minds but perhaps all of this can be justified for an income of $50,000, $75,000 or even $100,000 or more a year.

Then you might say to me, "Now Tobe, it's not all black and white . . . there is probably a gray in their somewhere". In my eyes where sickness and death are involved there should be no gray but unfortunately there is. For years, many years I went along with the belief that these people or organizations did not know the harm they did but I found out to my sorrow that I was wrong that they did know the harm they did. For example, there was a product called Nujol that was sold widely throughout America about 50 years ago. It was the most popular laxative in America and the oil people made millions on it even in those days. Then the thing crashed because some researcher discovered that when people used this product and thought it was wonderful for a laxative for it gave the imbiber regular bowel movements that were smooth as the purring of a kitten it also caused serious diseases by preventing the absorption of valuable nutrients by the body. O.K., this was conclusively proven. Absolutely without argument it was a positive, scientific fact and sales dropped to zero. As far as I know it was never completely off the market; they just didn't advertise it.

458

Now 50 years later they're back. These big shots just waited until the shouting and the tumult died and then they brought it back again to make many more millions. I could show you various repetitions of a similar nature. A drug is brought on the market and then found to be deadly . . . like thalidomide that caused all the troubles with the deformed children. Well, they are not letting thalidomide die, they just let it lie dormant for a few years and now they are bringing it back for supposedly other purposes and benefits . . . so don't tell me that these boys don't know what they're doing.

That's it, you have my story. They know what they do, they do it deliberately and also with the positive intent and idea of getting rich and they are getting rich and America is becoming sicker and sicker with each succeeding day. I'm standing here before you and am telling you, the day of reckoning is coming. Old fogeys like myself who have passed 66 will not commit mayhem. We're not tuned to violence but there is a younger generation coming up . . . they're the ones who are being harmed more than anyone because they haven't had a chance from the day that they were conceived, let alone from the day they were born. They owe all their misfortunes, all the harm that is being done to their bodies and to their minds to these purveyors of death, slow death, and I think that when the time comes they'll know how to handle these purveyors.

For me it doesn't make much difference but I have warned them . . . they'd best mend their ways before it is too late. But I know they won't and then it will be too late.

CHAPTER 76

NUREMBURG TRIALS FOR FOOD PROCESSORS AND CHEMICAL CORPORATIONS

If you are a member, either as an employee or an executive of any one of these corporations I am predicting that the day will come sooner than you think that you may be held to account for the crimes that you have committed. Now I'm speaking directly to all people who are connected with the food processing industry and the chemical corporations, be it agricultural chemicals or drug chemicals. Yes, the list will include soft drink makers, tobacco manufacturers, distillers, brewers and vintners as well as those who harm people by polluting the air that they breathe and the water they drink.

There were the Nuremburg trials after World War II. Most people, I think, have heard of these trials. Anyone connected with the war crimes was brought to trial and held to account for his part in the murder or the killing of millions of innocent people. I am

461

making a direct prediction in stating that such a trial will be held in the 1900's, maybe in a year or two wherein the people responsible for curtailing the lives of millions of Americans or causing them to die will be charged, brought to trial and punished for their crime against the American people. O.K., go ahead — you can laugh all you like and think that at last Tobe has gone berserk. But I'm telling you now and I feel it in my bones that these trials will be held and people will be brought to account and people will be made to pay for the crimes they committed and condoned. This will also include members of the government and government agencies who permitted this to happen. In fact, they will be more to blame than the processors because they could have prevented this horrible disaster.

It is my opinion that the crimes of the processors is much more serious than the crime of the war criminals. In the case of the war criminals there was a war on and it has been said here and there and everywhere that all's fair in love and war. Therefore, they committed these crimes in the heat of passion with war raging and therefore there is some form of excuse but what excuse do the food processors and the chemical corporations and the drug makers have? Ignorance . . . you know, they know and I know that "they know what they do".

They know what they do because they are spending billions of dollars apart from selling their wares to justify their actions. They are hiring the best mouthpieces and the best writers and commanding space in the best advertising news media in the world to promolgate the lie that the organic nuts, the raw fooders and the health nuts and the anti-polluters are wrong and crazy. I repeat, they are spending millions or billions of dollars to justify their actions. Therefore, they know what they are doing and this fact that I have mentioned just now will be the prime proof at the trials that they knowingly committed these crimes.

There are between 3,000 and 4,000 chemicals used in food as of the present day. It is admitted by the best authorities that more than half of them — and I say more than three quarters of them — have never been tested or proven for their safety or harm. Yet, the

Food and Drug Regulations permit them to be used in the food of infants, pregnant women, children, boys and girls, adolescents, adults and old people. The same situation exists with drugs that are used in medicine. The creators of these drugs and medicines do not try them on their own families and friends . . . no, they put them on the market and get paid for them and if and when enough people drop dead sometimes the Food and Drug ask the drug barons to remove them from the market and for your enlightenment this is not always done. The drug manufacturers frequently refuse to take the drug off the market in spite of the harm it does. With drugs there is some excuse, vague as it may be, but with food additives, with agricultural chemicals there is no excuse.

Of course the purpose of these products is apparent and obvious . . . to make money for someone. I do not object to people making money, I do object to people being poisoned, harmed, crippled and destroyed in the process. While I mentioned at the start that these people will be brought to trial, you may ask, "Well, who is going to bring them to trial?" Most certainly it will not be the present government. That is right, but the present government is not the government of tomorrow. The present thinking is not the thinking of tomorrow. The present legislators are not the legislators of tomorrow. Christ said, "The meek shall inherit the earth". It is the meek who will conduct these trials and when the sentence is brought down believe me, it will not be meek.

If I were a food processor or a manufacturer of agricultural or drug chemicals or one of the other manufacturers that do umbrage to the human frame I'd begin to worry. I mean exactly what I say. I know as sure as the sun rises that that day is coming soon, much sooner than they know. I think the Nuremburg trials have begun. The public is waking up and the more money these harm doers spend on justifying their nefarious practices the harder it will go with them.

I realize that most people will regard my prediction of the Nuremburg type trial that I have suggested as being a figment of my imagination. Say what you will, but in my mind's eye I see these trials already in the making and I am stating clearly that it won't be long now. Start building your defence now . . . you'll need it.

CHAPTER

77

FOOD ENRICHMENT

Just what does food enrichment mean?

To begin with, I am a suspicious individual. When somebody tells me he is going to make me rich, I clamp my hands on my pockets and become cautious. Perhaps that proves I am a non-cooperative member of society.

The most commonly used term of enrichment is for flour. Because I have a horticultural background, I know that it's impossible to improve upon the nutritional qualities of a seed. Whether the seed be large like a coconut or tiny like a petunia, I am just unintelligent enough to believe that man cannot improve upon either one. Perhaps if I had a university degree and my mind had been trained and brainwashed by brilliant professors I could have learned to accept the thesis that man can make a better job of things than nature. I am

465

convinced that it takes many years of study and hard training to take a young untrained student and change him into a dyed-in-the-wool believer in the magic of science.

A farmer takes a wheat seed and he plants it and maybe he gets 20 or 30 wheat seeds back for his investment and labor. His wife takes some of these wheat seeds and grinds them up and makes flour and from the flour she makes bread and that is eaten. The result is sound nutrition and a sound body and mind. The brainwashed scientist comes along and when he grinds the wheat he removes most or part of the outer coat and the germ and feeds this to the hogs and the rest is food for man. At first the people got sick and died so the scientist studied a little more and he came up with the idea that if he added some synthetic vitamins he could then balance things up and everything would be O.K. So he did that and today the world accepts enriched white flour as the thing to make bread with.

Now remember, science does all these fearful and wonderful things for the benefit of mankind — so it says. Anyway, we are supposedly enriched by the addition of these synthetic substances to our flour and we are supposed to grow stronger, bigger, healthier and live longer. And you are not supposed to doubt this . . . this is an established scientific fact. And if you say it isn't, then you're a dope, you're a dullard, you're a food faddist, you're a crank, you're a fink and you might even be a quack.

I have described the general process of the enrichment of flour to you but the same thing could be said of many other substances that have been likewise enriched. Margarine is another notable example. Plain ordinary farm butter made from unpasteurized milk from a healthy cow is, according to the scientists, not as good as fortified margarine. They tell us margarine is the "superior spread", whatever that is supposed to indicate.

Come with me and let's do a little rationalizing with my non-scientific, untrained, unschooled brain . . . and let's see what I've got to say.

466

(1) I maintain that if any substance or food, as they call it, requires enrichment or fortification, then it is not a fit food for man or beast. In simple terminology, it is a toxic substance or a poison.

(2) If and when a substance requires enrichment it is, in cold direct language, a tacit admission that the health of the public has been impaired, usually for many years, by eating this substance before it was fortified.

(3) If it has been fortified, then you have to contend with the toxic substances that were added. Remember, it is never a whole or wholesome food that is added, usually it is a synthetic chemical.

(4) When enrichment or fortification is mentioned or used it is a positive attempt by the processor to use leger de main to becloud an issue. Further it is an admission that something good was removed and something inferior was substituted.

(5) It is clear-cut that when they want to fortify anything, what might have been a food before is now a questionable food substitute.

(6) Enrichment or fortification indicates that the substance being fortified is an imitation or a counterfeit of a food.

(7) In my kindergarten days I was taught a rhyme about Humpty Dumpty who had a great fall and the tale related that all the King's horses and all the King's men could never put Humpty Dumpty together again. It is just as true that you cannot reconstitute a seed so that it will grow again, especially after you have removed or destroyed some of its parts, any more than a butcher can put together a dissected and dismembered animal and make it breathe again.

(8) In many or most cases the fortification or enrichment substitute is a synthetic chemical substance that cannot be properly absorbed, assimilated or metabolized by the animal body.

467

(9) The United States Department of Agriculture in 1965 published a bulletin called "Dietary Levels of Householders in the United States" in which it was stated that poor diets are increasing among the American people. I maintain that the food enrichment policy is at least partially responsible.

(10) The health of the nation would clearly indicate that the enrichment or fortification program has failed. Any informed, unbiased individual can plainly see it.

(11) They are now talking seriously of adding additional iron — synthetic iron, of course — to food or enriching our food with additional iron. I ask, "Why do they take the natural iron out in the first place?"

(12) It is further indicated in the food processing literature that they want to add vitamin E to foods, especially margarine.

This food fortification and enrichment program has been going on now for about 40 years. For them to come along now and suggest further fortification and enrichment, lets the cat out of the bag or should I say, permits a foul odor to permeate the atmosphere.

They have been telling us for years that the enrichment program builds strong bodies and what else and now they're admitting that they need further fortification and enrichment . . . which means that all along for 40 or 50 years we have been fooled. We have been made sick and our children have been harmed because the fortification and enrichment program did not do what it was supposed to do. Who is to pay for the millions of bodies that were damaged and their years of life that were lost?

O.K., let's face the situation fairly and squarely. If any one of you were naive enough to believe that a thief who held you up and robbed you would leave you with more money than you started out with, then you've got to be out of your mind, to say the least. Why would any processor or bandit enrich you to a greater extent than you were to begin with, unless there was a motive?

468

The story is as clear as crystal. They removed these substances from food to serve their own purposes ... in truth, to fortify and enrich themselves and their stock-holders and their directors. I do not suggest that making money and a profit in America is a crime but I do suggest that robbing our food of its vital nutrients and substituting a few synthetic chemicals is one of the greatest crimes of all time.

The statistics from the bulletin called "Dietary Levels of Householders in the United States" put out by the U.S. Department of Agriculture showed that in 1955, 15 per cent of the people in America were found to have poor diets. In 1965, it was 20 percent. In 1955, 60 percent of the people were supposed to have good diets. In 1965, it was down to 50 percent. Therefore, it must be admitted that our eating habits have changed for the worse ... and this does not only refer to low income bracket households. The high income households were affected every bit as much or more.

This would all indicate that by following the advice of the food processors, the government and the American Medical Association, our health is failing badly. Truth will out!

CHAPTER 78

SATAN'S BROWNIES — FOOD ADDITIVES

Are food additives really necessary?

I go on record as stating, boldly and lucidly, that no chemical additive should ever be used in food. This statement will be ridiculed and bombarded, I'm sure, from every side. But I still stand squarely before you and say that all food additives are either harmful or potentially harmful.

The opposition will immediately say that if it weren't for food additives we couldn't support our teeming populations nor could they have the variety or the quality or the color or the beauty or the attractiveness of the foods that we now are accustomed to. This is the same pitch that is given to justify the widespread use of chemical fertilizers, dusts and sprays. Well, with part of these assertions I will have to agree, but to completely counteract their

471

argument I would state that in America there are probably 100,000 people who live and enjoy life without having any additives in their food.

The number I mentioned is just a guess . . . it may be much, much greater, I am sure it is not less . . . but I am among that number. I would say that my diet for the past fifteen years has been 99% free of food additives. I emphatically maintain and claim that you do not have to have additives in your food.

I still get some additives when I eat some toast in a restaurant when I am travelling and I may get some additives in a bite or two of meat that I might eat when I am out.

Now I will go one step further and I will boldly maintain that no food additive was ever added for the benefit of the consumer. The opposition can bark themselves black and blue in the face but if they will allow me to enter the argument I can prove to any reasonable man or woman that no additive was ever put into food for the benefit of the consumer.

I maintain that, of the thousands of people who get sick every year in America due to food poisoning, in practically every case this food poisoning was due to the chemical additives in the food and the unusual bacterial changes rather than because the food was bad. When an individual eats a food that has turned or is beginning to putrefy, it will not poison him or kill him. The worst it can do is turn his stomach and his stomach knows what to do under such conditions . . . or he may get diarrhea. However, in most cases it will never reach his stomach because his stomach will refuse it.

I claim that no food was ever nutritionally improved by the inclusion of an additive. Yes, in this instance I am including such things as improvers or enriching agents. In the first place, most of the enrichers are synthetic chemicals and some or most of them are unassimilable by the human anatomy.

I claim no chemical food additive is without its harmful or

poisonous effects. Further, no food has ever been nutritionally enhanced or improved by additives. Therefore you have a right to ask, "What is the purpose of a food additive?" Of course the purpose is bold and clear . . . to make money for the processors.

No, I have absolutely no objection to anyone making money, as long as he makes it honestly and not at the expense of making his fellow man sick, or killing him outright. There is plenty of room for food processing without the use of chemical additives.

I would be willing to stake my life that if an edict were passed notifying the food processing industry that no chemical food additives would be tolerated within a two year period, they would have just as big a variety, they would have just as big a sale and they would have better foods and they would be preserved by natural means and methods. But it would take a little bit of adjusting, it would take a little bit of effort and perhaps a bit more watchfulness and care.

Chemicals do a marvelous job. They perform like a robot. When a chemical is put into a food, it has been tested to do the job it's supposed to do . . . whether it is to add color, to stabilize, to emulsify, to kill bacteria, to enhance flavor, to prevent oxidation, to acidify, to prevent caking or any one of many other functions. And they perform these functions to perfection. The only thing wrong with it is that each and every one of them causes harm of varying degrees and nature.

The U.S. Department of Health, Education and Welfare, under whom the Food and Drug Administration operates, makes the following statement in one of their little booklets, under the heading "Responsible Industry Helps":

"Law-abiding manufacturers and dealers need the protection of the law. It guards them against unfair competition by inferior or dishonestly labeled goods. The self-policing and voluntary compliance activities of the regulated industries contribute greatly to consumer protection. Coupled with effective enforcement, such activities help

473

to assure public confidence in the quality of American foods, drugs, and cosmetics — the best in the world."

This little "rider" that they have put in the bulletin sounds very nice and very good, but it doesn't tell you that this is actually a disclaimer and if you got sick or ill or died because of some food that you ate, the manufacturer could say that he met the Food and Drug regulations and standards and therefore you would have no claim against him. So you see, it's not protecting the public . . . it is, as I have contended for years, really protecting the food processor. Now get that straight!

In the same booklet, there is a group of laws and one states: "Sets safe limits on the amount of pesticide residues that may remain on food crops, and checks shipments to see that these limits are observed."

Well, everybody knows that they permitted the wide use of DDT and it practically polluted our planet. Are they the safe limits that the Food and Drug were talking about?

Another one of the laws states that the Food and Drug "Passes on the safety of colors for use in foods, drugs, or cosmetics, and tests and certifies each batch manufactured where necessary."

Does that mean that the deadly red dye that the food industry uses is not harmful? Why, it's been proven harmful time and time again, even by the Food and Drug!

Then you might ask why it is permitted. Because so much pressure is brought to bear upon the bosses or the heads of the Department of Food and Drug they cannot demand its removal. Yet the Food and Drug have the temerity or guts to say that it passes on the safety of colors for use in foods. That, I say, is a damnable lie!

Still, in this instance I am not blaming the Food and Drug. I am blaming those who permit those violations to occur. The Food and Drug do try to do a job.

The use of chemical additives in food has risen from 419 million pounds in 1955 to 661 million pounds in 1965 and 850 million pounds in 1970, and it is estimated that it will be 1.03 billion pounds in 1975.

It is my serious and informed contention after years of study and observation that thousands or tens of thousands of people die every year in America because of the cumulative effects of added chemicals in foods and drugs. Is there no one to say a word for these who pay with their lives?

I have been presenting this kind of an argument to people now for at least fifteen years. For ten of those fifteen years I got absolutely nowhere. I was ridiculed, I was laughed at, I was called a crack-pot, a faddist or a nut, but I knew I was right then as I am now and I persisted. Now as of the last few years the public and even the newspapers are becoming conscious that something is wrong and there seems to be a general re-awakening.

I am positively sure that many people believe that I hate everybody, including the food processors and the chemical corporations and the Food and Drug. Well, please believe me, I don't hate them at all. I may hate what they do but I'm not a hater, anyway. I have no quarrel with anyone without just and due cause.

I will agree that many of these processors and drug firms act in good faith. Still, I also know that many of them realize the harm they are doing but they permit themselves to be blinded by the fact that they are making a heck of a lot of money. For these people I have nothing but contempt and I regard them as despicable creatures ... and I know there are quite a few of them ... too many.

Believe it or not, I know people who were employed in these businesses and because of my writing and also the writing of others, they became aware of the evil that they were doing and they quit their jobs and found other employment. They have told me this and they said they were unhappy when they learned the truth and decided to do something that was not causing harm, degradation and

475

death to their fellow man. They went even further and said that they had nightmares because they felt that they had done harm to their friends, relatives and perhaps even to their own flesh and blood. Yes, one even made it a point to come and thank me for alerting him and he now has a job that allows him to live with a clear conscience.

Let's deal for a moment with another factor of this food chemical business. Would you be denied food that you enjoy or like because food additives would not be permitted? Well, go ahead and mention some of them and see if that is true.

Do you like ice cream? Well, you can make the best ice cream in the world by using only natural products and if ice cream is kept frozen, man, it should keep till hell freezes over without too much deteriorating. But who wants ice cream that is six months or six years old?

Take canned foods like tomatoes or peaches. By the simple process of heating the tomatoes or the peaches, they would keep for some years without any chemicals being added. Why do they put the chemicals in? No doubt there are many reasons ... to keep the product firm, to prevent it from losing its color or perhaps to improve its color. But we've all eaten peaches and tomatoes without these chemicals and they were good. So again I claim they are totally unnecessary.

Now let's take fish. Here is where I believe the additives do a lot of serious harm. Fish can be eaten fresh, fish can be canned and can be frozen. Fish forms an important part of my diet and I have used frozen fish for many long years without any trouble. I prefer it fresh but I'll accept the frozen if the other isn't available. Also, I will eat a can of sardines, herring or salmon. Why do we need additives? There is no legitimate reason that I can see, except as I said before to enable corporations to make millions.

The same applies to meat as to fish. But in these cases usually the meat is treated with chemicals to maintain or create better color. The public does not like dark colored meat, for example, so they put in the nitrates or nitrites to create the attractive bright red color. Well, I'd sooner eat dark meat without chemicals than red meat with chemical additives in it.

One of the most widely used and the most harmful of chemical additives is benzoate of soda. It is recognized as a deadly poison so they only allow it in quantities of 1/10 of 1%. But there is no inspector standing around watching that the percentage is not overdone. However I contend it is even deadly at 1/10 of 1%.

Well, they put the bit into the food — fish or jam, for example — and the benzoate of soda goes to work at once, killing every microorganism in that food and it is very effective at doing this job. So it has killed off everything in that food and the food is as dead as a doornail. You buy it and you eat it . . . so what? You eat dead food. You've eaten dead food before so that's nothing new. But . . . and there is a great big "but" here . . . the deadly benzoate of soda is very much alive. It only stops acting because it has killed off all of the organisms in that specific food, there is no more there to kill, but the moment it gets into your body it starts up again where it left off and continues its nefarious onslaught and begins to kill your body organisms . . . and that's where you begin to run into serious trouble. If you keep on eating a lot of food with benzoate of soda in it, you're going to find an awful lot of your essential organisms impaired, damaged or destroyed and it's apt to do the same thing to everyone who eats foods containing benzoate of soda.

Now this is a very simple example that I have given to you but it is absolutely true.

O.K., so you want to continue to eat food with additives . . . well, bless your dear heart, that is your privilege . . . continue to do so! But at least I have pointed out the dangers and also that they are completely unnecessary.

Now let me tell you something about the dollar value of these chemical food additives. In 1955 it was 172 million dollars, in 1965 it was 285 million dollars and in 1970 it was 400 million dollars. It is estimated that by 1975 the dollar value will rise to above 500 million dollars. This should clearly indicate why chemical food additives are so widely used in our food (not in my food if I can help it).

It is important to note that these figures do not include such widely used so-called food ingredients as sugar, salt and starch. These are not usually classed as food additives.

Records indicate that the food industry is the largest industry in America. The average American family spends more money on food than any other item on their budget.

To give the food processors' side in a short terse but adequate manner let me quote Dr. Emil M. Mrak, chancellor of the University of California.

"Convenience foods have literally disenslaved the housewife. They have permitted her to serve with ease a diversity of nutritious foods of consistent high quality . . . These great advances have been brought about through the work of chemists, their development of new processes, and the safe use of chemicals."

I take issue with the claim that these foods are "nutritious or of high quality or safe".

It is of importance to realize that besides the "intentional" chemical additives in food there are what is known as "non intentional" additives. These are such things as pesticides, plasticizers as contained in wrapping materials and packaging for food materials.

Let us seek a definition of a food additive. Here is what the Food Protection Committee of the National Academy of Science — National Research Council deems a food additive:

"A substance or a mixture of substances, other than a basic foodstuff, which is present in food as a result of any aspect of production, processing, storage or packaging".

You must agree that this definition covers a lot of ground and gives the processor tremendous latitude. Actually it means that he can use anything that his heart desires or that convenience and practice demands. Most certainly it does not offer the slightest protection or compensation to the user.

It is generally assumed that all the chemical food additives used in foods have been tested and proven safe by the Food and Drug Administration. This is not true – most of the chemical additives permitted in food have never been tested or proven safe.

There is another aspect of additives that you should know. It is what is known as "Gras" items. These GRAS (pronounced "grass") substances, which include pepper, cinnamon, baking powder, citric acid, monosodium glutamate, mono- and diglycerides, and about 575 other materials, did not have to undergo extensive or renewed animal testing to be approved as safe in foods. On the basis of somewhat tortured reasoning, these GRAS substances are not even considered food additives under the terms of the Food Additives Amendment.

To counteract such articles and attacks, for example like these that I write and make, the food processors state, "Under the poison per se doctrine, the property of being a poison is a characteristic inherent in certain substances. Some materials are poisons; others are not. The doctrine completely ignores the fact that every substance known is a poison to the human body if taken in large enough amounts. Drinking too much water or eating too much salt can kill you. The caffeine in coffee, the theobromine in cocoa, the oxalic acid in rhubarb – if taken in high enough doses – can be harmful, if not lethal. On the other hand, small amounts of arsenic (present in many natural foods) can be perfectly safe.

"Summing up the views of most scientists, Dr. Henry F. Smyth, Jr., an administrative fellow at Mellon Institute, says, 'There is no such thing as a class of substances that are poisons . . . A poison is simply too much.'

"The original Federal Food, Drug, and Cosmetic Act of 1938

479

naively supported the poison per se concept. It stated that no food would be allowed to contain an added substance if it was poisonous or deleterious (unless the substance was required to produce the food or if it could not be avoided in good manufacturing practice)."

To further illustrate what the food processors think of me I quote: "Obviously, a segment of the population does consider additives hazardous, if not in some cases lethal. They are all for eliminating additives from foods entirely. These are the people whom industry men frequently classify as crackpots, faddists, food quacks, or well-meaning but pitifully misinformed people. 'As far as knowledge of foods is concerned,' one company official bemoans, 'they are functional illiterates.'

"These are the people who automatically assume that natural foods are inherently good, but chemicals in foods are contaminants, adulterants, or poisons. They fail to realize, of course, that all food components are, in fact, chemicals.

"These are the people who, lacking knowledge, are driven by their wild, unreasoning fears. Often, these are fears aroused by books, magazines, or newspapers."

CHAPTER

79

FOOD FADDISIM IS HURTING
INDUSTRY IS FIGHTING BACK

I would like to discuss with you an article by Henry J. Heinz II who is the chairman of the H. J. Heinz Co. You might by accident know who they are.

He wrote this fine essay which is receiving wide publicity from the news media throughout America. I wonder if you could guess why. It could be that his company spends millions of dollars advertising but anyway it's getting a lot of publicity for free this time.

He tells us in the article that we are a nation of nutritional illiterates despite a wealth of scientific knowledge of nutrition. He tells us that many of us do not know what a balanced diet is. We have an abundant food supply, he goes on to tell us, our eating

481

habits are deteriorating and a U.S. Public Health Survey tells us that malnutrition has spread widely across the United States; in the case of children and infants food deficiencies are particularly serious and malnutrition in infants may cause permanent mental and physical retardation. He claims that we made tremendous progress as late as 1940 when the United States suffered from endemic malnutrition — pellagra, rickets and goiter and then by the 1960's he admits our progress not only halted but we began to slip backward.

Then he goes on to state "Our problem today is primarily one of ignorance compounded by a confusing array of unscientific books and articles, some very well publicized, giving poor nutritional advice. Food faddism is becoming a national problem". Then he tells us that "they want to improve their food intake, but they do not know or understand modern food science and technology and therefore, distrust processing and modern agricultural methods. We have extensive knowledge in nutrition today, but, unfortunately, the faddists and their converts are not benefitting from it.

"For those living in poverty more adequate federal food programs must be accompanied by meaningful education. For the majority, nutrition education is sorely needed, but they are not getting it today. There are, to be sure, many programs on nutrition education in effect in the United States, but they are too dispersed: the Department of Agriculture has thousands of "nutrition aides" who give basic nutritional advice to mothers; it prints and distributes literature on the subject; a few school systems and universities provide some training in nutrition. But most do nothing. And nowhere, to my knowledge, is there a coordinated approach to teaching the subject of nutrition."

Anyway, I've given you the gist of what Mr. Henry J. Heinz II has said and is so concerned about. Now I'd like to tell Mr. Heinz a few things that either he doesn't know or doesn't want to know or deliberately ignores. The tomato, before he cans it, is an excellent food but when he puts it in the can, cooks it along with the innumerable chemicals it has about as much nutritional value as red ink. The children and infants that he is so concerned about whose

482

food deficiencies are so particularly serious are in reality being fed with his and other food processors' canned foods . . . yes, the same canned baby and other foods that his company and other companies turn out by the millions. If instead these self-same children and infants ate the whole, raw vegetable and fruit they would no doubt be healthy and suffer no deficiencies but the canned pap that he sells them, loaded with salt, monosodium glutamate, and other permitted chemicals can only bring ill health and untimely death to those children and infants that he is so concerned about.

If Mr. Heinz doesn't know, someone should tell him that no food, no natural food created by nature can be improved or made more nutritious by canning or processing. It is a positive undeniable fact that invariably its nutritional value is lessened and often, in fact, most often poisonous chemical substances are added which can only cause sickness and untimely death, too. Yet, I realize that this good man is worried, seriously worried and he has good cause to be worried because one of these days America will rise en masse and put an end to this skulduggery that has been going on with the food of the nation for many, many years. Only when we return to the way of proper eating, that is, raw vegetables, raw grains and raw fruits and nuts without processing of any kind can the health of the people be assured and maintained. I know it is difficult, I know it won't come without a terrible struggle but I think even Mr. Heinz in his heart knows that that is the answer.

All the college professors and scientists on earth with their Ph.D's cannot improve on nature and on our natural food. They know it and you should know it but that doesn't mean they admit it, for a man will do anything for a buck and anything plus for a lot of bucks. This is the whole reason why raw food is slow to take hold.

If the universities and the government, industry and financiers are ready to teach the truth it will take only one generation to wipe sickness, disease and untimely death off the map and all fields of healing, hospitals, medicare, drugs will be erased with them along with the chemical fertilizers, chemical food additives, food processors, brewers, vintners, distillers and drug manufacturers. I predict, that the

483

day is coming when this actually will take place. People will not forever allow themselves to be lullabied to an early grave so that large corporations can make millions.

CHAPTER 80

I KICKED SMOKING

This article is addressed to smokers and right from the start I want to tell you that I smoked for many years . . . although not to excess. Luckily I broke the habit and to prove that I licked it I will light a cigarette and then throw it away. I could also take a puff to show my contempt for it but why should I defile my body? If I can do it then you can do it.

How do I know? Because I am no better a man than you and maybe not as good. I have no more will-power than you. So why can I do it and not you? Well, I'll tell you . . . you just don't want to do it and I did want to do it. I said to myself, "Rather than be a slave to tobacco I'd rather be dead!" In fact, any man who is a slave or is addicted to any of these things, in my opinion, would be better off dead.

485

So, seeing I wanted to live, I am alive and because I gave up these enemies of mine, I'll probably live to be much older. In fact, had I continued along the paths that I was following 20 years ago, I would have been dead and buried a long time ago. And I'm as sure of that as the fact that the sun rises and sets.

Now my main purpose in writing this article is to make smokers as mad as hell. I'm writing this to them and I'm trying to wave a red flag in front of a bull. I'm telling these men who smoke that they are not men . . . they're puppets, they're dope fiends, they're bums, they're weak, puny creatures who have no right to be called men. Any man who would defile the good body that parents and a mighty God gave him is not worth that good body or worth worrying about.

My most beloved brother who was two and a half years older than me died from smoking a few years ago. I say he died from smoking and I will repeat it again and again. The doctor said he died from cancer but the cancer was caused by smoking, I'm sure, but the doctors wouldn't say that. The tobacco people might not like it and besides, they want to make it sound as though God took him. The hell God took him . . . he died because he was addicted to cigarettes. Even almost to his last breath he was sucking on a cigarette, much to my disgust.

He was the brother who was closest to me and whom I loved dearly. But he wouldn't give up smoking. He wouldn't give up one puff of one cigarette in order to live. That's how much he was addicted. Yet this brother was intelligent enough to keep his two sons from smoking. He said to them when they were just young lads, "Smoking is a dirty filthy rotten habit. I am addicted to it. Don't let it get you!" Neither of his two sons ever smoked. He died because he loved his cigarette but he brought this point home to his two boys.

I smoked my first cigarette when I was eight years of age and when I was a kid we used to "bang butts," as we called it . . . that is, pick up the butts that people threw away and we'd open them up, throw away the paper and re-roll the tobacco in newspaper or toilet

486

paper. Then we'd smoke them.

I was lucky. Smoking bothered me. I was allergic to cigarettes somehow or other and they used to make me dizzy and sick. Even when I grew older I could never smoke, although I kept trying. I felt that everybody else smoked and that it was sort of a sophisticated thing to do, so I tried to smoke. But it didn't matter when or where I tried to smoke it always made me woozy. No I didn't smoke much but I did smoke four cigarettes a day or sometimes more . . . two of them when I was on the can and somehow I believed it seemed to help me have a better bowel movement and also to help me relax and fall asleep at night very quickly.

I do not attempt to deny that I enjoyed the few cigarettes I smoked even though they made me woozy but in any event I decided to give up smoking. It was quite a sacrifice for me to give up those few measly cigarettes. In fact, for weeks after I said I'd quit I went through the motions of smoking even though I didn't light the cigarette because once I vowed I'd never smoke again I meant what I said.

What I am trying to say is that I was addicted, I liked smoking and I enjoyed it very much, but I refused to be a slave to it and I knew that it was doing me some harm. So I said, "Enough!"

Without fear of contradiction, most people recognize that smoking is not a good habit and that it does do harm of various kinds to the smoker. However, I go a few steps further and make this clear-cut emphatic statement and I address this to all smokers and drinkers, "A non-smoker and non-drinker has a higher I.Q. than a smoker and a drinker. He has better reflexes. He has better eyesight. He has better hearing. He has better digestion. And he has keener perception. Therefore, the harm that smoking and drinking do to a human being is bordering on the calamitous."

I have for more than 50 years watched the behaviour of smokers as compared to non-smokers and I have never in my whole life seen one single man or woman who was better in any way

487

because he or she smoked. Sure, I recognize the fact that some men are bolder and brasher and more nervy when they have a cigarette . . . and probably that's the reason some men use tobacco. But I don't need a cigarette to make me bold and brave.

On many occasions I have had people say to me, "Well, if I had to give up smoking, I'd rather be dead."

My reply invariably is, "As far as the world is concerned, you would be a lot better off dead. If you are a smoker you stink up everything around you and become a problem to everyone."

Apart from that I think that smoking is an evil dirty habit. Smoking makes you smell like a plugged up sewer. Your breath, your body and your clothes smell.

I still have some friends who smoke because I've learned through the years to love them in spite of their bad habits.

Occasionally I have an individual come in to see me and we chat for a while about any one of many things and then sometimes he pulls out a package of cigarettes from his pocket and as he goes to light it, I say to him, "Up until now I thought you were an intelligent man. Now I know you're not!"

A very good friend of mine, who is an addicted smoker, told me that he gave up smoking for nine months and then he went back to it. He said that without his cigarette he was miserable and also miserable to everyone around him and he made life difficult for those he worked with. And even though he licked the habit for nine months, he went back to the bad habit because he didn't want to inflict his miserableness upon his associates . . . yet he recognizes that tobacco is his enemy and not his friend.

In this day and age surely no one can kid himself or make himself believe that tobacco is not harmful or deadly. Yet I meet people who still claim that it is not proven that smoking causes lung cancer, heart disease and emphysema. Well, I don't bother to argue the point. If you want to smoke, that's your business and if you want to kid yourself, that's your business, too.

In any event, if you are not man enough to give up smoking you're not much of a man — so why should anyone worry about you?

CHAPTER
81

ANGEL OF DEATH'S ASSISTANT — DIETHYLSTILBESTROL

I have done a great deal of fighting about the refining and chemicalizing of our food and drugs. One of my most important targets has been diethylstilbestrol. I started fighting this cancer-causing female hormone or estrogen about fifteen years ago and although it seems as though I am fighting a losing battle, I've never given up. I believe I have been the foremost opponent of the use of DES in America and because of this I have made many strong, important, powerful enemies. You see, billions of dollars are here involved.

I have enough evidence accumulated to prove to anyone who has an open mind that diethylstilbestrol is a cancer-causing chemical. I am also of the opinion that most of the people who are at all acquainted with the subject know that I speak the truth. In fact, some of them knew it long before I did. Yet little or nothing is done

491

about it and at times it seemed as though I was fighting the battle alone!

No, I am not going to give up the fight . . . I'm going to keep on, whether I win or lose or whether I drop dead in the attempt. I could say that it is one of the worst offences against mankind but to me every one seems to be the worst one, so I don't want to sound like a broken record and I will not make that statement in this case. I just want to say it's harmful, its dangerous and it's deadly, and it's probably one of the most widely used of all the harmful chemical synthetic substances in America today.

In spite of the fact that it is widely recognized as being deadly and harmful, from time to time I see articles in various newspapers, magazines and research reports that tell how wonderful and how great and how beneficial this diethylstilbestrol is. In fact, I hold in my hand at the moment a copy of Science News, (Vol. 92, October 7, 1967) and on Page 343 there is an article with the heading in big bold type, "Estrogens Double Life," and there is a sub-heading, "Physicians are prescribing for morning-after birth control a variety of compounds designed for other purposes."

Now I know that Science News was a little tiny puny publication but somehow they seem to get bigger and smarter and have put on a new front. And maybe the publishing of such articles might have been the means of acquiring this expansion.

No, I am not suggesting that they were bribed or paid off and I have no malice in the matter at all . . . that's definite. Nevertheless, this article appeared and they certainly were doing diethylstilbestrol a heck of a lot of good.

This article starts off by telling you, "The Food and Drug Administration lays down the law for drug companies, telling them what they can and cannot claim their products will do. But it has no authority over a physician's prescribing habits."

Then they go on to give a lot more information about this

and talk about other drugs and further on down the page they make this statement:

"In limited trials with women, Yale University researchers last year demonstrated that an estrogen compound called diethylstilbestrol — approved for a variety of other purposes — is an effective morning-after drug. Patient use during the year since that initial report confirms the fact that 25 milligrams of diethylstilbestrol are 100 per cent effective in preventing pregnancy when taken within six days after intercourse, according to Dr. John McLean Morris, who headed the team. Other estrogen compounds are also effective in proper doses. Even the combination estrogen-progesterone oral contraceptives may be effective if a month's supply is taken at once, he says, but it's not to be recommended lightly.

"None of these drugs are available without a doctor's prescription; frequent use is considered hazardous, and the drugs should not be taken without close medical supervision."

With every mouthful of meat or fowl that you eat you are probably getting a good dose of diethylstilbestrol, commonly referred to as DES or an estrogen or a female hormone. This is made synthetically today but it was supplied from natural sources before. Its main reason for being is that it was found that when injected into animals in various ways it increased their weight more rapidly and also induced the animals to eat less food. Therefore, it is used to fatten animals quickly, to make more profits for the farmer or the cattle raiser. The most reliable evidence in America clearly indicates that diethylstilbestrol does cause cancer and I quote from the 7th edition of the Merck Index. Read it for yourself.

DIETHYLSTILBESTROL

"Human Toxicity: Large doses may cause anorexia, nausea, vomiting, abdominal pain, diarrhea, headache, dizziness, lethargy, paresthesia, skin eruptions, breast engorgement, uterine bleeding (including bleeding following withdrawal of drug), amenorrhea, loss of libido in males, dysuria, edema, congestive heart failure, mammary

493

carcinoma in males. May cause or contribute to mammary or genital carcinoma in females.

"Caution: Hepatic disease. Benign prostatic hypertrophy. History of mammary or genital carcinoma or familial history of these. Should not be employed for uterine bleeding unless possibility of carcinoma has been thoroughly investigated.

"Vet. Use: Chemical caponization of poultry."

Now if we had no other shred of evidence to indicate that diethylstilbestrol was harmful, I think you have enough there to make it so that no human being who can see, read or understand, would ever use the product. But there are tons and tons of other evidence that points out the harm, the danger, of diethylstilbestrol.

I am sure any normal human being will ask this question, "If what you have pointed out is true − and it must be true because you have quoted the authoritative Merck Index − then how in heaven's name is it still allowed to be used?"

Well, I shamefacedly must tell you something else . . . it is probably the most widely used drug in the world today. It is used in the feed of practically all animals in America. It is used by the physicians throughout America and perhaps the world in the treatment of cancer. It is used quite heavily in the "pill" − that is, the pregnancy-preventing pill. It is used to make animals sterile. If they have a wolf plague somewhere, they put out bait treated with diethylstilbestrol and it makes the males sterile. It's universally used, evidently, for many, many things.

The Food and Drug permit the use of diethylstilbestrol in practically any quantities. From my investigations there are no rules governing the quantity fed to animals. In fact, only a short time ago they permitted the farmers to double the amount of diethylstilbestrol fed to animals in spite of the objections of a large segment of our society. I have never seen any rule as to what the amount is. The Food and Drug claim that most, if not supposedly all, of the DES is excreted by the animal and is not found in the carcass. On the other hand, reliable researchers claim that a large portion of the DES is found in the meat and organs of the animal both before and after butchering. This statement of fact is now admitted.

The supporters of DES claim that it saves the American meat buyers millions of dollars and that it makes better profits for the farmer. The merry battle has been raging for about 25 years. The sales of diethylstilbestrol are said to bring in almost 500 million dollars to the chemical corporations and they have no intention of permitting that volume of business to be lost.

I have contended for years that when the DES is added to the animal feed it causes the animal to become diseased and a cellular expansion to occur which adds weight because of the greater retention of moisture. This I maintain is lost in the cooking and the housewife winds up paying more for her poorer, diseased meat.

It was because of diethylstilbestrol that I curtailed my own meat eating. I have all but eliminated meat from my diet. I further contend that it impairs the flavor and quality of the meat and the wind-up is that the only people who make money out of DES are the chemical corporations and those officials and men in authority whom they bribe to maintain their product in good standing.

This should make you see the pattern. Millions of dollars are involved and not only the manufacturers make these millions but all down the line ... distributors, wholesalers, retail outlets, hospitals, doctors, salesmen and employees. They all benefit from these millions of dollars and that tells the story. That is why it is difficult, if not downright impossible, to get it removed.

I maintain that it is harming and killing not hundreds, not thousands, not tens of thousands, not hundreds of thousands, but actually millions. But millions of dollars are more important than millions of people. Besides, they're still breeding babies and they claim there is a danger of a population explosion, so maybe its use is justifiable. Who am I to judge?

There is no question about it. The tremendous rise in the chicken industry of America is due to DES. It makes the chickens grow rapidly and they are ready for market in a few short weeks. But of course every chicken is diseased and it has been established that DES definitely causes cancer in the chickens but as none of the chickens are permitted to live out their normal span of life they do not die of cancer. By arrangements with the Food and Drug it is permitted to remove these cancerous parts and they are then used in bologna or in weiners or other ways and the rest of the chicken can be used in the regular manner. If you think this is just a figment of my imagination I want to stress that news of the cancer caused in chickens and the story I'm relating was published in most of the newspapers in the United States a few years ago.

. . . .

It appears as of the time this book goes to press that our side has won the fight . . . DES has been banned, with certain conditions. So obviously someone else did recognize the deadly harm of DES.

However, this is no time to celebrate and stop fighting because I assure you "the enemy" is not beaten, he is just rearranging his forces and he will break through in another field and then the fight or proceedings will start all over again.

Then it will take another two, five or ten years to catch up with them and the merry-go-round will go round and round and round. Gold coins are round too, and that is the story.

CHAPTER

82

"THE PILL" WILL KILL MILLIONS

While the birth control pill has only been on the market for about 10 years I have been acquainted with it for something closer to 17 years. Yes, I have actually been following the development of the pill since Dr. Gregory Pincus announced the first idea of using the pill. If you dig back you will find that the tests started back at least 17 years ago. At that time I made fairly close and exhaustive studies when most people didn't even know there was such a thing in the air. As a matter of fact, the earlier trials with the pill were made in some foreign countries. Those who pioneered in this field were Drs. Gregory Pincus, John Rock, Celso-Ramon Garcia, M.C. Chang. Strange to relate, Dr. Pincus was interested in preventing conception, whereas Dr. Rock was interested in inducing conception in sterile or barren women . . . somehow they got together, but that is a story in itself.

The more I study, read and dig into the scientific literature on the pill the more ridiculous the situation becomes and the more terrifying because of the tremendous danger it poses for the women who use the pill. The point that I want to bring home now is the same point that I sought to emphasize about 17 years ago and that is that monkeying with the sex apparatus or reproductive organs of the female is a mighty dangerous proposition . . . one that is fraught with serious danger, much more serious than most responsible people realize and unfortunately most medical doctors minimize it. I'm suggesting that they are playing not only with dynamite but something worse than the atom bomb.

No one can deny that the pill is effective. In fact, it's almost fool-proof and therein lies one of the grave dangers — its effectiveness. In order to be totally effective it must drastically or totally affect the woman's whole being, especially her organs of procreation and they include things like the fallopian tubes, the ovaries and the uterus. Now I only mention here the main organs that are affected but there are many other functions and tissues involved.

I am suggesting that in order for the pill to perform its functions it must create havoc with all of the organs involved in procreation. These organs must in some manner be prevented from performing their normal functions. I am fully aware that young people who fear the disgrace or the inconvenience of pre-marital pregnancy are not too much concerned about future damage or uncertain harm, especially when the drug and medical interests assure them that there is no danger. They are interested at the present moment in enjoying sexual relations promiscuously without the dread fear of becoming pregnant. When I was a young man fifty or so years ago my young girl friends and I also had grave fears about their becoming pregnant and I found that most of the girls who would have loved to enjoy intercourse were just frightened to death and the most I could get out of them was some torrid lovemaking. When I was given the opportunity to enjoy sex it was with grave concern on both of our parts and even then we took such precautions as were known and available to us 50 or so years ago.

Today a woman has several well known preventive measures she can follow. Of course the first is the pill. Then there is the intra-uterine device and the diaphragm and the vaginal suppository and the vaginal douche. However, those who can afford it prefer the pill because it is not messy and it doesn't involve medical manipulative assistance.

The main components of the pill are the estrogens. Estradiol is the oldest of them. It was first isolated in 1936. Exactly when it was first synthesized I am not certain but the closest date that I can find is 1941. The other estrogen is diethylstilbestrol. The literature does not tell me when it was first isolated but the first synthesis was made in 1943. The hormone that is used most extensively today, at least they are starting to use it more extensively, is progesterone. It is not listed under the estrogens but it is a female hormone. According to the dictionary it is a steroid hormone obtained from the corpus luteum in crystalline form, occurring in two isomeric forms, alpha and beta. It was first isolated from the corpus luteum of pregnant sows in 1934. It probably was synthesized shortly afterwards. There are numerous patents for the synthesized progesterone.

Now I want to stress that the gravest danger facing the girl or woman who uses the pill is cancer. The danger of cancer to women using the pill has not been stressed and seldom even mentioned. In truth, the drug and medical groups pooh-pooh the idea of cancer and even worse they actually suggest that the pill will reduce or prevent risk of cancer. They do mention occasionally that there is a danger of thrombophlebitis, pulmonary embolism and other heart problems but this occurs only in rare cases. Many other complications are mentioned but seldom, if ever, do they mention the word cancer and of course I know why. The danger of a heart attack and other conditions doesn't frighten a woman too much and she is willing to take the risk but if ever the word got out that it might cause cancer this would no doubt seriously affect the sale of the pill and that is one thing that these drug companies do not want to see happen. In every book about the pill written by a doctor, invariably he goes to great lengths to assure you that there is no danger whatsoever of cancer. As Shakespeare might have said, "He doth protest too much,

499

methinks.'

Here and now I'm being very emphatic and stating the gravest and the greatest danger of the pill is not a heart condition, phlebitis or other comparatively minor conditions, but cancer. I stress again that I do know what I am talking about. Anyone who has read any of my writing should know by now that I do not make unwarranted or unfounded statements.

The drug companies know full well that the estrogen pill has proven successful. That is, it definitely does prevent conception. However, the way things are moving at the present moment they are "running scared". Evidently, evidence is piling up to indicate that the estrogens cause cancer, especially cancer of the breast. Therefore, they want to get out of the estrogens before the house caves in on top of them, but they are reluctant to give up the billions of dollars profit that can be made in the estrogen pill so they are switching to progesterone whose cancer-causing qualities are yet not established. So they feel they will get another five or ten or more years on the progesterone pill before its damage mounts up and the evidence against it becomes clear. My advice to women is to shun the use of the pill, be it estrogen or progesterone. I maintain that both will cause cancer in a few years, as well as other dangerous, harmful conditions.

Estradiol in the body is converted to estrone and estriol. It is believed to be the true ovarian hormone, also known as dehydrotheelin, dehydroxyestrin.

Another very important factor I wish to bring to light and that is when the doctor team that first created the pill was working on it they knew full well that these estrogens did cause cancer as evidenced by anyone who is willing to take the time to investigate because it's found in the Merck Index, edition 1960 which means that the knowledge contained therein was known years before. This knowledge clearly indicated as you read here that these estrogens did positively, scientifically cause cancer.

500

However, in the 1970 edition of the same Index all reference to cancer and other diseases has been carefully expunged. I do not feel that any further indictment is necessary. The women of America and their husbands if they are interested can take it from there. I am not an accredited scientist, I am not a healer of any kind, I'm not a biochemist but I am a researcher and what I have brought before you is from my investigations and studies and it is all presented for you to investigate and then you can go further if you so desire.

While no mention is made it appears that Diethylstilbestrol is the synthetic form of the natural hormone estradiol. The toxicity is identical as are many other factors.

I'm giving you the human toxicity of estradiol and diethylstilbestrol. You'll also find the human toxicity of progesterone.

ESTRADIOL

"Human Toxicity: Large doses may cause anorexia, nausea, vomiting, abdominal pain, diarrhea, headache, dizziness, lethargy, paresthesia, skin eruptions, breast engorgement, uterine bleeding (including bleeding following withdrawal of drug), amenorrhea, loss of libido in males, dysuria, edema, congestive heart failure, mammary carcinoma in males. May cause or contribute to mammary or genital carcinoma in females. History of mammary or genital carcinoma or familial history of these. Should not be employed for uterine bleeding unless possibility of carcinoma has been thoroughly investigated.

"Caution: Hepatic disease. Benign prostatic hypertrophy."

The human toxicity of Progesterone: side effects rare, headache, exhaustion, syncope, uterine bleeding may occur.

O.K., girls and women and people who are interested in girls and women, I gave you my warning in the strongest terms at my command and from now on it is up to you.

Let it be known that I claim there is a clear link between various forms of cancer in women and the estrogen intake be it of a therapeutic nature or in food. Something that has not been recognized in dealing with various forms of cancer is the effect and impact of DES. It must be understood and realized that every women is getting an extra dose of the estrogen in her daily diet whenever she eats a piece of meat be it chicken, beef or lamb. Therefore, those who eat meat and who take the pill are getting doses far above that which the body can in any way cope with.

From the best information that I am able to dig up DES or diethylstilbestrol is not used in the pill. Estradiol is used in the pill but estradiol per se is the natural hormone made from sow's ovaries but which can also be made from mares' and stallions' urine. Diethylstilbestrol appears to be the strictly synthetic form of estrogen, although estradiol is also made synthetically. It is my belief that whether it is estradiol or diethylstilbestrol only the synthetic form is used.

Further, I state that the big difference between the natural estrogen and the synthetic estrogen is that the body can eliminate rather readily the natural estrogen whereas it has difficulty or perhaps finds it impossible to eliminate the synthetic estrogen by normal urination or through the bowels.

I wish to emphasize that as of this writing – October, 1972 – considerably more than 12 million women of child-bearing age are taking the pill. To this number must be added those hundreds of thousands or millions of women who take hormones or are prescribed hormones by their doctors. This is to aid them in menopausal problems and also in an attempt by women to remain forever young or forever feminine.

The medical profession is fostering these myths and of course is encouraged, supported and no doubt financially assisted in this endeavour by the drug corporations who are the ones who profit enormously.

This traffic in human life, this traffic in the lives of women is a giant compared to the white slave traffic which was fought so vigorously by the various churches. Where are the churches now when actually millions of women are being done to death?

Now I'm trying with every power at my command to bring this proof to the attention of the authorities or the government or the medical profession or whoever else can help prevent this terrible disaster that will occur. But I don't have much hope in that direction. My real hope is to get to the young people themselves and to direct them to believe me or at least have them check on what I say to see whether or not I speak the truth . . . and I swear to you that I do speak the truth.

Here is a list of some of the best known brands of the Pill along with the main functional ingredients:

OVRAL	—	d-Norgestrel Ethinyl Estradiol
NORINYL-1	—	Norethindrone Mestranol
MICRONOR	—	Norethindrone No Estrogen
ORTHO-NOVUM	—	Norethindrone Mestranol
ENOVID	—	Norethynodrel Ethinyl Estradiol
NORIDAY	—	Norethindrone No Estrogen

The following is a description of some of the ingredients of the various pills available on the market.

Estradiol is an estrogenic hormone therapy. The most potent natural hormone.

Norethindrone is an orally active progestogen, with estrogen as the oral contraceptive. It is a constituent of Norlestrin, Etalontin, Prolestrin, Primosiston tablets and Anovlar 21. (17-Hydroxy-19-nor-17a-pregn-4-en-20-yn-3-one).

Norethynodrel is an orally active progestational agent with Mestranol as the oral contraceptive. It is a constituent of Enovid, Enavid, Conovid and Prevision.

Ethinyl Estradiol is an estrogenic hormone therapy.

Mestranol is an Estrogenic agent. ($C21H26O2$) It is a constituent of Enovid, Enavid, Conovid, Norinyl, Ortho-Novum, Previson, C-Quens, Sequens, Metrulen, Ovulen. (3-Methoxy-19-nor-17a-pregna-1,3,5 (10)-Trien-20yn -17-ol).

You will note that 4 out of 6 of the leading contraceptive pills contain "estradiol". Estradiol is positively known to cause cancer and this has been known by all the foremost authorities for at least 15 years. Yet they permit women to indiscriminately take this cancer-causing drug almost every day of their fertile lives because women who want to avoid pregnancy have to take these pills at least 20-odd days every month. Well then how can they avoid getting cancer? This is something most people haven't thought about.

Let me tell you the difference between the estrogen pill and the progesterone pill. Now the estrogen pill need only be taken for 21 of the 28 day menstrual cycle, consecutively . . . 21 of the 28 days. The progesterone pill must be taken continually starting during mentruation if it is to function efficiently from then on.

I have here advertisements for five of the well known birth control pills. The 6th, Enovid, I do not have an advertisement for. I'm quoting them in entirety and if I were a girl or a woman or anyone interested in a specific girl or woman I would study this

504

carefully and after I'd studied it I would decide whether the use of these pills is worthwhile or whether it is too dangerous. You will notice that nowhere is the word cancer or carcinoma mentioned although the dangers of many other conditions are given, which bears out what I said earlier in the chapter.

OVRAL*

Each white tablet contains 0.25 mg. of d-norgestrel (0.5 mg. of dl-racemate in which only the d-enantiomer is biologically active); and 0.05 mg. of ethinyl estradiol.

Contraindications: Patients with thrombophlebitis or a history of thrombophlebitis or pulmonary embolism. Liver dysfunction or disease. Known or suspected carcinoma of breast or genital organs. Undiagnosed vaginal bleeding. During breast feeding due to possible transmission of steroids to the child. Young patients in whom bone growth is not complete.

Adverse Effects: The following are some of the reactions which have been observed with varying incidence in patients receiving oral contraceptives. Nausea, Spotting, Vomiting, Change in Menstrual Flow, Gastrointestinal Symptoms, Breakthrough Bleeding, Amenorrhea, Edema.

The following occurrences have been observed in users of oral contraceptives: Thrombophlebitis, Neuro-Ocular Lesions, Pulmonary Embolism. Please consult Product Monograph for full information.

Warnings And Precautions: Discontinue medication pending examination if there is sudden partial or complete loss of vision, sudden onset of proptosis, diplopia or migraine. Withdraw medication if papilledema or retinal vascular lesions occur. Safety of Ovral* in pregnancy has not been established. If two consecutive cycles have been missed, pregnancy should be ruled out before continuing the regimen. Consider the possibility of pregnancy at the time of the first missed period if prescribed schedule has not been followed.

Pre-treatment examination should include special reference to breast and pelvic organs as well as a Papanicolaou smear.

Endocrine and liver – function tests may be affected. Pre-existing fibroids may increase with estrogen-progestogen therapy. Some degree of fluid retention may result. Use with caution in patients with history of cerebrovascular accident.

In cases of undiagnosed vaginal bleeding, adequate diagnostic measures are indicated. Patients with a history of psychic depression should be carefully observed. Diabetic patients should be carefully observed.

Supplied: Ovral* is available in compacts of 21 white tablets and in refill strips of 21 white tablets. Ovral* 28 is available in compacts of 21 white tablets followed by 7 pink inert tablets and in refill strips of 21 white tablets followed by 7 pink inert tablets.

NORINYL-1

Norinyl-1 – The low potency pill. (1 MG Norethindrone, 50 MCG Mestranol).

Dosage: Norinyl-1 (21's) – Initial Cycle: Start the first cycle of medication on Day 5 of the menstrual cycle (counting the first day of menstrual flow as 'Day 1') by taking one white tablet daily for 21 consecutive days; no tablets are taken for the next 7 days.

Subsequent Cycles: The second and subsequent cycles are begun after seven tablet-free days, regardless of whether bleeding has finished or not. Each cycle consists of 21 days of medication and a 7-day interval without medication.

Norinyl-1 (28's) – Start the first cycle of medication on Day 5 of the menstrual cycle (counting the first day of menstrual flow as 'Day 1') by taking one white tablet daily for 21 consecutive days, followed by one orange tablet daily for 7 days, thus completing a 28-day course of medication. On the following day (day 29) begin

506

another 28-day course of medication and repeat for all subsequent cycles. A pill is taken every day regardless of whether menstrual bleeding has appeared, is continuing, or finished.

Contraindications: Contraindicated in patients with undiagnosed vaginal bleeding; carcinoma of the breast or genital tract; history of cerebrovascular accident; presence of exophthalmos or migraine; thrombophlebitis: thrombotic phenomena; significant liver dysfunction or hepatic pathology; ocular lesions associated with neurovascular disease (i.e., partial or complete loss of vision, visual field defects or diplopia): incomplete epiphyseal closure; patients who are nursing; suspected pregnancy.

Precautions and Warnings: Prior to drug administration, a thorough physical examination should be given, with special attention to the breasts and pelvic organs. Pre-existing uterine fibroids may increase in size. The conditions of epilepsy, migraine, asthma, cardiac or renal dysfunction should be carefully observed, since progestational agents may cause mild fluid retention. Observe patients with a history of psychic depression and discontinue the drug if depression continues or recurs to a marked degree. When breakthrough bleeding occurs, consider the possibility of nonfunctional causes. Pregnancy or other causes should be ruled out before therapy is continued in any patient missing two consecutive menstrual periods.

MICRONOR

Contains Progestin alone. By eliminating estrogen, Micronor reduces estrogen-related side effects. Each Micronor tablet contains 0.35 mg. of norethindrone (17 alpha-ethinyl-17-hydroxy-4-estren-3-one).

Contraindications: 1. History or presence of psychic depression. 2. Hormonal imbalance causing oligomenorrhea and oligo-ovulation. 3. In the presence of undiagnosed vaginal bleeding. 4. Carcinoma of the breast or genital tract. 5. Women breast feeding their children. 6. Pregnancy, actual or suspected. 7. Marked liver

507

dysfunction and disease.

Warnings: 1. Although the following adverse effects have not been reported with Norethindrone alone, such effects have been associated with the use of oral contraceptives containing estrogens and progestins and should be kept in mind when prescribing Micronor tablets.

(i) Thrombophlebitis or pulmonary embolism. (ii) Neuro-vascular Lesions of the eye or visual disturbances such as partial or complete loss of vision, defects in visual fields or diplopia. (iii) Cerebrovascular accidents, transient aphasia, paralysis or unexplained loss of consciousness.

If the patient develops any signs of phlebitis involving either superficial or deep veins, or embolic complications, or any of the other conditions listed above, medication should be discontinued. Also, any patient developing migraine while on therapy should discontinue medication.

2. The pretreatment physical examination should include special reference to breast and pelvic organs as well as a Papanicolaou smear. Adolescent patients should be assessed for adequate physical development prior to medication. 3. The first follow-up examination should be done within six months following commencement of the oral contraceptive and thereafter at least once a year. At each visit the examination should include all tests done at the initial visit. 4. In the presence of scanty bleeding or in the absence of a menstrual period for 45 days, pregnancy should be ruled out. If the pregnancy test is negative, another pregnancy test should be done at 60 days and the appropriate action taken. 5. Patients with pre-existing fibroids, epilepsy, asthma, should be carefully observed.

Precautions: Micronor contains a low dosage of a progestin without the addition of an estrogenic agent. Some of the side effects of oral contraceptives have been associated more with the estrogenic component. Nevertheless, until further evidence becomes available, Micronor should be used with caution in the following conditions. 1.

In the presence, or history, of cardiac or renal disorders, which might be adversely affected by fluid retention. 2. Frequent or prolonged breakthrough bleeding may not be related to the medication, therefore investigations for other causes should be considered. 3. In metabolic or endocrine disease, careful clinical evaluation should precede medication. Physicians should be alert to recognize evidence of adrenocortical or thyroid suppression, although the risk with Micronor appears to be minimal. 4. The influence of prolonged therapy on pituitary, ovarian, adrenal, thyroid, hepatic or uterine function is unknown. Follow-up studies are in progress to determine possible effects. 5. The pathologist should be advised of therapy with Micronor when relevant specimens are submitted. 6a. Diabetic patients or those with a family history of diabetes should be followed closely for any decrease in glucose tolerance. b. Those patients who exhibit signs of latent diabetes may be given Micronor, but only under close supervision. c. Overt diabetes in the younger age group whose disease is of recent origin, well controlled and who do not exhibit hypertension or other signs of vascular disease such as ocular fundal changes, may use Micronor for a limited time, at the discretion of the attending physician.

7. Patients with essential hypertension may be given Micronor, but only under close supervision. If a significant elevation of blood pressure occurs at any time in either hypertensive or normotensive patients during the administration of Micronor, cessation of medication is necessary. 8. As the effect of Micronor on the endometrium is unpredictable, it is advisable for patients to discontinue medication every two to three years and resume only after normal ovulatory cycles and menstruation have been re-established.

Clinical Studies: Clinical studies to date with Micronor tablets involved 2,963 patients who completed a total of 26,713 months of use. In this group, 55 pregnancies occurred. Twenty-seven resulted from failure of the method, resulting in a corrected pregnancy rate of 1.2. Twenty-eight were attributed to failure of the patients to take the tablets correctly, resulting in a patient failure pregnancy rate of 1.3. The over-all pregnancy rate was therefore 2.5.

Dosage & Administration: 1. With Micronor, the first tablet is taken on the first day of menstrual bleeding. One tablet is then taken every single day until the Dialpak tablet Dispenser is empty. Without missing a day, Micronor tablets are continued from a new dialpak. Micronor tablets are taken every day — even during menstrual bleeding. 2. Tablets should be taken at about the same time each day, either morning, afternoon, or evening. This routine makes it easier to remember to take tablets and also ensures maximum protection. Close adherence to the regimen is important. 3. If tablets are taken incorrectly, an additional method of birth control should be used along with Micronor until menstrual bleeding occurs again.

Packaging: Micronor is available in a 35-day dialpak tablet dispenser, containing a five week supply of tablets.

ORTHO-NOVUM 1/50*

Unique Formulation: By combining the progestin (norethindrone) and the estrogen (mestranol), Ortho-Novum 1/50 is composed of two of the lowest activity hormones used to prevent conception.

Lowest Progestational Activity: Norethindrone, as used in Ortho-Novum 1/50, has the lowest progestational activity of the progestins used in 50 mcg. estrogen tablets.

Lowest Estrogenic Activity: Mestranol, as used in Ortho-Novum 1/50, has the lowest estrogenic activity of the estrogens used in oral contraceptives.

Composition: Each Ortho-Novum 1/50 tablet contains 1 mg. norethindrone (17-alpha-ethinyl-17-hydroxy-4-estren-3-one) with 50 mcg. mestranol (ethinyl estradiol-3-methyl ether).

Clinical Studies: Clinical studies to date with Ortho-Novum 1/50 tablets have involved 4,977 patients through 51,544 cycles of use. Ortho-Novum 1/50 has proven virtually 100% effective in these studies.

Dosage and Administration: For the first cycle only, have her take one tablet a day for 3 weeks, starting on Day 5 of her menstrual cycle. At the end of the course of Ortho-Novum 1/50, she stops the tablets for one week.

From now on, she simply completes each course of tablets, stopping at the end of each course for one week. The tablets should be started whether or not menstruation has occurred or is finished.

If spotting or bleeding should occur while taking Ortho-Novum 1/50, the tablets should be continued in the regular manner.

Duration of Use: As long as physician feels is desirable.

Precautions and Contraindications: Since it has been suggested that there may be a causal relationship between the use of progestin-estrogen compounds and the development of thrombophlebitis, physicians should be cautious in prescribing Ortho-Novum 1/50 tablets for patients with thromboembolic disease or a history of thrombophlebitis.

Patients with pre-existing fibroids, epilepsy, migraine, asthma or a history of psychic depression, should be carefully observed. Pre-treatment examination should include a Papanicolaou smear.

Ortho-Novum 1/50 should not be taken: In the presence of malignant tumours of the breast or genital tract: In the presence of significant liver dysfunction or disease: In the presence of cardiac or renal disorders which might be adversely affected by some degree of fluid retention: During the period a mother is breast-feeding an infant.

Packaging: Ortho-Novum 1/50 Tablets in Dialpak* Tablet Dispensers of 21 and bottles of 500.

NORIDAY

Composition: Each Noriday tablet contains 0.35 mg of norethindrone (17-alpha-ethinyl-17-hydroxy-4-estren-3-one).

Effectiveness and Clinical Studies: Clinical studies to date with Noriday tablets involve 2,963 patients who completed a total of 26,713 months of use. In this group, 55 pregnancies occurred with an overall pregnancy rate of 2.5 which is higher than conventional oral contraceptives, 27 resulted from failure of the method, resulting in a corrected pregnancy rate of 1.2; 28 were attributed to failure of the patient to take the tablets correctly, resulting in a patient failure pregnancy rate of 1.3

Mode of Action: The mechanism of contraceptive design is multicausal primarily at the local pelvic level and secondarily at the systemic level. The hormonal effect is mainly progestational.

Pelvic effects include changes in the cervical mucus and endometrium. Systemic effects involve mainly the inhibition of secretion of pituitary gonadotrophins which in turn prevents follicular maturation and ovulation.

Contraindications. 1. History or presence of psychic depression. 2. Hormonal imbalance causing oligomenorrhea and oligo-ovulation. 3. In the presence of undiagnosed vaginal bleeding. 4. Carcinoma of the breast or genital tract. 5. Women breast-feeding their children. 6. Pregnancy, actual or suspected. 7. Marked liver dysfunction and disease.

Warnings: 1. Although the following adverse effects have not been reported with norethindrone alone, such effects have been associated with the use of oral contraceptives containing estrogens and progestins. It should be kept in mind when prescribing Noriday tablets. Thrombophlebitis or pulmonary embolism; Neurovascular lesions of the eye or visual disturbances, such as partial or complete loss of vision, defects in visual fields or diplopia; Cerebrovascular accident, transient aphasia, paralysis or unexplained loss of consciousness.

If the patient develops any signs of phlebitis involving either superficial or deep veins or embolic complications or any of the other conditions mentioned above, medication should be discontinued. Also, any patients developing migraine while on therapy should discontinue medication.

2. The pre-treatment physical examination should include special reference to breast and pelvic organs, as well as a Papanicolaou smear. Adolescent patients should be assessed for adequate physical development prior to medication.

3. The first follow-up examination should be done within six months following commencement of the oral contraceptive, and thereafter at least once a year. At each visit the examination should include all tests done at the initial visit.

4. In the presence of scanty bleeding or in the absence of a menstrual period for 45 days, pregnancy should be ruled out. If the pregnancy test is negative, another pregnancy test should be done at 60 days and the appropriate action taken.

5. Patients with pre-existing fibroids, epilepsy, asthma, should be carefully observed.

Precautions: Noriday contains a low dosage of progestin without the addition of an estrogenic agent. Some of the side effects of oral contraceptives have been associated more with the estrogenic component, nevertheless, until further evidence becomes available, Noriday should be used with caution in the following conditions:

1. In the presence or history of cardiac or renal disorders which might be adversely affected by fluid retention.

2. Frequent or prolonged breakthrough bleeding may not be related to the medication, therefore, investigation for other causes should be considered.

3. In metabolic or endocrine disease, careful clinical evaluation should precede medication. Physicians should be alert to recognize evidence of adrenocortical or thyroid suppression, although the risk with Noriday appears to be minimal.

4. The influence of prolonged therapy on pituitary, ovarian, adrenal, thyroid, hepatic or uterine function is unknown. Follow-up studies are in progress to determine possible effects.

5. The pathologist should be advised of therapy with Noriday when relevant specimens are submitted.

6. a) Diabetic patients or those with a family history of diabetes should be followed closely for any decrease in glucose tolerance. b) Those patients who exhibit signs of latent diabetes may be given Noriday, but only under close supervision. c) Overt diabetes in the younger age group whose disease is of recent origin, well controlled and who do not exhibit hypertension or other signs of vascular disease such as ocular fundal changes, may use Noriday for a limited time at the discretion of the attending physician.

7. Patients with essential hypertension may be given Noriday, but only under close supervision. If a significant elevation of blood pressure occurs at any time in either hypertensive or normotensive patients during the administration of Noriday, cessation of medication is necessary.

8. As the effect of Noriday on the endometrium is unpredictable, it is advisable for patients to discontinue medication every two to three years, and resume only after the normal ovulatory cycles and menstruation have been re-established.

Adverse Reactions: The administration of Noriday causes irregularities of the bleeding pattern in terms of frequency and duration. The intervals between those bleeding episodes, sufficiently intensive to require sanitary protection may vary from less than nineteen days to over sixty days. Seventy-six percent of these inter-bleeding intervals fall between 19 and 60 days.

The following adverse effects have been observed although a cause-and-effect relationship has neither been proven or disproven: spotting, amenorrhea, migraine, breast symptoms, headache, depression, dizziness, nervousness, G.I. symptoms, cystitis-like syndrome.

Treatment of Overdosage and Accidental Ingestion: In case of over-dosage or accidental ingestion by children, the physician should observe the patient closely although no medication is required. Gastric lavage should be given only if considered necessary.

Dosage and Administration: 1. With Noriday, the first tablet is taken on the first day of menstrual bleeding. One tablet is then taken every single day until the MemoretteR tablet dispenser is empty. Without missing a day, Noriday tablets are continued from a new Memorette. Noriday tablets are taken every day even during menstrual bleeding.

2. Tablets should be taken at about the same time each day, either morning, afternoon or evening. This routine makes it easier to remember to take tablets and also insures maximum protection. Close adherence to the regimen is important.

3. If tablets are taken incorrectly, an additional method of birth control should be used along with Noriday until menstrual bleeding occurs again.

Packaging: Noriday is available in a 28-day Memorette tablet dispenser, containing a four week supply of tablets.

. . . .

There appears to be mountains of evidence to indicate that girls whose mothers took a synthetic hormore when pregnant — be it diethylstilbestrol or estradiol — are now developing a rare form of vaginal cancer. Now do you understand what I'm saying? There are probably today thousands, perhaps hundreds of thousands of girls who will or are developing a rare form of vaginal cancer because their mothers took or were treated with the synthetic forms of estrogens . . . diethylstilbestrol as found in meat or as administered by a doctor for menopausal problems, or as a replacement therapy in estrogen deficiency or for mammary carcinoma or for urinary bladder malignancy or suppression. Believe it or not diethylstilbestrol has long been used in Acne vulgaris, in plain ordinary acne and for premature labor. It has also been used in vaginal suppositories or ointments. It is important to note that diethylstilbestrol has been used in literally hundreds of ways and therefore the damage done is incalculable.

I am stating that most of the cases of vaginal cancer and other forms of cancer found in young women of child-bearing age is due to diethylstilbestrol administered by the physician during, before or after pregnancy. Here I quote an article concerning this.

"Girls whose mothers took diethylstilbestrol DES or any other form of synthetic estrogen while they were carrying them were urged Saturday to have a thorough pelvic examination as soon as they begin menstruating, no matter how young.

"The hormone has been linked strongly to a rare and, if untreated, fatal form of vaginal cancer in the daughters of mothers for whom it was prescribed to prevent threatened miscarriage. The finding, first reported last year by Dr. Arthur L. Herbst, a Harvard University gynecologist, led the Food and Drug Administration to ban its prescription for this purpose in November 1971.

"Herbst, here to participate in the 14th annual science writers' seminar of the American Cancer Society, said his plea applied not only to girls whose mothers are known to have taken the hormone during pregnancy, but also to those who experience heavy vaginal bleeding or staining. Medical records and parental memories are not always infallible, he explained, so that some young women may be unaware that they were exposed to the drug in the womb.

"Radical Surgery — Vaginal adenocarcinoma, as the cancer is known, can be cured by radical surgery in which the uterus and the lining of the vagina are removed. Although the patient then does not menstruate and is incapable of bearing children, she can be rehabilitated through reconstructive surgery. Several have married and have successful sexual relations, Herbst said.

"Asked whether 'pap' smears weren't sufficient for examination purposes, Herbst said the test by itself isn't sufficiently sensitive to this kind of tumor. Although many physicians and parents are reluctant to have teen-agers undergo the more thorough procedure usually reserved for adults, he added, the seriousness of the risk offers no alternative.

" 'This kind of examination must be approached with tenderness in these girls,' He said. 'Perhaps one should not do it right away. It might take several office visits. But with time and patience, it can be done thoroughly and must be. This is a lethal disease.'

"The link between DES and vaginal adenocarcinoma first came to Herbst's attention when seven cases of the rare cancer were found at the Massachusetts General Hospital between 1966 and 1969 among women 15 to 22 and an eighth was discovered at a nearby hospital. The cancer had never been seen in patients so young and had only rarely been reported in older women.

"Since then, about 70 additional cases have been reported in this country and abroad, Herbst said. Most, like seven of the original eight, were in girls whose mothers had taken DES or a related hormone during pregnancy.

"Registry Established — Herbst said he has established a registry supported by the American Cancer Society and the National Institutes of Health to collect information about this form of cancer and is tracking down the sons and daughters of 800 women known to have taken synthetic estrogens during pregnancy.

"This study may help scientists to discover whether the drug is potentially harmful to male as well as female offspring of such women and to determine whether less radical surgery can be curative.

517

"Asked by a reporter whether the DES residues that sometimes remain in meat after cattle have been fattened on the drug may also injure the human fetus, Herbst said that he had no information on the subject, but that the possibility cannot be ruled out.

"DES is also used as 'a morning-after' pill if birth-control measures have not been taken or have failed. Again, its results with respect to the fetus are unknown. However, women who do not abort after taking it usually are aborted by other means, he said.

"Meanwhile, said Herbst, the FDA has counseled doctors not to treat women threatened with miscarriage with estrogen unless absolutely necessary and to use natural rather than synthetic hormones for this purpose in any case. The reason for this, he explained, is that the safety of even the natural substance is in doubt."

Here you will find some more information that may be of interest.

"Breast Cancer Cure Unknown — Nicosia, Cyprus April 14 — A leading British cancer surgeon said today that despite great technical advances virtually no progress has been made toward successfully treating breast cancer in the last 30 years.

" 'We are making no dent at all into the mortality rate of breast cancer', Professor Harold Ellis of Westminister Hospital told the British Medical Association's 15th annual clinical meeting here."

"Congressman Delaney calls DES the 'Judas' Chemical! Congressman Delaney termed DES a 'Judas' chemical that may betray the health of future generations:

" 'The Agriculture Department which' Delaney says, 'is not an unbiased source of information, told the House Intergovernmental Relations Subcommittee last June that the use of DES is saving each person in the U.S. around $3 per year in the cost of meat. That's 30 dimes. Thirty pieces of silver we are being offered to betray the health of future generations.' "

Here are 26 different names by which Estradiol is known. It is all the same product.

Estradiol	Gynoestryl
Cis Estradiol	Oestergon
Estratriene	Ovastevol
Epidyhydroxyestra triene	Diogyn
Dihydrofollicular Hormone	Estrovite
Dihydrofolliculin	Macrodiol
Dihydroxyestrin	Ovahormon
Dihydrotheelin	Oestroglandol
Dihydromenformon	Primofol
Dimenformon	Profoliol
Ovocylin	Lamoiol
Ovocyclin	Femestral
Progynon-Dh	Gynergon

Primofol = c18h24o2 — A crystalline steroid possessing estrogenic properties.

The following excerpts will give you a little more food for thought.

" . . . no physician can feel completely confident that long-term use will prove safe for all patients."
— *The Medical Letter, June 10, 1960.*

"Twenty years may go by before we can be sure about the safety of the present oral contraceptives; and, in a fortunate and well-fed country where other methods of contraception are available and effective, it seems sensible to restrict their use to those menstrual irregularities that must be corrected or to those circumstances where other methods of contraception are impossible or ineffective."
— *The Lancet, June 2, 1962.*

"It may be many years before we really know about their safety . . . Meanwhile, it should be quite clearly understood by everyone, and I include husbands here, that if a woman takes drugs of this kind for social rather than therapeutic reasons they are taking part in a mass experiment — call them guinea pigs if you like . . . "

— Dr. E. A. Garrard, in his inaugural address on becoming
president of the British Medical Association, 1964

"In the opinion of MWN's (Medical World News's) Moscow correspondent, the recent Soviet decision to mass-produce IUD's (intra-uterine devices) fits in with their generally conservative approach to medicine. 'They favor a mechanical device over a chemical one because its effects are limited to the uterus. But they do not want to miss out on something that might prove to be better, so they are proceeding cautiously in many directions. Meanwhile, the Western world is their guinea pig for The Pill."

— Medical World News, January 10, 1969

CHAPTER

83

X RAYS . . . GOOD OR BAD?

It was in 1895 that William Conrad Roentgen, a German physicist, discovered the X ray. Then it was called the short-wave ray and later it was called the Roentgen ray but today it is best known as the X ray. This great discovery really was an accidental one but I'm not trying to detract from Roentgen's work because he was a well known physicist and did mighty good work in science. For the discovery of the X ray he was given the Nobel Prize in physics in 1901. He was born in 1843 and died in 1923.

As you know, the big user of the X ray is the medical profession. They jumped into it like a dog to a good bone and have expanded the use of the X ray continually since it was first discovered. The dental profession, seeking to emulate the success of the medical profession, followed suit and between the two of them they really made hay out of the X ray. Yes, I'm not using the wrong word . . . they really made hay and they are still making it in stacks.

In truth, upon studying various aspects of the X ray — as much as I can learn and find — I feel it is not a bad creation. I think it has its place, I think it is a valuable contribution to mankind. But due to the way it has been used and abused, mainly by the medical and dental professions, it has now become an actual scourge on mankind and it is doing harm out of all proportion to the little bit of good that it does. It is like many other things in life that are good but are so badly abused that they become deadly, harmful enemies. That is just exactly what has happened to the X ray.

At the time of the discovery of the X ray it was not recognized that exposure to this extraordinary ray invariably caused damage to living cells and this means harm to all human or animal tissue. I stress, this was not recognized at the time of the discovery of the X ray. The sale of X ray equipment now runs into the hundreds of millions of dollars and probably the manufacturers and the sellers of the X ray equipment are as much to blame for the scourge that exists today as any segment of the business or professional world. The official American government journals tell me that the widely used chest X ray is now on its way out. Also, they are trying to get rid of the inefficient X ray machines and the outmoded and sloppy techniques as well . . . the techniques that fail to protect the parts of the body not being examined from X ray beams.

It is recognized by the American government that "the genetically significant dose," (a measurement of how exposure of the population to X rays may affect future generations,) dropped more than one-third from 1964 to 1970.

They go on to tell us that complete protection from radiation of course is impossible because man is exposed to natural background ionizing radiation from cosmic rays and from the earth's crust. The mean annual dose from these natural sources is about 120 millirads. A millirad is a unit of absorbed radiation dose. Humans are also exposed to radiation from nuclear testing, nuclear power plants, radioactive drugs, industrial use of radiation, and therapeutic and industrial use of radium.

It is recognized that radiation, no matter from which source it comes, affects even those yet unborn. In medical use, the X rays strike the genital organs of the male or female. Obviously the X rays have an affect upon the genes and therefore future generations will be affected by the X rays taken today. Geneticists feel most mutations represent defects in the evolutionary process and that any agent which produces unnatural mutations should be avoided when possible.

The U.S. Government Publication, "FDA Consumer" states that the full impact of any damage to the genetic heritage may not become evident for many generations.

Health experts generally agree that the amount of radiation exposure needed for diagnostic X ray examinations is acceptable, but that any unnecessary exposure should be avoided. Now the latest figures that I have cover 1970 and it shows that 210 million people were exposed to either medical or dental X rays. The number of X rays have been increasing steadily since the ray was first discovered.

The FDA and the American College of Chest Physicians and the American College of Radiology in cooperation issued a joint policy statement urging that the use of mobile X ray equipment for mass screening of the general population for tuberculosis should be stopped. They are also taking steps to make the equipment manufacturers improve their machines and their components for safer examinations.

There were 650 million films taken. This means that 650 million people were exposed to X rays. Records seem to indicate that on a per capita basis one out of every two people in America had been X rayed for health reasons. The use of X rays is still increasing. It is suspected that X rays may be causing a significant number of avoidable deaths each year. Poor techniques and faulty equipment are

523

partly to blame but the most shocking aspect is that much diagnostic X ray exposure, at least 30%, is unproductive. And it has been estimated that deaths due to X ray-induced diseases run around 4,000 or more annually.

The big worry, it appears, is the danger of X ray damage to the reproductive cells of mankind and this is giving great concern to radiation experts. It is known that the X ray's damage can cause genetic defects in the offspring, from mental retardation and blindness to a number of deadly genetic mutations.

Radiation biologists now know that any X ray dose to the gonads — no matter how insignificant — carries some risk of causing genetic mutation. The sickening aspect of this is that X ray doses are cumulative and Dr. K. Z. Morgan, Director of the Health Physics Division, Oak Ridge National Laboratories estimates that as many as 30,000 malignancies, stillbirths, and spontaneous abortions may occur each year because of genetic damage caused by X rays.

We must recognize that X rays are not a toy and they are not entirely "do-gooders" either. The X ray has a tremendous amount of energy and the damage it does to tissue and components of the human body is staggering. It damages delicate walls. It alters metabolism. It is known to cause leukemia. We know that these X rays are used in the treatment of cancer yet it is a positive, recognized fact that they do cause cancer.

X rays are positively known to have a life shortening effect. It is known today that most of the childhood cancers are the result of X ray exposure of the mother prior to and after conception. It is known that the reproductive organs of the female are altered by X rays in such a manner as to include a cancer as a part of the unborn child's genetic inheritance . . . and to make it worse this may be passed on from one generation to another.

Animal experiments have clearly proven that X rays of the reproductive organs and embryos of guinea pigs, mice and rats have created deformities in the offspring. Furthermore, it has changed the sex ratio of newborns, induced cancers, and caused developmental retardation and early death. There is no reason to believe that it does not have the same effect upon man.

The International Commission on Radiological Protection has issued warnings and recommendations but still pregnant women are knowingly and unknowingly exposed to X rays. The Commission strongly recommends that all radiological examinations of the lower abdomen and pelvis of women that are not in connection with the immediate illness of the patient be limited to the 10-day interval following the onset of menstruation. It is in this period that pregnancy is least likely.

It is a known fact from a Harvard study that with 700,000 infants in 39 U.S. hospitals a 40% increase of leukemia and cancer of the central nervous system had occurred in children whose mothers were X rayed during pregnancy.

The tremendous increase in X rays and the natural increase of the disastrous effects of these rays can be partially laid at the door of physicians and dentists who have their own equipment. This equipment costs a lot of money and must be paid for and the easiest and the most business-like way to pay for it is to take X rays for which the patient always pays and thus X ray-taking is very, very profitable but the medical and dental hierarchy are well aware of the situation and are trying to slow it down or stop it.

Some patients are smartening up, too, and malpractice suits against physicians and dentists are on the increase and physicians and dentists who are addicted to taking X rays are being a little more cautious now. It is claimed by one authority that because Medicaid and local programs pay as much as $15 to $25 per X ray many dentists and doctors have turned their X ray machines into money printing machines and there is no danger that they will be charged for counterfeiting by any authority.

Dr. John L. McClenahan, in an editorial in the magazine Radiology stated "It is easier to order an X ray examination than to think". Besides, most doctors are too busy to think.

Drs. Russell S. Bell and John W. Loop of the University of Washington School of Medicine did some research on 435 patients who were treated for head injuries and in the procedure were X rayed in hospital emergency rooms, in spite of the fact that preliminary examinations did not indicate a fracture. The report discovered they did not find a single patient whose treatment was significantly different as a result of the X ray.

From all of this you can readily understand why both doctors and dentists almost invariably order or take X rays. It appears that the dentists are worse offenders than the medical men.

Perhaps you'll recall that 10 or more years ago practically every shoe store had an X ray machine so that you could see how your foot fitted into your shoe. This practice was discontinued because of warnings of the danger of X rays and a mighty good thing, too, that it was discontinued. However, the use of X rays by medical men and dentists has been increasing phenomenally.

So where do we go from here ... abandon the X ray? No doubt there are times and places when it has some use. I can honestly say that in my lifetime as it applies to me I have not known one useful thing that it has done for me, although I have been X rayed on a few occasions ... but not in recent years since I've been alerted. The part that worries me is this cumulative affair. How many hours or days or years will these X rays cost me in my span of life? From the information that I have reviewed and read and studied there is not a shadow of doubt that even the slightest X ray kills body organisms and as I spend my life and eat with the intent of building body organisms and keeping them alive I consider any X ray a deadly enemy.

Whether or not you permit X rays in the future is strictly your own affair. I'm suggesting that you avoid X rays like you would a plague because X rays either are a plague or can cause a plague.

CHAPTER
84

TOILETRIES, ACCESSORIES AND NECESSITIES OF LIFE

I've always felt that primarily food and drink were the necessities of life. Of course, this is strictly a limited viewpoint.

In our present civilization I have learned that there are many, many other things that are considered necessities. We'll start off by enumerating some of them. Here is my list, and I want you to know I use none of them and consider them totally unnecessary and, with few exceptions, harmful to varying degrees . . . mouth washes, throat gargles, shaving cream, shaving soap, after shave lotion, breath purifiers, deodorizers, deodorants, detergents, perfumes, tooth paste, tooth powder, hair rinse, hair shampoo, hair set, hair oils, hair creams, depilatory creams, eye shadow, eye mascara, lipstick, rouge, cold cream, face powder, talcum powder.

The shining or polishing of one's shoes is a necessity today.

Wearing good clothes is essential. Having clean laundry and underclothing is hygienic and considered a part of our way of life.

Of course, today in America women consider a hairdresser a most vital part of their existence, as well as beauticians who fix up their beautiful or not so beautiful faces. And of course, this means that a wide range of cosmetics are recommended and used. Then we have things like tooth brushes, tooth powders and tooth pastes. And of course, we can't for a moment omit soaps, with their various fragrant odors both for the face and the laundry. Nowadays most laundry soaps are made with detergents . . . this might even include facial soaps.

Besides all this, a very vital part of a women's toilet is a deodorant. It plays a much more vital part than most people ever recognize. And there is a very good reason why women today need anti-perspirants or deodorants. If man depended upon his sense of smell, as all other animals do, in order to find a mate, I'm afraid there would be no copulation and no childbirth and our birth rate would drop to zero.

Today women do not depend upon their spoor to attract a mate. Instead they use mini-skirts, cosmetics, beauticians, hairdressers and all such other means. Even if a man did have a keen proboscis and an alert sense of smell, it wouldn't help him a darn bit because any woman who calls herself a woman disguises any odor by the anti-perspirants, deodorants and such. Furthermore, I am so nasty and mean as to suggest that most of the odors or effluvia that emanate from the female species bear no relationship to sex and I am sure that by a natural arrangement the female of the species has a gland (a sort of pouch like the musk deer) that gives off a scent that is so very, very alluring and interesting and delightful to the male. Or is it vice versa?

What I am trying to convey to you is the simple truth that the odor that emanates from women is not one of sweat because I don't know of any women today, especially in business life, who have any cause or reason to get themselves into a sweat. But the

528

odors that do emanate are unpleasant odors that are caused by the chemicals in the food they eat, by the cigarettes they smoke and by the artificial chemical odors that they use under their arms and under their ears and on their hair and on their bodies in general.

No woman would dare take the risk of leaving her various cosmetics on overnight. So they have to bathe and use caustic soaps and detergents to remove the coat of paint or enamel that they put on their faces and bodies. Then, of course, in order to step out again into the field in the morning they have to put the same stuff back on again. So you see, it's a never-ending vicious cycle.

I am one of these peculiar, stupid individuals who suggest that a woman never smelled any better than she did when she allowed nature to take its course. I, for one, have never found the odor of honest sweat painful or offensive. I feel that a man should smell like a man and a woman should smell like a woman ... and not use artificial smelling agents to disguise one from the other or make them both smell alike.

I would take all the beauty concoctions, all of the fragrance enhancers, all of the breath purifiers, all the tooth pastes and perfumes and cosmetics and hair sprays and, no, not dump them all in the ocean where they could do serious harm to the denizens of the deep ... but I would go to the highest active volcano in the world and dump them down into its crater. That is the only way you could prevent any other part of the world from being seriously contaminated.

"Horrors!" you say. "How could we live without tooth pastes and tooth powders and abrasives and mouth washes?"

I have lived without them for more than fifteen years and my dentist still allows me to sit in his chair and he works over me, my wife hasn't left me, my friends have not hung up the 'not welcome' sign, my business associates still continue to associate with me and even my staff don't go around with masks or clothespins on their noses. In fact, I would be willing to wager with you, you

529

honey-dipped prude, that the odor, if any, that emanates from my body is less offensive than the odor that emanates from yours after you have smeared all that junk over you.

Yes, I do bathe daily, or more often if I work on the land, without the use of soap and have done so for many years. I use a scrubbing brush and plenty of good warm water. The only soap that I use is some on my hands if I have been working outdoors and some on my face when I shave. In fact I have stopped using soap on my face and use only water and no lotion or after-shave. In case you don't know it, using lots of soap prevents the proper absorption of vitamin D and you can do yourself serious harm by getting insufficient vitamin D. If I do use soap it is the simplest — preferably castile.

Just the other day the following appeared in a popular American weekly newspaper.

"Unwashed men stand less chance of picking up skin disease than housewives with a compulsion to stay clean and deodorized, a leading skin specialist says.

"Dr. Knox, chairman of the dermatology department at Baylor College of Medicine, Houston, Tex., said in many cases men who have not washed their hands are actually more germ-free than the average housewife with her keep-clean mania. The use of a body deodorant is especially bad, because it blocks the openings of the sweat glands.

"Dr. Knox added that 'bathing twice a day is ridiculous, and persons over 40 should not bathe every day in winter.

" 'Bathing takes away the valuable skin oils which nature intended to be there, or else evolution would have done away with them,' Dr. Knox said."

Yes, I would also avoid the use of talcum powder of any kind. All it tends to do is plug up your pores and that's the last thing that a healthy body requires.

Sure as shooting, the cosmetic manufacturers and the cosmetic stores and counters and the manufacturers of such things as eye paint and eyebrow pencil and fake eyelashes and mascara will not cheer Tobe on to victory. Well, to me those spell injury and destruction to the human anatomy.

My wife does not use much make-up. She does use some, even though I plead with her not to use it. I tell her in all sincerity that she never looks better than when she uses nothing but plain water with which to wash her face.

No doubt there are women whom the camouflage helps. Oh, by all means I see the necessity for the use of these cosmetics, in fact, in great quantities for some of the women I have seen and known. Not every woman was born beautiful although I think there is something beautiful about every woman. You know, beauty is as beauty does. Besides, when you are in love beauty is in the eyes of the beholder. Granted there are reasons and times when cosmetics are needed like on the stage or for performers. For such occasions I would not seek to banish cosmetics.

But for all of you beautiful women with the skin you love to touch, with hair like gossamer and with eyes that sparkle and cheeks that glow, you have no need for these harmful, caustic, detrimental camouflaging items. Besides, when a man sees a woman plastered with make-up he is apprehensive about what lies under that built-up facade.

Now just a word about babies. I know mothers who scrub their poor little babies with soap and then bathe them in oil and then cover them with talcum. You know, with such treatment, it is absolutely astounding that any baby lives to grow up.

For years I have watched mothers soap their babies' heads until a rash and a crust appeared and they kept rubbing and rubbing and the more they rubbed the worse it became ... never realizing

531

that the rubbing with soap was the complete cause of the trouble. Then of course they go and pay the pediatricians high fees and buy expensive drugs to correct the condition that required nothing but being left alone or being washed with plain ordinary water.

You'd be astounded if you knew the number of people who suffer from no other condition but the over-use of these beauty accoutrements. If the use of these accoutrements were stopped overnight, a third of all the conditions that afflict women would no doubt disappear from the face of the earth.

Why not stop using these problem creating cosmetics?

CHAPTER

85

THANKLESS JOB

I have frequently been taken to task because of my distrustful attitudes and my expressions of doubt and lack of confidence in practically all of our institutions, establishments and ways of life, but never have I been attacked so bitterly, so forcibly and so earnestly and viciously as I was attacked by a person whose first name was Jenny.

Actually I think Jenny liked me and even liked what I was doing but after a discussion with me when I kept tearing down everything she believed in and respected she exploded "Have you nothing good to say about anybody or anything? You're always tearing down, attacking, and destroying . . . anybody can do that. What is needed is something constructive. Your rantings and your ravings and your writing are too morbid and too depressing. I can no longer read it, I don't want to read it, I don't want to hear about

533

it . . . even though I think you are right on most things . . . you are carrying it too far. You've left me nothing to cling to, nothing I can believe in".

I was genuinely affected by Jenny's attack and also by the way she felt and I just had to stop and do a little thinking and some deep, profound soul searching. Let me tell you this . . . I don't derive any joy or pleasure out of the work I'm doing. There are many people in this world who have a job to do and do it well and yet their hearts and their souls are not in it. They'd rather be doing something else but this is something they do well and there aren't too many people who are willing to relieve them of the responsibility and do the job as it should be done. That's the boat I'm in.

If it were not for the fact that I have seen the results, the benefits of my labors I would not be able to continue because it is even too demoralizing for me. I am steeped in and surrounded by a sea of corruption and evil and even though I fight it off and have alerted millions of others to the dangers, still it's beginning to seep into my bones and when someone like Jenny comes along and sinks her talons into my back I feel as though I want to get out, that I want to run away, that I want to go to some place or somewhere where I can sing and say nice things about people and feel that the world is a grand and glorious place with clean air and good wholesome people.

Still I can hear Jenny's voice ringing in my ears "Is there no good food left in this world? Are there no honest, decent medical doctors, are there no loyal, dedicated scientists, are there no respected decent government officials, are there no uncorrupted universities, are there no decent, honest food processors, bottlers, butchers and bakers left in this world? Are there no farmers left who grow decent crops? Are there no clergymen who are sincere and dedicated? Are there no reliable, well run institutions left in our country?"

So I must reply to the challenge and state that the only decent food I know of in America today is that which you grow in

534

your own garden by your own hands. The M.D's are tied to the drug industry, there are a few M.D's who don't like it and even the great American medical association is having a partial revolution on its hands. As for scientists, most of them are employed in industry or by government or by universities and they do as they are told. As for honest, decent politicians and government officials . . . well, if they were honest and decent their position would be untenable and the few that do exist are finding their position untenable and they are besieged from all sides.

As for honest food processors and producers, I don't know one single one. Oh yes I do, one name comes to mind but I can't give it here because there may be others and I don't want you to feel as though I were playing favourites. Generally speaking, concerning food processors the word 'process' itself tells the story. If it is processed it is not fit to eat and there are just bad processors, worse processors and worst processors.

As for farmers, they raise the kind of beef that the packers want. They grow the kind of crops the shippers and the chain stores want and these are not the kind of meat and not the kind of crops that the farmers themselves eat.

Clergymen? What priest, minister or rabbi listens or pays any attention to the poor or to the hippies of his congregation or his parish? He caters to those who make the big donations and contributions and ignores those who would change the present order of things. Speaking of our institutions they are a part of the government and the government is controlled by the doctors, scientists, food processors and the farmers and the clergymen. So what can you expect from that array?

This is what I'd like to say to Jenny . . . if I could live with myself after I did it I would be glad to throw in the sponge and end it all and go about growing roses or chrysanthemums and singing love songs and writing poetry. But that damnable voice within me keeps saying "Sure, go ahead, throw in the sponge, have fun and enjoy life, you selfish bum . . . and let millions be poisoned, die untimely deaths

535

because you, you rotten skunk, knew and didn't tell".

So there it is Jenny, you old witch. You got it off your chest and I got it off mine but . . . I've got my problems too as you can plainly see and if you can spare the tears — weep for me — I've none left to shed.

CHAPTER
86

WHY THERE ARE DOPES AND BRIGHT CHILDREN

Animals instinctively know what is right for them and perform most functions so that the species can be continued in good health from one generation to another, ad infinitum. Now this does not apply to domesticated animals whose feeding and living habits are controlled by man. Where man interferes, the animal invariably deteriorates. This applies to cattle, dogs, cats or race horses. A race horse may run faster than he did in the good old days (I'm not even sure of that) but he is certainly not as healthy as a horse on the range.

Man has lost his sense of instinct and now he must rely upon his brain if he is lucky enough to have one. If a person has brains it is a gift from the parents, mainly from the mother. If you are intelligent or if you are stupid you were made that way by your mother . . . not your father. Your father had little or nothing to do

537

with it. Don't misunderstand, a father makes a contribution but he has little to say about the brain power of the infant.

If a young couple wants to be sure to have a healthy, intelligent offspring care should start some months before pregnancy. Proper food should be eaten by both would-be parents and a mode of life followed that would be conducive to giving birth to a healthy offspring. Smoking and alcoholic beverages are 100% taboo for parents who would create healthy offspring. The use of coffee is condemned, the use of all drugs is emphatically condemned. A wholesome, uncontaminated, unchemicalized raw food diet would be ideal and if such were followed there would be no danger whatsoever of having anything but a perfect and intelligent offspring.

So now we have two healthy young people . . . an intelligent, alert female and an active, alert, capable male. Sexual intercourse takes place and they give themselves heart and soul to each other, a climax is reached and the process begins. From here on out the food eaten by the pregnant female is of vital importance to both the mother and the unborn child. It is even of greater importance to the unborn child because any serious damage that might result will be much greater in the child than in the mother. Furthermore, any damage due to impaired nutrition will only affect the mother to a degree that can be corrected but for the unborn infant in most cases any problem or deficiency caused by lack of proper food will affect the child for its entire life and in most cases it is irreparable. Thus the mother-to-be is solely responsible for the mental potential of her child. This is the very, very important factor that must be considered by every would-be mother.

It is necessary that the mother make sure that during the entire period of pregnancy she has proper food so that the fetus will be properly nourished. Scientific evidence clearly states that among body organs the brain is first to complete its growth. It is further learned that the most rapid period of growth is from the 5th fetal month to the end of the first year and it is during this period where nutrition deficiencies can be deadly serious.

Here is another very, very important factor to realize and that is that by the end of the first year of life the brain develops to 70% of its adult weight. Furthermore, by the end of the second year the development and growth of the brain is practically complete. Now you can understand why improper or undernutrition during that rapid growth period would not only inhibit brain growth but would probably result in irreparable damage to mental activity. Therefore, I stress that the pregnant mother should take no risks whatsoever. She must be sure that she will be properly and adequately nourished during the entire period of pregnancy. Then it is essential that the child be properly fed for the first two years of its life.

Now here enters another vitally important factor . . . breast feeding. The only sure, the only positive way that you can be certain that your child is properly nourished is by feeding him from your own breast. At the same time be sure that you in turn are properly nourished. Furthermore, you must breast feed this child for the two-year period. Then, and then only will you have a healthy and an intelligent child. Of course I realize that two years is a long period but from the information that I have and from my own observations I know that it can be done, it has been done and it is being done . . . granted, by the rare few. If you love your child and if you want to have the joy of raising a healthy offspring into childhood and manhood then you should be willing to devote the first two years to its proper upbringing. Remember you still have 50 or more years to go and you'll probably be in close contact with your offspring, thus the 2 year period does not seem so long and enduring. Imagine having a retarded or palsied child due to your neglect and facing this for 50 or more years.

I fully realize that most pregnant women are under the care of their medical doctor. However, most girls do not go to their doctor before conception takes place. Many of them do not go to their doctor until they have reached the final month of pregnancy. No doubt the average obstetrician and gynecologist is well trained in pathology and various medical techniques but most of them are ill-equiped to handle nutritional problems. In fact, it is a well known fact that most doctors have had little if any nutritional training.

Furthermore, I do not know of any medical doctor who will warn the would-be mother that she must not take any drugs whatsoever and avoid coffee, tea, alcohol and tobacco.

A qualified medical doctor told me 15 years ago that to the best of his knowledge there were no truly healthy babies born in America and from all accounts and observations this statement appears to be true. From my actual experience, discussion and reading with and of doctors I know that most of them ignore — or do not consider — nutrition a factor in disease.

I am sure that the medical profession has access to the information that I have given in this chapter but whether they accept it or follow it is another matter. Obviously doctors do not regard drugs as being harmful, otherwise they would not prescribe them so flagrantly. Obviously they do not regard nutrition as being important. Therefore, you cannot expect the average medical doctor to give you sound nutritional counselling.

There is only one sure safe way to have a healthy, normal, intelligent child and that is by following the procedures that I have outlined. My advice is, don't trust to luck. Nature still knows how to produce healthy babies but you must give nature a chance and cooperate with her. You must in no way block nature. Healthy, intelligent babies can be yours for the asking.

CHAPTER
87

HELP THE CRIPPLED, THE PALSIED AND THE
RETARDED CHILDREN

I have been a member of a service club for about 30 years. I like the work service clubs have been doing for their fellow man. I like it because it is without thought of payment or benefits to ourselves that we do this work. It is always for the benefit of others. Can anyone deny this is noble on the part of service clubs and their members? They go out and they raise funds due to their own efforts. They spend their time, use their automobiles and even spend their money . . . all to raise funds so that they can contribute to the welfare of society and especially to help young children — blind, crippled, retarded children. Each service club selects its own kind of work or contribution to society. There are many of them, many different organizations with many members and they all help carry out this noble and beneficial work.

The members of the service clubs in America run into the millions and now they have them in practically all countries of the world. Can anyone deny that this is meritorious and commendable work? I, too, have given of my time and my efforts and even of my money to help in this work and was proud of my contribution.

Now after a third of a century of membership and activity in a service club I feel that I have not done enough. In fact, I feel as though I have let down those whom I tried to help. I know in my own heart that there are millions of crippled children in America today who need not have been crippled if I had been more honest with myself, bolder and stronger and willing to fight.

Give me some men who are stout hearted men
Who will fight for the right they adore,
Give me some men who are stout hearted men
And I'll soon show you ten thousand more.

Had I, along with many thousands of members, had the courage to stand up against the government, the medical profession and the drug and chemical corporations, the food processers, the tobacco companies, the distillers and the brewers and say, "We will not allow you to create crippled, palsied and retarded children," none of them would have been born. Instead they would have been healthy, straight and of good mentality.

It was because we were weak, ignorant, fearful and lacking in courage and guts that these children were born. Whether we like it or not we must bear the responsibility of helping create them or bring them into being in the condition in which they exist today. We cannot hide behind the thin curtain that we tried to help them and raise money to give them pleasure. What a puny satisfaction that is . . . what a despicable substitute for a strong body, limbs and mind which were their heritage and which were denied them because we would not stand and fight for them. They would not be in that condition if we had acted like men should act or were we tranquilized by booze, tobacco and coffee?

542

Here I singled out service clubs because they do try to contribute to the welfare of their communities. My complaint against them is that they do not do enough. They should act to prevent the tragedy and not step in only when the tragedy has occurred. None of us are blameless. We are as guilty as those who actually perpetrated or created the outrage. The creators, the causers, those responsible directly are the governments, the medical profession, the food processers, the chemical manufacturers, the drug corporations, the tobacco producers, brewers, distillers and the vintners.

While all of these corporations and groups actually created and caused these things, we, the rest of the population – poor, puny people – stood by and permitted it. We neither spoke up nor did we use the means at our disposal to stop or prevent it. Therefore, we are all accessories to the fact. No man is innocent. We are all guilty . . . it is just that some are more guilty than others. Each of us should hang his head in shame and writhe in agony with a guilt complex . . . even with the present knowledge we know it is being done and we still do nothing to stop it. We do not deserve to be free men. In fact, I doubt if we are men at all.

We deserve to be drowned in a sea of spit from the mouths of the children whom we permitted to be created and born crippled, palsied and retarded. The hockey and baseball players give of their time to play for them, the service clubs buy them toys and wheelchairs and take them to circuses. Actors entertain them, politicians pose with and embrace them . . . all for show. Big hearted, public spirited, noble minded citizens! But where were they when the bodies and minds of these yet to be born children were being desecrated . . . having fun, enjoying the bounties of life and living.

Yes, and in spite of the many millions of these unfortunate children as a sign and proof of our errors not a finger is lifted or pointed at the perpetrators and more thousands of the same are born every day and all we do is shrug our shoulders and say "It is God's Will" and go along arranging benefits for the games, wheelchairs and circuses . . . we, the noble citizens of America.

CHAPTER

88

ABOUT SLEEP

I have not been able to find many studies on sleep. The one study done a year or two ago indicated that men who slept 7 hours or less had fewer heart attacks than men who slept 8 hours and more. This made sense to me because I feel that most of us spend too much time in bed.

In the past 20 years I have curtailed my sleeping hours from 8 or 9 down to 6 1/2 hours daily but this was not because of a heart condition. Occasionally I will sleep 7 or 7 1/2 hours and occasionally only 4 or 5 hours. But as a rule I try to get my full 6 1/2 hours sleep. However, I do this in two batches. I try to take a rest after my evening meal, dinner to us, which is taken usually between 6 and 7 in the evening. I usually stretch out on the living room rug and get about 1/2 an hour to an hour and a half of sleep. Then I start to work again at 9 or 10 or 11 o'clock and work until 2 and 3 in the morning. In the morning I usually arise at 8 and have breakfast when we have company around 8:30. Normally, I have my first meal at noon.

Most people I know try to get 8 hours sleep. Most of the older people that I know try to get more and usually do sleep anywhere from 8 to 12 hours a day. My mother always claimed that sleep was a thief and if you permit it it will steal your life away. My father did not sleep many hours. He usually got a nap in the afternoon but he arose every day at 6 or before and never got to bed until the wee hours of 1 or 2 o'clock in the morning. I doubt if he ever slept 8 hours at a stretch in all the years that I knew him.

I have noticed of recent years that most of the people who have passed their 60's or 70's tend to sleep more and I consider this one of the causes of aging. Yes, I certainly believe that long hours of sleep do cause aging.

The normal sleep rule or regulations that I was taught indicated that infants should sleep most of the day, the children should sleep about 12 hours, that young people should sleep at least 10 hours and that normal adults should sleep at least 8 hours every day. I can find no scientific or logical basis for these hours of sleep. I think it is absolutely wrong to allow or encourage infants to sleep most of the day and night. Yes, I fully realize that chickens begin to roost before the shades of night start to fall and begin to awaken or stir about as the dawn is breaking.

I also know that a dog and a cat will sleep when there is nothing else to do and most dogs and cats will sleep away many hours. I think this is due to the fact that they are well fed and do not have to spend any time foraging for food. So I don't think we can judge or take an example from most domesticated animals, although in many cases we can learn something from their habits. It is my conviction that a man need only sleep long enough to regenerate his batteries. Sleeping more than sufficient to rest the body and mind is totally unnecessary and can even be harmful. I maintain that long hours of sleep by older folks contributes to senility.

From my actual observations I feel that those people who sleep long hours are not as active or as spry or as mentally alert as those who sleep fewer hours. Try and investigate by checking with your friends and people that you know as to the number of hours they sleep and see whether or not my investigations and findings are correct. I reiterate that those who are most active, those who are the most mentally alert are those who sleep less than 8 hours.

I'm not trying to deny the necessity of sleep but 6 or 7 hours of sound sleep are, in my opinion, all that any active human being requires and more than 7 hours is detrimental to health. Of course spending 8 hours in bed does not necessarily mean that you get 8 hours sleep. I've also learned that I can miss a night's sleep, that is I get only 3 or 4 or 5 hours, without any serious effects. I can even do this for two or three nights running but beyond that I'll feel it and show it on my countenance. I recognize the need for sleep and I advocate adequate hours of sleep.

For more than 20 years I have tested various hours of sleep and I find that I do best, I work best, I am most productive when I average 6 1/2 hours sleep per day and the better I maintain this average, the better is my performance physically and mentally.

While most of my work is sedentary I still maintain a high degree of activity but even when I do a fair amount of strenuous physical work the same number of hours of sleep is maintained.

CHAPTER

89

WE EXAMINE BABY FOODS

There was quite a big to-do about monosodium glutamate in baby foods. To me this was a crying shame . . . to think that two of the largest food processors in the world lowered themselves to the state where they would jeopardize and injure our children, our infants, for the sake of making a few bucks.

Actually the MSG was totally unnecessary in the food but they put it in because the mothers usually taste the food and the MSG does make the food taste better and therefore they would buy it for their infants.

I have had a long experience with MSG . . . probably a greater experience than most people in the world. I am not bragging about it but I had some unhappy findings about MSG and therefore I am well acquainted with it. And to think that any corporation would so

549

injure our infants so they could sell more baby foods! I can't put my thoughts into words.

MSG has been positively linked with impairing the mental faculties of mice in tests and I am positively certain it would affect our infants. That's how much you can trust our great and huge food processing industry.

Anyway, a chap who worked for one of these large baby food manufacturers came into my premises to make a purchase and somehow we got to talking. I've never been in love with food processors of any kind and when he mentioned that he worked for one of these processors, I suggested that they made foods that harm the people. He claimed that this was not so and that his company had a strict policy to allow no chemical additives in the food that they made for children. I said, "I'm very, very happy to hear that and if what you say is true, I'll recommend your products to every mother that I know." And so we parted.

Well, that day or the next I hiked to the supermarket and went to the section where they sell the canned baby foods and I studied the lists of ingredients on the labels of that certain company's baby food. I found that basically what he said was true. I could see no food additives listed on the labels but I did see in one case "tomato paste" and in another case "flour" and then I knew the jig was up!

A few days later, on the weekend, the same chap turned up and I said to him, "Are you still positive that your firm does not use any chemical additives in their baby foods?"

He said, "Yes, I checked it out again with my superiors and it is a positive fact that we add no chemicals to our baby foods."

So I said to him, "Where do you get your tomato paste?"

He said, "We buy it from one of the larger paste manufacturers."

Then I went in and got my copy of the Food and Drug Manual and flipped the pages to tomato paste. There in clear bold type was the fact that it contained a harsh and harmful chemical preservative. My friend paled at this allegation.

I said to him, "Where do you buy your flour that goes into your baby foods?"

He said, "We buy it from one of the largest mills in the country."

Then I flipped the pages of the Food and Drug manual to flour and when he looked at the list of chemicals permitted in the flour, he almost turned green. I think there were 17 of them at the time . . . 17 chemicals added to flour. And that was the flour that was put into their baby foods and they said that none of their foods contained any chemical additives.

Well, I didn't expect any results from this because after all he had a good job with this company and he wasn't going to jeopardize his job just because Tobe pointed out that his company was a fraud and a quack. But I presume they meant well and they didn't realize that the flour contained these chemicals or that the tomato paste contained them. I am also sure that many, many other commodities that they use or buy also contain chemical additives . . . even if they don't add any themselves.

The World Health Organization is concerned about baby foods and they said, "Require separate consideration from all other foods as regards the use of food additives and toxicological risk."

The WHO were talking good sense, based on sound logic. They claimed that additives should be kept out of baby foods because infants just do not possess the fully developed systems that adults do to eliminate poisons from the body. Therefore, the committee was most strong in its urgings that baby foods should be prepared without food additives. But they added "if possible."

However, the American baby food processors evidently do not agree. Sodium nitrite is widely used in baby foods that contain cured ham. The purpose of sodium nitrite is to preserve and produce the pink color in cured meats. A sister compound, sodium nitrate, has for years been implicated in blue baby disease. It is claimed that a safe nitrate level is about 45 parts per million, but the sodium nitrates have a habit of being converted into nitrites in the human body.

It has long been suspected that these nitrates and nitrites are seriously harmful and the Food and Drug of Canada intended making a deep investigation into these compounds that have been used in the food industry for well over 50 years. But evidently the food processors regard the addition of the nitrates and nitrites as being so valuable that they had their lobbyists pressure the government to get the Food and Drug off the backs of the nitrites and nitrates, so nothing was done. Evidently they like that bright pink color of the meat and for that they would sacrifice the health of our babies and the ultimate well-being of our nation. Nice people, no?

CHAPTER

90

CELLULAR REGENERATION

We know that the body is composed of cells, billions or trillions according to the best authorities. Cells keep dying and new cells are being made by the body from the food that is supplied to it. It's strictly a matter of replacement.

As long as the cells are replaced by food, physical health is maintained at a steady or high level. I consider cellular regeneration the most important function of the animal body. There is nothing to compare with it. Upon it depends our health, our very way of life. Cells have been called by one great authority "the carrier of life."

The cell's function is unique. It knows how to sustain itself and follows the pattern of proper assimilation, interchange and excretion. If we are sick it is our cells that are sick because the great accumulation of trillions of cells is you. You are as healthy or as sick as your cells.

I'm sure some of you have heard of Dr. Paul Neihans. He has been using cellular therapy or cellular forces since 1920 and has more than 30,000 successful treatments to his credit and he has treated some of the most famous and most renowned men of this century.

His method of treatment is the injection of live cellular tissues, usually taken from an unborn lamb (it is sometimes claimed that he uses a calf). It is also claimed that he has treated practically every known disease with marked success. He is now an old man and at the present day living in Switzerland. Someone told me he had passed away but I have not seen the report. There are thousands of his articles which appeared in the press throughout the world as well as books. You can get information about him very, very easily and it's worthwhile knowing. The point is that by the use of this live cellular tissue from other animals he has accomplished cures and benefits that have astounded the world. The medical profession called him nasty names, they refused to recognize him, they probably cursed him but he stands unchallenged in his field. The medical profession cannot claim to even remotely match his achievements. Neihans is, of course, a fully qualified medical practitioner.

Please understand that I am not a convert to Paul Neihans nor do I support or approve his treatments. I'm just relating as a reporter what I know, what I have read and what I'm told about Paul Neihans. I have been acquainted with his work and his activities for more than 25 years. I have been puzzled, I have been dismayed, I have been worried about his means and methods but no one on earth can deny that they have been almost 100% successful. No healing science has matched or can match Paul Neihans' success. I have never read of a failure by the Paul Neihans live cellular tissue injection treatment.

Please now, don't run off immediately to Paul Neihans or think that I am sending you there. I'm telling you my story so please listen.

554

Of course you must recognize that the drug profession have been watching the antics and success of Dr. Paul Neihans very carefully because as soon as possible they'd like to latch on to his method and incorporate it in a drug or an injection or whatever other means the drug people use to sell their wares. The pharmaceutical or drug industry has produced a purified hormone of synthetic origin to be used for injections for various conditions by medical doctors. They have also crystallized various hormones for implantation. However, they have not been able to copy the success of Dr. Paul Neihans for their synthetic crystallized hormones have not yet proven successful but you can bet they are still trying with might and mane.

Many famous doctors and professors have checked and double checked on Neihans' method of treatment but they could find no negative reactions whatsoever from his methods and they also found that his treatments were invariably not only successful but permanent. I trust you got the message . . . permanent. What conventional medical doctor ever accomplished that?

For the past 25 years I have read and reread anything pertaining to Dr. Neihans. I have been impressed, I have been convinced that Dr. Neihans treatment is successful because it is alive and it is not treated or involved with any synthetic drugs or chemicals. Niehans, by his great work, has managed to bring down the treatment of disease to its simplest common denominator. If you had a disorder of the eye he would take the eye of an unborn lamb, mascerate it and then inject it into your blood stream. The same treatment would apply to any other organ of the body. As I stated before, the greatest authorities have learned that this method does not produce any negative reactions whatsoever and it almost invariably improves the organ that has been damaged and which is being treated, in an unbelievably short time.

Now you may ask what has this all to do with Tobe, with the Golden Treasury, with raw food and with proper living, so let me tell you. Any seed, large, medium, small or tiny contains all the components that are found in the human body or the animal body. The seed has the same ability to regenerate that is contained within

555

the fetus from which the gland or the organ is taken. It is my belief that eating raw grains, raw root vegetables, raw green, yellow and red vegetables, fruits and nuts gives the body the opportunity to strengthen, to replace and to regenerate any organ or part of the human body.

The requirements are simple . . . you must use only fresh, viable, raw, unchemicalized, unheated, untreated seeds, plants and roots. Only they have the ability to reconstruct cells to perfection. It is my belief that the genetic code operates for miniscule insects or animals or bacteria as well as for plants, and for animals and for humans. Now whether you call it DNA for Dioxyribonucleic acid or Ribonucleic acid or you call it cell regeneration or the genetic code or cellular therapeutics or cellular enzyme action I do not care . . . to me it is all one and the same thing.

I further maintain that this genetic code of cellular regeneration will function if the natural treatment is followed and the body that is being treated still has sufficient enzymes to fulfill and carry out the treatment. You cannot expect cellular regeneration to function immediately if it is applied to a human body that has abused itself for 50 or 75 years and then suddenly changed over to raw foods. It just will not work because there is no harmony, there is no cooperation and the ground has not been prepared.

Just what it takes to correct the condition or make it function I am not prepared to say and I don't think anyone knows but the wheels should be set in motion at the earliest possible time.

If you want to try this method of raw food eating start immediately and some reactions may be felt because a person who is not used to eating raw food may run into many problems. The body may react in various ways. You may have aches, you may have pains, you may have intestinal disturbances or even other disturbances because you can't just change over from eating cooked, processed, chemicalized and otherwise refined and mutilated foods and start eating raw seeds and raw vegetables and raw fruits in abundance at the snap of your fingers. Almost invariably some form of disturbance is manifest but it only lasts for a day or two and perhaps sometimes maybe weeks or months with those who have had heavy drug treatments or were preponderantly users of cooked foods.

The adjustment of the body and organs is sometimes difficult and slow but it can be done and is being done by people even in their mid-eighties and some that I know in their mid-nineties. This is not an exaggeration; it is a positive statement of fact that can be substantiated but again I state that the older the individual the more difficult the transition may be. It is not always true . . . some of them make the transition quite readily and easily and with little or no trouble.

I contend that any disease known to mankind can be treated by means of a raw food diet and it will bring better results than Paul Neihans live cellular tissue injection. Please understand clearly I am not knocking his method or treatment . . . how can I with the miraculous results he has achieved? The advantage that Neihans has is that he injects his tissue directly into the bloodstream and therefore the action is much more rapid. He also has the advantage of not having to sell his patients a bill of goods on the raw food diet which most people, especially older people would find difficult, repugnant or even impossible. They pay Neihans big, fat fees as you can readily understand and they are willing to pay these big, fat fees as long as they don't have to endure personal inconvenience and discomfort which will be the case if they have to change their diet drastically. This would also change their way of life, their standard of living and seriously affect invariably their social life. When people are very wealthy and famous all of these things are actually more important than health or life itself.

Lest you think that this cellular regeneration system used and made famous by Niehans is something new let me assure you that it has been used by mankind for thousands of years, even in pre-biblical times. There are positive records that this treatment was used more than 4,000 years ago. Even native aborigines of various countries have used this treatment in various ways and it has been handed down since time immemorial. When the chief of a cannibal tribe captured

557

an enemy who had a strong heart he ate his enemy's heart. When an enemy had a strong spear throwing arm he ate that arm or when an enemy chief had a reputation for promiscuous virility he ate his genitals.

If you cannot see, believe or accept cellular regeneration brought down to its simplest, most logical and most natural terms . . . by the eating of raw foods, you have my deepest sympathy. If you can see it, accept it and use it . . . you will indubitably improve your health and greatly increase the span of your life. It all depends upon you, your cells and the cells in the food that you eat. Can it ever be simpler?

CHAPTER
91

AIR AND BREATHING

I felt that a book on health would be incomplete without a discussion or an investigation of the merits of air and breathing. I found that I have seldom discussed the merits of breathing in my writing and I sincerely believe that I have been remiss in my duties. I have known a few men, some who are my good friends, who studied breathing, who practiced deep breathing and who were strong advocates of its merits and benefits. I'd like to mention them here.

First and foremost is Clarence Eklund who has for years hammered away at me, emphasizing the tremendous value of oxygen. He claimed it was a food, not only something to breathe. He is now in his mid 80's.

Another is Herbert Angus Mowat, a friend of many years standing, who in spite of serious World War I injuries has regained and maintained superb health up until the present day. He also is in his mid 80's.

Now there is Dean Bosserman who is the most ardent and compulsive advocate of the merit of air and breathing of any man on earth today. He is convinced that deep, deep breathing is the foremost answer to health and long life.

There was also my old friend George Clements (Professor Hilton Hotema) who passed away at 92 years of age. For many years he stressed and emphasized the tremendous value of air and deep breathing. No doubt there are many more who advocated the merits of deep breathing and air and if I have forgotten or neglected them I apologize.

Friend Bosserman pointed out to me some very pertinent things about the lungs. For example, he stated that the lung's surface if placed on a flat plane would comprise approximately 2,000 square feet. Approximately 7 tons of blood are propelled through the lungs every 24 hours by air or as he calls it the 'Life Force'. He claims that the lungs are by far the largest organ in our body, practically filling the thoracic cavity.

Scientific studies indicate that man uses about one fifth of his lung capacity. Dean Bosserman suggests that only one fifth of the poisons generated by the living processes are eliminated and only one fifth of the vital life substance – air – is taken in to carry on the living process. This means only one fifth capacity operation of the most vital of all body functions and it should be put to much greater use.

According to him here is what takes place in the lungs. There is an exchange of the death cargo, which has been picked up in the capillaries, for a cargo of life sustaining air, through a membrane as thin as the skin of a soap bubble in a flash of brilliant color, ready and on its way to exchange this cargo of life for the death cargo the cells have developed in the capillaries. We know no more today how this process is accomplished than we did 50 years ago. This function must not be interfered with and pure air must always be available in the lungs or we are soon in trouble. There is no mechanism in the body to neutralize bad air — only the cilliary hairs and mucous membrane in the nose to prevent larger particles from penetrating the lungs.

Everything that lives must breathe. There can be no life without this process. Even those animals that hibernate must breathe or die. The major component of the air that we breathe is nitrogen. Oxygen makes up about twenty-one percent. It is estimated that there are approximately a billion air cells in the lungs. Every person requires 3,000 cubic feet of air every hour.

So much for my friend Dean.

Air is the invisible, tasteless, odourless mixture of gases surrounding the earth. Air is called the breath of life. Its composition is actually approximately 21% oxygen, 0.8% argon, 78% nitrogen. The balance is composed of aqueous vapour, carbon dioxide and traces of ammonia, helium, neon, krypton, zenon and other rare gases.

Let us discuss now for a moment the different kinds of air involved in breathing. One is Alveolar which refers to the air in the alveola which is involved in the pulmonary exchange of gases between the air and the blood. Its content is determined by sampling the last portion of a maximal expiration. Two, is the Complemental — the amount that may be breathed in over and above the tidal air by the deepest possible inspiration. Three, Dead space — the volume of air that fills the respiratory passageways and which is not available for exchange of gases with the blood.

Four, Functional residual is the volume of the air left in the lungs at the end of a natural unforced expiration. It is the sum of expiatory reserve volume and residual air.

Five, Residual. The amount of air remaining in the lungs after the fullest possible expiration. It amounts to approximately 1500 cc.

Six, Supplemental. This is the amount of air that may be forcibly expired after quiet expiration. The amount is approximately 1600 cc.

Seven, Tidal. This is the amount of air that flows in and out of the lungs with quiet respiration. The average adult male uses about 500 cc which is approximately one pint.

The claims made for the benefits derived from proper breathing and inhalation and exhalation border on the utterly fantastic. Some maintain that if we learned to breathe properly and had access to pure air we could live in perfect health without food. It is claimed that no man can live more than three minutes without access to air. It is unfortunate that most of us seldom think of the value of good fresh air until we find ourselves in a position where breathing conditions are so bad that we are almost stifled. We just take air and breathing for granted because it is provided for us automatically and because breathing is an involuntary action on the part of the body.

Many people have foul breath and according to an eminent medical authority this indicates any or all of the following . . . improper diet, constipation, lack of exercise, use of drugs, alcohol or tobacco, stomatitis, necrosis of the jaw, caries of the teeth, tonsilitis, diphtheria, gangrene and abscess of the lungs, fetid bronchitis, bronchiectasis, pyothorax, catarrh, diabetes, kidney disease and other disorders. If there is a urinous odor it indicates uremeia. If there is a sweetish odor like that of ripe apples it indicates diabetes, especially during coma.

Breathing exercises should be practiced at least twice a day upon arising and again before retiring. The lungs should be filled to capacity and the exhalation should be as complete as possible.

Here is the breathing exercise advocated by Dean Bosserman:

"The simple breathing I advocate is, first and most important, get the dormant, stagnant air out of the lungs as much as possible,

562

using the diaphragm and rib cage in a squeezing operation to accomplish this. This requires considerable effort and is the most tiring part of conscious breathing.

"After this has been accomplished the inhalation of clean pure air can reach the air cells properly supplying them with the life essence. Without the exhalation of the dormant, stagnant air first, this miraculous process cannot take place properly and the body suffers proportionately.

"At the depth of the exhalation and peak of inhalation it is good to hold the breath for a second or two, tensing all of the body muscles, even the facial muscles. Do this every eleventh or twelfth breath or as one desires. It will supply adequate exercise for most, especially those who are working toward an all fruit diet. Their bodies not requiring the violent exercise, most 'general livers' have to move the poison mass most colons are subjected to.

"It is also good to occasionally, while holding the inhaled breath, pull the diaphragm down or push it down consciously, thus activating dormant air cells in the largest part of the lungs.

"No doubt all rhymic breathing exercises taught have merit but our immediate concern is to remove the stagnant air and get fresh air to the greatest amount of air cells in the lungs — rhythm can come later.

"We must have all of the air cells functioning, doing their job in the proper manner, to receive the benefits we are entitled to from this most important body function."

CHAPTER

92

KEEP YOUR TONSILS AND OTHER ORGANS

I am one of the few lucky individuals. My parents were too poor to have my tonsils removed. We didn't have money to pay the doctor and we didn't have money to pay the hospital bills or a nurse . . . so I've got my tonsils. And, friends, that's the only reason I've got 'em, please believe me. Yes, and I believe that most folks of my age who have their tonsils, adenoids and appendix have them because they were too poor to pay the surgeon's fee.

The medical profession — or I should say, a segment of the medical profession — has been for years very vociferous about having children's tonsils removed. If I had my way I would punish those who remove tonsils, just as I would a criminal.

So you see, poverty isn't always the bad wolf it is cracked up to be. In fact, I've learned that poverty can be a blessing. Now when

565

I say this, you can believe me, for I have been poor all my life and it has only been in the last few years of my business life that I have been able to pay my bills almost on time. It took me forty-odd years to achieve even that little miracle.

I've never been able to afford the best of anything and I've always had to make do with the second or third or fourth best. I don't think that I have one best item in my home. But I'm happy and healthy and look bravely and hopefully into the future because of it. So let it be said that poverty does have its attributes, slim though they may be . . . you can only go up.

When I was about 13 or 14 years old I was working for a means of existence and I couldn't afford to go to high school. So I did my high school going at night and held down a job during the day. One day a peripatetic purveyor of mental pabulum (book salesman) came in to see me and he offered me a beautiful big gazeteer-atlas free, as well as a mighty fine, good sized dictionary. Of course, I accepted them with open arms but then he informed me that I would have to contribute just a few cents every couple of weeks to buy a magazine called Collier's. I didn't want to give back the big dictionary and the big gazeteer-atlas, so I accepted and I became a reader of Collier's magazine and remained one for close to 40 years, until they went out of business.

The same salesman later sold me a set of the Harvard Classics and then a set of the Harvard Shelf of Fiction. I will be grateful to that peripatetic salesman for the rest of my life. He is the man who is responsible for the education that I attained. And I know that I have earned half a dozen Ph.D. degress through the knowledge found in those books, plus tens of thousands of others with this acquired knowledge. I am ready to help my fellow man and my poor and rich friends.

Now what's this all got to do with tonsils?

Well, just wait a minute and I'll tell you . . . although I had to go in a rather roundabout manner to get to it.

I read every issue of Collier's, from cover to cover and I recall an article about tonsils. The editor evidently sent out a reporter and he had a group of doctors on each side give their views — pro and con on why you should or should not keep your tonsils. And believe it or not, even in those days there were a lot of doctors who were strongly opposed to tonsilectomies. I read both sides and I was convinced that the fellows who said "no tonsil operations" were right and from that day on I have been responsible for many hundreds, if not thousands of people keeping their tonsils. Remember this goes back over fifty years.

The usual question that people throw at me is, "What are you going to do if your tonsils are infected or inflamed? You have to have them out, don't you?"

I say, "No, friend. If your tonsils didn't get inflamed, it would be some other part of your anatomy that would be suffering worse. Your tonsils are there to do that job and they're doing it. It's like hiring a bodyguard. Along comes a thug and he beats up your bodyguard after a tough battle. By then the police have come and your bodyguard has time to recover. Sure, he got beaten up but you escaped unharmed. That's just the way it is with your tonsils."

If your children get attacks of tonsilitis, then rest assured that the tonsils are doing their job and that your children are being exposed to toxic substances or harmful conditions. So correct their diet and correct their way of life and correct what they drink and what they are doing and the tonsils won't have to be fighting all the time to prevent the body from being injured.

The reason tonsil operations became so very popular was because practically any doctor, even just out of medical school, could perform the operation with little danger of serious harm being done to the individual and collect $25.00 or $50.00 for doing it and then he could claim he was a surgeon, too. Today it would cost you more than that for the anaesthetist alone.

I recall back 50 years ago and even less the doctor used to

567

line up or arrange a whole block of kids, 20 or more, to have their tonsils removed. Come Saturday he'd do them all in assembly line fashion at from $25.00 to $50.00 a head, depending on their ability to pay. So even in those days a smart young guy with a medical shingle could knock down $500 to $1000 for a day's work. In case you have any doubts about the veracity of my statements . . . don't . . . they are absolutely true.

I have been checking casually over a period of many years and I find the healthiest and the longest lived people usually have their tonsils, appendix, gall bladder and all their innards. So if your doctor suggests or advises a tonsilectomy for you, your offspring, or any member of your family check, double check and then see another doctor.

Here are a few references you may find of interest.

Dr. J. P. Reev, assistant clinical professor of New York Medical College, made this statement: "Numerous studies in the literature failed to reveal the usefulness of this operation except in most unusual or extraordinary circumstances."

Dr. L. P. McCorkle and associates, from Western Reserve University School of Medicine, reported from a study of 230 children: "Attack rates from the common respiratory diseases in the present study were no lower among the children who had had their tonsils removed than among those who had not had this operation."

Also, "The 26 children who had a tonsilectomy while under observation were found to have had a higher than expected rate of common respiratory diseases both before and after operations."

Dr. Jane Colter Mertz, from a study, stated: "After age 40 the incidence of illness among persons with tonsils removed was higher than among persons with tonsils present."

Dr. J. H. Paton from a study of 909 girls, proved that: "Removal of tonsils increases the susceptibility to respiratory

568

infections and that the adenoid operations are followed by increased susceptibility to middle ear inflammation."

CHAPTER 93

YOU CAN IMPROVE YOUR EYES,
YOU CAN GET RID OF YOUR GLASSES

At this writing I'm past 65 years of age and even at the expense of boring you I am going to tell you my "eye" story, and how I used myself as a guinea pig.

Back more than 20 years ago I found that my vision wasn't as good as it had been and with great reluctance, fear and apprehension I decided that I'd have to see an optometrist and get myself a pair of glasses. To me this was sad because I'd had my eyes examined through the years and had been told in absolutely every case that my eyes were as perfect as eyes can be. This is not a boast, this is a simple statement of fact.

Well, reluctantly I had my eyes fitted for a pair of reading glasses and they were weak glasses. The optometrist said that I didn't need them very strong. I was reluctant to use them and used them only when there was small print that I couldn't see too well or when the light was bad. Under normal circumstances and conditions I read without my glasses. However, as the years progressed I found myself using them more and more and more until I had to wear them for most of my reading. Then I also began to notice that sort of a cloud was forming over my eyes and spots were appearing frequently. This also gave me cause for concern and I was a bit perturbed.

I had a nephew who was then an optometrist and he said that it is only natural that as we get older our vision fades a bit and we first begin to notice it when we look in the telephone book for a number and he said, "I'm quite accustomed to people who say, 'Boy, they must be making the type smaller in these telephone books because I don't see it very well.' And that seems to be the first definite indication that your sight is fading."

My nephew was definitely of the opinion from his studies and what he had been taught that this was to be expected and as you get older your eyes become weaker and this is a sign of age and you've got to get glasses and from then on periodically you had to have your glasses strengthened.

However, I don't accept everything that is told to me, as you well know, and I began to massage my eyeballs every day and I found it most convenient to do this when I was washing in the morning and also whenever I thought of it I would carefully and firmly massage my eyeballs. Somewhere I had read or heard that if you could keep the eyeballs elastic and keep them from hardening that you could retain your vision longer.

Now as health and food conscious as I am and have been for many years it had never once occurred to me that food could be a factor in better sight. What is even more strange is that during the war years we often read stories about feeding the airmen lots of carrots because it improved their vision but for some unexplainable reason no connection between nutrition and vision entered my mind.

Nevertheless, I continued to massage my eyes and I did what every eye doctor or ophthalmologist, optometrist, optician or oculist warns you not to do and that is I deliberately strained my eyes. In the back of my head was the thought that no muscle becomes strengthened unless you give it a little bit of extra work so I felt that by straining my eyes every now and then that it would give them some exercise and strengthen them. Now even at this moment I still think that was one heck of a good idea and probably one of the most important factors in maintaining my vision.

I doubt very much if any ophthalmologist or optometrist in America tells his patients to eat proper food so that they will not require glasses. This is common sense. After all, if the optometrist or a doctor sent his patients home to eat proper food and told them to come back in 6 months and then he'd see if they needed glasses he'd find that he wouldn't sell many pair of glasses because when they came back their vision would have improved. If any eye doctor would make such a suggestion, the patients would think he was crazy and would go to another eye doctor to get their glasses.

When I look around me and see the number of people from practically infancy upwards wearing glasses I am appalled. Being a creature of nature I am convinced that most of these eye crutches are not necessary. Don't condemn me if I have a feeling that the eyeglass profession have just done a mighty sweet job of brainwashing us.

When I was a lad if anyone in a classroom said that he had a headache or some such thing, immediately the teacher insisted "You must have your eyes examined, you're probably straining your eyes." And that would go for any headache that any child would complain of and this was a standard procedure. Ever since I was a little boy I've heard that selfsame story that if any young child had some eye problem immediately it was assumed he needed glasses and soon he was fitted with glasses. I think the optometrists have done the best brainwashing job of any group on earth. I don't believe a half or a quarter or a tenth of the people to whom they sell glasses really need them. Boy, will the "eye glass" profession and the manufacturers love me for this . . . just like the medical doctors and food processors love

573

me.

Someday I'd like to make a test on this and have 100 different people whose vision tests A—1 go to an optometrist for an eye examination and tell the optometrist a little lie that they have a little headache or a little bit of strain and I'll bet you 99 out of 100 will come back from the optometrist wearing a new pair of bifocals or something of that nature. No I'm not insinuating or suggesting that the optometrists are dishonest . . . no, no, perish the thought. I'm just suggesting that perhaps they are a wee bit over zealous or unduly concerned about the good and welfare of the eyes of the populace.

For the record let it here and now be understood that I feel sure that the people of America have eyes that are not what they should be. To maintain good eyesight the first and foremost thing is that we must have adequate vitamin A and it has been established and proven that not one person in 100 in America has adequate quantities of vitamin A or carotine. Anyway, what I'm saying is that not one in 100 get adequate quantities of the substance required to maintain healthy vision.

Agreed, there are many eye conditions and eye diseases. I can't even suggest or wouldn't dare suggest that all of these were due to wrong feeding and living habits. To say that food was the only factor would be nonsensical because I know full well that even such things as smoking and the use of alcohol and coffee and tea and such harm most of the organs of the body and I'm sure that they also contribute their share to eye damage.

Now, really, wouldn't it strike you that if someone exposed to the smoke of cigarettes for a few hours a day would in the period of 20, 30, 40 or 50 years have some damage done to his eyes, apart from any other part of his anatomy? I have watched hundreds of people through the years smoking and more than half of them, in fact, most of them allow the smoke to rise and of course a share of it enters their eyes. Just how much this contributes to eye damage I am in no position to say but it must be substantial.

Now how much damage is done by watching television is another factor that needs some investigation. There are no positive tests made along these lines but again common sense will quickly indicate that damage could range from a little bit to a lot. I'm pointing this out to you so that you'll understand that there is definite damage to your eyes from television and the more you watch and the closer you are to your television set the greater the amount of the damage.

Also, there are many occupations that contribute to the degeneration and deterioration of the eyes. Even smog is a serious contributor.

Very few people worry about damage to their eyes because it's so easy to get glasses fitted and of course you can always have your glasses strengthened. So, most individuals really don't concern themselves too much . . . not until it becomes quite serious and some day they'll walk into their optometrist and find that he can no longer increase the strength of their glasses, that the limit has at last been reached.

I recall back when I was just a boy, probably under ten years of age I saw an odd old lady take a piece of orange peel, bend the peel and hold it near her eyes and juice from the peel would squirt into her eyes. She did this every time she ate an orange. Well, when I saw her do it and since she was old I thought that she knew what she was doing, I did the same thing and I did it for years. I've learned, of course, since that orange peel contains various valuable nutrients and whether or not the eye or the body can absorb them when squirted into the eye I'm not sure but I don't think it did my eyes any harm. I wouldn't be a bit surprised if it did them a lot of good. It probably would have done me more good had I eaten more oranges or learned earlier to eat the peel. But who eats orange peel, except me? Nowadays if you ate the peel it would probably poison you with the various sprays and deadly substances which are used, especially on Florida oranges. In those days, going back 50 or more years, there was little or no spray used and it was comparatively safe.

Now let's look at the eyes from the nutritionists' angle. They suggest the use of vitamins A, C, D and riboflavin, all of which contribute to the health and welfare of the eyes. Adequate intake of vitamin A is positively, absolutely essential if you are going to have good vision. The best researchers in the world have claimed that vitamins A and D given together have a greater prophylactic value than either given alone. It is definitely established that the most clearcut effect of lack of vitamin A is night blindness which often occurs suddenly after total exposure to a day's bright sunlight.

Bicknell and Prescott state, "Night blindness can be cured, often in 12 hours, by eating food rich in vitamin A such as liver. The dramatic witness both of the onset and the cure explains why liver has been used for centuries for night blindness."

Bear in mind that even though you may eat fats that supposedly contain vitamin A, Bicknell and Prescott state "many fats when heated develop an 'anti-vitamin A' factor which destroys the biological activity of vitamin A. Whether this is a chemical or biological effect is unknown."

I'd like to illustrate the value of vitamins in the health of the eyes. Please do not misconstrue my statements. I am no pill pusher for any brand or any organization. I am not suggesting or stating that you must buy vitamin supplements or vitamin pills of any kind, I am just stating the importance of vitamins in your food and their effect upon your eyes. I advise and strongly recommend you get your vitamins from natural wholesome food. Evidence for the role of riboflavin deficiency in the production of cataracts is very conflicting.

"P. L. Day and associates as well as other observers have described its occurrence in several species deprived of riboflavin and its arrest in 89% of the animals treated by the administration of riboflavin in doses of 120 U.G. twice weekly."

"Riboflavin appears to play an important part in the nutrition of the eyes. Conjunctivitis and keratitis occur in animals on riboflavin free diets within 7 to 8 weeks followed by a dullness of the eyeball

576

and finally, according to some observers, opacity of the lens. Twilight blindness or aknephascopia was considerably relieved by riboflavin."

"The work of Kimble and Gordon suggests that riboflavin may be necessary for the proper utilization of vitamin A."

"Snow blindness may be due to riboflavin deficiency. This blindness is attributed to riboflavin deficiency because the diet is poor in riboflavin and the light reflected from the snow being very strong and causing local destruction of riboflavin in the eye."

"The importance of vitamin C in eye health is best illustrated by the following references. Researchers Friedenwald, Buschke and Michel claim that vitamin C plays an important part in nutrition of the ocular tissues. According to these workers vitamin C deficiency in the guinea-pig causes a disappearance of vitamin C from the ocular tissues long before any symptoms of scurvy appear. The healthy lens of the eye has been shown to be particularly rich in vitamin C, the amount of which is greatly reduced or entirely absent in the lens that has developed cataract. According to Bellows, patients with cataract also show lower vitamin C levels than do control patients in the same age group and economic status. He has also shown that the onset of the cataract that develops in rats fed on large quantities of galactose can be delayed by the administration of vitamin C."

Also, "It is possible that vitamin C is in some way essential for the metabolism of the lens, but there is no convincing clinical evidence that it arrests the progress of cataract in the human eye, although Josephson believes that the administration of up to 300 mg. of vitamin C a day to patients with cataract causes marked improvement within a week."

I cite these examples taken from the best researchers in the world to illustrate how important is nutrition and how it affects your seeing ability.

Furthermore, all the vitamin C, the vitamin A and the riboflavin needed can be found in good foods, especially raw green and yellow vegetables, raw wholesome, fresh seeds. Riboflavin is widely distributed in plants and in animal tissue. Among the best sources are yeast, milk, white of the egg, fish roe, kidney, liver, heart and growing leafy vegetables. Grain and legumes, although they contain riboflavin are not particularly rich sources. However, when the seeds germinate or sprout the riboflavin content increases.

Therefore, if you would improve your eyesight the first and the most important consideration is to eat better food, mostly uncooked.

CHAPTER

94

THE TRUTH ABOUT CONTACT LENSES

Back about five years ago I wrote a few articles attacking contact lenses. I must admit that I didn't know anything about contact lenses and I didn't know anything about how it affected the eye but logic and horse sense clearly spelled out that there was grave danger in forcing a piece of glass or plastic over the retina of the eye. That is why I denounced them as being harmful, an insult to the body and stated that no one who knew anything about nature or health would ever permit or condone such treatment of the human body. Imagine a wearer of contact lenses of his own free will and accord, permitting a foreign object to be placed in contact with what are probably the most delicate and sensitive tissues of the entire human body.

As a child I learned that even a tiny fragment of dust could cause serious pain and disturb the functions of the mechanism of the eye. I am sure there is hardly a person alive who at one time or another has not had a particle of some kind lodged in his eye. Now if you put a large object in or on top of the eye, it stands to reason and is only common sense that the body will do its best to rid itself of the intruder. So it will be with every person who wears contact lenses. Contact lenses will create a condition in which the body is continually fighting to clear out the irritant or source of trouble.

Therefore, apart from any other considerations, you have in simple language the reason why I profoundly believe that contact lenses will definitely do serious, and often irreparable harm to the eye. It must also be conceded that contact lenses are worn mostly for reasons of vanity. It is not my wish to condemn vanity because to a degree vanity has its place in our society . . . we all like to see a man or a woman who takes pride in his or her personal appearance, because it leads to cleanliness, neatness, personal appeal and magnetism. Thus I feel that a person should possess a degree of vanity.

Yet it is a fact that most people wear contact lenses because of vanity. When we allow vanity to harm and cause dysfunction of the body, then I think it is being overdone, to say the least.

From the best sources that I can locate it would appear that contact lenses — that is, the modern version — were first introduced in about 1948. It is estimated that today more than 9,000,000 people wear contact lenses.

I must admit that for some people contact lenses are a boon or even a necessity . . . that is, for example, athletes, politicians and performers or actors. While I feel that it is not 100% necessary it probably is to their advantage to wear contact lenses so the world won't know that their eyesight is impaired.

The ophthalmologists will defend contact lenses to a degree, stating that in cases of cataract, the use of contact lenses is not only justifiable but essential. That is, when you have had cataract surgery it is absolutely essential to have some form of lens, be it glasses or contact lenses.

Here is another little bit of information about contact lenses that is not generally known. Believe it or not, they were used back in the 1800's but then they were known as scleral lenses. In those days they covered most of the exposed eye. The sclera is the white of the eye. In those days the scleral lenses were made of glass and they were very expensive and they were most uncomfortable.

The modern contact lenses actually cover only part of the eye, the cornea, which is the transparent membrane of the eyeball. They are tiny curved discs which are half an inch in diameter. Today they are made of plastic and they can actually be snapped or broken by the pressure of your fingers.

Some years ago the Federal Fair Trade Commission had to step in and prevent the false advertising that was being used to sell contact lenses and they passed a law making it illegal for any advertiser to make the following statements about contact lenses:

(a) That they are suitable and safe for all persons, regardless of their age, health or eye condition.

(b) That they can be worn satisfactorily and without discomfort by all, or nearly all persons.

(c) That they can be fitted without any discomfort.

(d) That they can be worn for any short or long period without discomfort unless the advertisement clearly reveals that practically all persons will experience some discomfort when first wearing them and that in a significant number of cases the discomfort period may be prolonged.

(e) That they can be worn all day without discomfort by any person except after that person has become fully adjusted thereto and unless such is the fact.

(f) That they will completely replace eyeglasses in all, or nearly all, cases, or will provide better correction of vision than eyeglasses in all, or nearly all, cases.

(g) That contact lenses which are bifocals are as satisfactory to the wearer as prescription eyeglasses having bifocal lenses.

(h) That they will correct all defects in vision.

(i) That they will stay in place under all conditions.

(j) That they are unbreakable in all circumstances.

(k) That they can be adequately tried without financial obligation, unless such is the fact.

(l) That they will protect the eyes unless such representation is limited in application to the portion of the eyes covered by such lenses and does not denote or connote a greater degree of protection to such portion, than is in fact the case.

(m) That they do not rest upon, or have contact with the eyes.

Isn't it strange that in spite of the above warning by a government agency, the optical people who sell contact lenses are still selling millions of them? The public are willing and eager to buy.

It should be pointed out that as many as 25% of those who buy contact lenses possibly will find them too troublesome or uncomfortable to wear.

Here is a quotation referring to corneal contact lenses, from a British Medical Journal:

"Whatever its type or the material from which it is made, a contact lens must be considered a foreign body on the eye. Ideally it should fit the anterior segment of the eye, and allow respiration of

582

the cornea and a free flow of tears either round the material or through it. In addition it must provide a fairly rigid front surface to correct the patient's vision. Such a lens should be wearable day and night without being removed and not be a source of contamination by virus, bacterium, or fungus to the eye and lids. Furthermore the material must not undergo degenerative changes, with the production of toxic substances.

"Contact lenses with all these qualities have yet to be made."

Here is another reference that appeared in the Southern Medical Journal, as written by a Florida physician, Thomas S. Edwards:

"Fairly frequently the defective equipment is the contact lens itself. (It) may be found to have cracks and chips and spurs on the edge which will give circular corneal abrasions as the contact lens moves about the eye. Sometimes the specially constructed vents, grooves and ledges will cause corneal abrasions. Further, the edge of the corneal lens may be improperly ground, giving a sharp edge, or too thick an edge, above or below. These may cause numerous fine scratches in the peripheral cornea and sometimes the limbal region of the sclera. If the thickness is such that it irritates the upper eyelid it may, at times, actually remove epithelial cells from the lid . . . "

One of America's leading experts on contact lenses, Joseph M. Dixon, M.D., a professor of ophthalmology at the University of Alabama Medical Center, says that everybody who uses contact lenses will suffer eye damage and in many cases the damage will be permanent. "You would be amazed," says Professor Dixon, "at the number of ophthalmologists who wish contact lenses had never been invented. Our job is to help people see better, and glasses will do that with fewer complications."

Professor Dixon goes on to say that they will cause injury, however slight and however remediable, in the eyes of every single one of the 9,000,000 people who wear them.

One of the most important studies of the consequences of wearing contact lenses was supervised by Professor Dixon (A.M.A. Journal, 3/14/66). A survey was made of the country's 8181 opthalmologists, and 1904 reported on their experiences with 49,954 wearers of contact lenses during one year.

There were 7607 cases of eye damage reported in which the patients recovered without permanent defects. Medication, eyepatches, as well as hospitalization in many cases, were required.

There were 157 cases of permanent damage by scarring or other injuries.

There were 14 cases of eyes lost or blinded. All 14 had infections, 10 from bacteria and 4 from fungi.

Now something new has been added . . . a soft contact lens.

This was invented in Czechoslovakia in 1960. This new lens consists of a sliver of porous plactic slightly larger than a regular contact lens, that becomes soft and pliable when it touches the tears of weak-eyed wearers.

Because of its pleasing flabbiness the soft contact lens can be fitted in one sitting as compared to 4 sittings for hard contact lenses.

Ophthalmologists throughout America agree that the soft variety is more comfortable and less likely to become scratched, or to pop out unexpectedly, than the hard kind.

Nine million people in America due to near or far sightedness wear contact lenses. Yet there are actually more than 90 million people in America who use glasses. Millions of these glasses users have tried contact lenses but were forced to give them up because of various conditions and irritations of the eye.

The soft contact lenses are being put on the market in America by Bausch and Lomb and they are confident that the soft contact lenses will take hold in America because they are usually non-irritating and will undoubtedly win the large share of the 400 million dollar ophthalmic market.

They are calling their lens "Soflens".

From reports emanating from leading ophthalmologists it has been stated that the soft lenses have some disadvantages. For example, they provide less visual acuity, and they cannot correct extreme astigmatism. Due to the porous plastic of which they are made, which absorbs moisture like a sponge, the soft lenses are more difficult to keep sterile.

The wearers of the soft lens are advised to boil the lens for 15 minutes each night in salt water. They do not recommend the use of table salt because of the iodine content. Nor do they advise the use of tap water because of the many impurities contained. Therefore each pair of "Soflenses" comes with a bottle of salt tablets and an electric sterilizer that resembles a baby bottle warmer. The user is advised to procure his own distilled water.

A very interesting sidelight has arisen with these soft lenses. Some ophthalmologists suggest that the soft lenses are potentially dangerous because "the instant and continuous comfort may be a treacherous element in the soft lens".

"If you get hurt by the hard lens you usually know it immediately." A soft lens may mask the warning discomfort of an eye's injury, suggests the same expert.

Already serious injuries have turned up. One hospital has seen 3 complications involving experimental soft contact lenses. The patients later required cornea grafts.

To illustrate the merits or demerits of soft lenses, I want to quote this from Time magazine, May 31, 1971.

" 'I intend using the soft lens on every patient I possibly can', said Dr. Mary Young, who maintains a 3,000 patient a year Optometrical practice in Braintree, Mass. Until she tried on a pair herself at a Bausch and Lomb seminar last week, she had gone, red-rimmed and bloodshot, through 17 pairs of hard contact lenses."

From my continued study of the situation, I echo my continued warning — all users of contact lenses, either soft or hard, are endangering their vision and their eyes. Many will suffer serious incurable injury or damage. If you can get by without contact lenses do not use them, unless you want to be blind in your old age.

There are huge files of further records revealing the danger and the harm involved in the use of contact lenses. In spite of all the evidence that I have presented and I say there is scads and scads more, if you still want to use contact lenses, well, my advice to you is this . . . be extremely careful and remember, you're probably going to injure one of the most valuable human attributes or possessions — your eyesight!

CHAPTER

95

ABOUT SEX HORMONES — PLANT AND ANIMAL

During the past 40 or so years we in America have been taught quite a bit about sex hormones. Prior to that time the average person had probably never heard of the term.

First I should establish the meaning of the word "hormone", and according to the Oxford Dictionary it is "a substance formed in an organ and serving to excite some vital process as secretion."

Here we are dealing with sex hormones.

It is known that men have mainly male hormones and women have mainly female hormones but it is granted that we do also secrete hormones of the opposite sex. The male hormones are referred to as Androgenic and include testosterone, androsterone and dehydroandrosterone. The female hormones are referred to as

Estrogenic and include estradiol, estrone, estriol and progesterone.

Then many years ago it was found that when women having trouble with their menopause were injected with female hormones they received considerable benefit. Hormone therapy was quite expensive because it appears that the hormones were hard to come by. Then some research scientist found that stallions in heat and pregnant mares excreted vast amounts of the female sex hormone in their urine. So a thriving business sprang up — for example, in Quebec where they had mares and stallions by the hundreds — and the urine was run into drums and barrels and shipped to the drug manufacturers where they extracted the female hormone. This in turn was supplied to doctors and hospitals and injected into women and it supposedly helped them in overcoming disorders connected with the menopause.

Then about ten years later another research scientist came up with the synthesis of a strictly chemical female hormone.

The most important male hormone is known as testosterone, but not much is said or known about this. Evidently men aren't as important as women. Some claim that testosterone will tend to make men virile, but it is a natural secretion of males.

So now you know about the female and male sex hormones but what I want to tell you here is that while most people know about the male and female hormones, very few people know that there is such a thing as sex hormones in plants. These are, believe it or not, almost identical to those of humans.

Now the reason I am delving into this angle, which my readers may think is rather peculiar, is that I have a positive purpose . . . and the purpose is this. The world in general would have us believe that we have to kill to eat, that we have to raise animals for our food and for other reasons. It is assumed that mankind just can't get along without animals and that animals like cattle, sheep, goats and hogs are a part of our existence and way of life. It was generally assumed that if we needed sex hormones we had to get them from other animals.

However, they are now making synthetic ones, too, but generally speaking we know that the synthetic ones aren't as good as the natural ones. So when I come up and tell people that you don't have to go to animal sources or synthetic chemicals for sex hormones and that nature provides them abundantly in plants, well, that comes as sort of an extreme shock to some people. But this does not alter the fact that it is absolutely true.

It appears that a scientist from the California Institute of Technology found that the female sex hormone, estrone, is readily available in the pussy willow, as well as seeds of the pomegranate and date palm. Now anybody with a grain of knowledge or who is a bit alert will quickly recognize that every seed that exists on the face of this earth must contain adequate quantities of both the female and male hormones, otherwise the seed is never going to be able to germinate and make a plant. Even my simple brain grasped that long before the scientists said that it was so.

Then these scientists went on to discover that the male sex hormone, testosterone, could be isolated from a plant known widely in the desert as the jimson or jimson weed, which is actually a corruption of the word "jamestown". The article I read gave the name as jimmy weed, which I am sure is in error because it is definitely not called that, but evidently the name got twisted in the reports. I am well acquainted with the plant and therefore I have checked through and found that it was the jimson weed, properly known as Datura stramonium. It grows throughout the United States but is most frequently found in California.

The scientists, in attempting to confirm the identity of the plant hormone with the animal estrone, injected small quantities of the plant hormone into female mice. It was found that the changes in the uterus were almost exactly the same as those occurring when caused by the animal's own estrone.

The researcher, Dr. Erich Heftman, also discovered cholesterol

589

in the pollen of the date palm whereas for years we have believed that cholesterol was strictly an animal product.

It appears that the sex hormones have more than just the one function for estrogen is definitely involved in water retention and it maybe makes sense because plants are continually threatened by water loss. The estrogen prevents this and this is another role for this hormone.

After a lifetime of working with plants and trees and seeds, I am firmly convinced that there is a parallelism here . . . with plants, animals and humans.

CHAPTER

96

SEXUAL VIRILITY

If this book were called how to maintain sexual virility past 40, past 50, past 60, it would become an instant best-seller. However, I don't seek sensationalism. I'm not even interested in a best-seller. I'm just interested in keeping people healthy and helping them save their lives and in keeping them from kicking off before their time.

Man has been seeking the fountain of youth since time began. I presume that when Ponce de Leon went out in search of the fountain the kind of youth he wanted and was seeking was sexual prowess. There are few things that men throughout the civilized and barbaric world strive for more than virility.

Aphrodisiacs are the most sought after commodity in the world and they are sought by primitive people, the ordinary people, right up to the highest echelon of our society. Everybody, yes, even

591

homosexuals, are seeking to maintain, to regain, or increase, their sexual output.

The best authorities on health in America, along the American Medical Association lines, will tell you that there are no aphrodisiacs that actually work. One of the best authorities that I know, years ago told me that there are drug ways of getting an orgasm at the expense of 2, 3, 4 or 5 orgasms of the future. In other words, drug induced orgasms whip the body into a frenzy and you are less capable of performance thereafter. So obviously, drug induced orgasms are not the answer, as if you didn't know.

I am well acquainted with the usual run of the mill aphrodisiacs like Spanish Fly, Damiana leaves, Ginseng, oysters and a thousand and one other supposed sex inducers.

Now, I'm telling you this. You can preserve your fecundity, you can foster it, you can feed it, you can improve it . . . by the simple expedient of eating proper food. And the proper food for sexual virility is seeds — fresh, wholesome seeds — untreated, uncontaminated and uncooked.

The big trick is to make these seeds palatable. Oh yes, I know you'll eat 'em, even if they aren't palatable, as long as they will produce the sexual stimulation.

But I'm suggesting that you need not suffer their tastelessness. I can show you a way that you can not only make them taste good, but you'll cry for them like babies used to cry for Castoria. I'll tell you something else, that you can't over-do, or over-eat, or over-indulge, on these wholesome raw seeds, because they are natural and when you are full, you'll know you're full and you'll stop eating them.

Now when they want a bull to perform his function, that is the actual function for which he is created, they feed him corn, oats, wheat, barley, rye or any grains that he'll eat. Of course, if he is out roaming about and they are available he'll get them without anyone feeding them to him.

The same applies to a stallion. Neither a stallion or a bull will perform at his best on grass alone. They need the seeds. In case you wonder why grains, I'll tell you. It's simple. Seeds and grains are loaded with sex hormones. The grains, or the factors in the grain, stimulate and regenerate the endocrine glands. No, you don't have to have monkey glands grafted into you. Just get yourself regular quantities of fresh untreated grains.

Nuts are all right too but grains are better in my opinion, and they cost you a lot less, too. Perhaps nuts are a little more palatable. Probably you'll run off and you'll get yourself cashew nuts because they taste so good. But if you do, you won't get results because cashews are dead.

Now besides the grains in your diet, make sure you eat the seeds in your apples, in your pears, in your oranges, in your watermelon, in your grapes and if your teeth are good enough you can crack your cherry and plum pits. I've eaten them for a long time.

No, you don't need wheat germ or wheat germ oil. You don't need shots. You don't even need girls with mini skirts to give you ideas. What you need is fresh, wholesome seeds.

On Page 177 you will find my recipe for 3-V Cereal.

To balance your diet properly I would also recommend that you eat a lot of complete vegetables like turnips, beets, carrots, lettuce, fresh green peas, radishes, cucumbers, green and red peppers, celery and tomatoes. In fact, the best vegetable is where you eat the whole root and some greens and the whole food like tomatoes and cucumbers where you also try to get the benefits found in the seeds.

Whether you believe it or not at this reading, I assure you it works better than any other means or method on earth and it's cheap and readily available. You'll be a better man or woman for the inclusion of seeds in your diet.

CHAPTER 97

THE LESSON OF HUNZA

No book on natural health would be complete without some references to the healthy Hunzans. I made four trips to that country as a guest of the Mir — in 1959, 1961, 1963 and 1971. Each time I went it was with a purpose and I went, I saw, I learned and I observed.

My first trip was the most profitable one. I learned more on that trip than I learned on all the other trips together. But on the subsequent trips I kept my eyes open for certain things that I might have missed on the previous trips.

Where is Hunza located? It is the northern-most part of Pakistan and is a part of Kashmir. It borders Afghanistan, India and China and a narrow strip of Afghanistan 8 miles wide separates Hunza from the Soviet Union.

Hunza is in the Karakorum mountains and not in the Himalayas — no matter what other writers claim. I am probably the only writer who states emphatically that Hunza is in the Karakorums, not in the Himalayas. If you check your maps closely you will find that what I say is geographically true and that the other writers have not taken the trouble to find out where they were when they visited Hunza. So I repeat, Hunza is in the Karakorums, not in the Himalayas and the Karakorums are not a part of the Himalayas but are a mountain system of their own.

Hunza is located in what is known as the Pamirs which means "the Roof of the World". In the Hunza region there are more than 100 mountain peaks taller than 20,000 feet. I have visited most of the mountain systems throughout the world and I believe that Hunza is in the most beautiful mountain area that exists on the face of the earth. Nothing compares with it.

I wish that I were able to say that all of the stories told about the people of Hunza were true. Fortunately most of the things are true but one author in particular from California has made so many ridiculous statements that I have felt it my duty to try and set things in their true perspective.

This author claims that there are innumerable people in Hunza who are more than 100 years of age. In fact, she makes it sound as though everybody in Hunza lives to be over 100 and she claims that they play volleyball when they are 90 and 100 years old and makes all kinds of other ridiculous unwarranted statements. On my four trips to Hunza I found only two people who were more than 100 years of age.

I consider the Hunzans the healthiest people in the world. I consider them intelligent, capable and reliable. They are certainly healthier than any other people of that area or for that matter any other people in the world.

Things had not changed very much from the time I was there on my first trip in 1959 to my last trip in 1971. Some weaknesses have crept in. For example, they no longer mine their own salt which was a wholesome salt containing many elements and they now use a salt which is brought in from the bigger cities and is similar to the salt we use in America. Many of the citizens have now learned to smoke and I believe they drink more wine than they used to.

Many of the younger Hunza lads go into the Pakistan army and they learn the ways of civilization and they bring these ways back with them when they come home on furlough or when they have finished their stint in the army. Although the Mir is trying to maintain the good health and ways of the people of his country I am fearful that some deterioration will take place.

The greatest changes that I noticed actually took place in the Mir himself (the ruler of Hunza). I consider him a very fine person and with each meeting I like him more and understand him better and appreciate him more. I actually compare the appearance of the Mir with the appearance of the natives of Hunza. Now I made it a point to talk with and observe the people from the first trip to the second, to the third and to the fourth and I noticed that the natives changed little if at all during those 13 years but the Mir has changed. He shows his age and he is not nearly as robust today as he was in 1959. "Well," you might say, "what do you expect? He's 13 years older". Yes, but all the other people of Hunza are 13 years older too and they show little or no change.

What is the answer? Why? Really it's quite simple. Right from the start I think that I told in my book "Hunza: Adventures in A Land Of Paradise" that the Mir and his family did not eat the food of the people of Hunza. After all, he is their ruler, their king and he eats of the king's food and drinks of the king's wine and most of this is brought in from the outside world. So the food on the king's table is not the food of the people. Besides, the Mir smokes, drinks alcoholic beverages, drinks coffee and tea and partakes of conventional foods just as we do. Does that explain the situation? I don't think I have to say any more about that aspect.

Now it is clear, crystal clear, that the people of Hunza today

597

are the healthiest people I have ever seen in my life and I have travelled extensively to observe such things. So the same question that is asked a thousand and one times comes up, "Why are they healthier than other people?". Or more specifically, "Why are they healthier than we here in America?"

To begin with, they don't have an over-abundance of food nor do they have the variety that we have nor do they have our food processing or our food stores. Now don't misunderstand, they do have variety but it is all in the form of the natural and the whole, like seeds and various vegetables and grains, milk and cheese and bread or chapatties and only a small variety and quantity of animal foods.

They do not eat much meat because grazing is a problem. They just do not have the pasture required for raising cattle but there are some cattle and goats and many sheep. In the higher altitudes they have yaks and of course these are used both for milk and meat. Because of the lack of pasturage meat does not constitute an important item of their diet.

When the milk is used it is usually clabbered and what they call butter is what we would refer to as cheese. It is cured by keeping it underneath the conduits that carry the water from the glaciers to the different villages. The spread they use like butter they call "Gee" which is butter that has been heated. They have chickens and thus eggs, but they have no honey because they do not have many bees. Their apricot trees are fertilized or pollinated by the wind.

Fish is very restricted. The only fish they get is that which is caught from stocked streams. They do not have our means of sanitation. There are no phones, there is no electricity except in the Mir's home. Only the Mir has toilets or bathrooms as we know them or even running water. They have only a small hospital in the whole of Hunza and one doctor ... very few drugs and practically no surgery. There are no refined foods, although I did see a package or two of some foods on the shelves of the shops in Gilgit. Remember, Gilgit is 64 miles from Baltit, the capital of Hunza, and Gilgit is not in Hunza.

It must be stated that in recent years some refined salt and refined sugar have been finding their way into Hunza.

There are no motor cars or other means of transportation although they have jeep service from Gilgit to Hunza. But jeeps are not used in Hunza by the populace. There are practically no modern conveniences. Moving hay and animal foods and other transport is still by means of loading it on the individual's back. Men, women and children are the transport system. There is very little level ground. You are always either going up or going down.

The total population of Hunza is approximately 30,000 people and it is not increasing. Their diet is frugal, their homes are simple — the adobe style with an upstairs balcony that is usually used only in the summer. Heat is a problem. They just don't have any fuel. Wood is the only source of fuel and it is hard to come by because the surrounding mountains are not timbered and the wood has to be brought from a great distance. Keeping warm in the winter poses a serious problem.

There is no contamination as yet in the air they breathe or the water they drink. As yet there are no commercial chemical fertilizers used in Hunza. They still use human excrement and animal manures and all wastes are returned to the soil. There are still no sprays or chemical dusts used.

How Hunza has been able to maintain its sovereignty and its way of life is still difficult to understand but remember it is well nigh impossible to get into Hunza. The government now allows excursions into Hunza of groups of 15 or more. You are flown into Gilgit from Rawalpindi and from Gilgit you are taken by jeep to Karimabad in Hunza but you are only allowed to stay over night in a special hostel provided for tourists. You get a glimpse of the beauty of the country and then you are whisked back in the jeeps to Gilgit and flown back to Rawalpindi. But these groups must arrange their transportation well in advance and no one is permitted to linger. You are taken, you spend the night and you are out again.

To get a permit to stay more than a couple of days is practically impossible and it is just as hard for natives of Pakistan to get in as it is for outsiders. The reason I have managed to get there four times is that I have many good friends in Pakistan and they consider me a good friend of their country . . . and I am a good friend because I try to further the interests of that country and will continue to do so.

That the Hunzans are secluded and isolated goes without saying but that could not be the only reason for their health because there are many, many countries or places on the face of the earth that are just as isolated and inaccessible. For example, we went to Skardu which is even more isolated and to Khaplu which is even more remote again but the health of the people is not to be compared with that of the people of Hunza and I make comparisons and watch this carefully.

Obviously the ruler, the Mir, has something to do with it. He watches over the health of his people far better than he watches over his own or that of his own household. He will not permit them to get or to eat the foods that he eats and obviously previous rulers, his father, his grandfather and his great grandfather did likewise. To me the people of Hunza were better looking, healthier looking, stronger, more intelligent, more capable than the people of the adjoining countries. There are many so-called tribes or independent peoples in places like Nagir, Punial, Chitral, Dir and Swat. There are others too, but none of them are like the Hunzans.

What is the answer? What is their secret? I admit I don't know nor do I believe there is any special mystery or secret but perhaps you can see the answer in what I have related. I must admit that my four trips through that charmed land have failed to give me any clear cut answers that I have been seeking, yet it must be obvious to all thinking people. It must be a combination of many things like natural foods, unpolluted air, unpolluted glacial water, the absence of stress and complications, the continued activity, lack of noise and the rat race, the absence of chemicals in their food and their environment, the absence of motor vehicles and the absence of processed and refined foods.

I have sought to give you the picture as closely and as completely as possible without frill or fanfare. I have not exaggerated nor have I told lies which most authors who visit Hunza seem to do. I'm not casting reflections or trying to belittle anyone, I'm just relating the truth. You can form your own conclusions from my story.

CHAPTER
98

THE ANSWER TO LONG LIFE

This I consider to be the most important chapter in the book. If I have never contributed anything to the welfare or benefit of mankind before in my life I believe that this chapter will be my contribution. I believe what I have to relate here is not only important news, it's probably the most worthwhile bit of information I can ever hope to present to mankind. It is furthermore, I believe, the greatest contribution towards the lengthening of the life span of human beings ever formulated or devised. For more than twenty years I have been seeking the answers to long life not only in intensive studies and research but by means of travelling to all countries of the world to which I can gain entrance.

Granted, I did find the areas on the face of the globe where men tend to live longer than in any other place and that location is in the higher mountain reaches and it does appear as though men as a group live longer and remain in better health in the higher mountain regions than any other place on earth. The reasons are not immediately apparent but it has something to do presumably with the sustained physical activity that is characteristic of those who live in the higher altitudes. This ties in with the accepted concepts. Remember that every step taken in the higher altitudes is either up or down which does create greater physical effort than walking on a flat plane. It is also my finding that people seem to require less food or actually eat less in the higher altitudes.

Another very important consideration is that the water supply is definitely better at the higher altitudes because the lower down it goes the more polluted it becomes. In this case I am not referring to pollution in the modern concept of industrial, chemical, or atomical but in the physical sense that as it goes lower it is used by more people and therefore pollution of this sort takes place because of human useage. Understandably, where water begins — at its source, from a glacier — it has not been used by man and therefore is in its most pristine condition.

So here we have air, exercise, food and water being involved. Another consideration I bring forth that has not been before suggested is that smog or accumulations of waste or industrial by-products tend to collect or aggragate at the lower altitudes. It seems that the particles filter out at the lower levels and at the higher levels the lighter air rises and the heavier comes down so I believe that the air is definitely better at the higher altitudes. I don't know of any factories or pollution creators or industries located at levels anywhere above 8,000, 9,000 or 10,000 feet, so the air at those altitudes ought to be comparatively clean. This may not hold true above the large industrial cities like Chicago, Detroit, Pittsburgh, Los Angeles, Toronto, Tokyo, and others.

For centuries man has sought to increase his years or span of life by means of physical activity even at advanced ages. It was felt that by keeping himself physically fit and by eating proper food he could maintain his health and thus attain long life. Never before anywhere in my reading or my studies has it been stressed or

604

emphasized that mental activity was a factor or could even be a consideration. It was always the physical aspects that were stressed. It has been the way of life through all countries since time immemorial that as we get into the fifth or sixth or seventh decades of life we tend to shed our mental load, to relinquish responsibility and any engagement that would tax our intellect.

In my lifetime, when dealing with my associates and relatives and those with whom I was acquainted, it was always the story of youth taking over from old age, having youth come in and pick up the mental burdens so as not to strain the intellect or the brain of the older person. You know, this is the greatest mistake that mankind or humanity has ever made and I have recognized this for many long years. I wept and cried and moaned when I heard that people who were physically and mentally alert and active were compelled to resign or retire when they reached 60 or 65. In fact, some of the largest organizations in the world compel their executives to retire at a fixed age. This is mankind's greatest travesty. I know of no single error in man's conduct or reasoning that is as great as this major blunder.

Obviously, in our present system a man is not retired because of inability or because of too great a workload or because of ineffectiveness but only because of age. I have boldly stated on many occasions that it is a tragedy to take a man with knowledge, with experience, with sagacity pertaining to all facets of his business or his enterprise and push him out into retirement, senility and death.

Now let me digress here for a moment. Studies and discourses concerning the brain or the intellect of mankind have been made frequently throughout history and the general conclusion seems to be that a man's brain has never been used to anything resembling its capacity or abilities. This even applies to men like Einstein, Voltaire, Newton, Plato, Socrates, Aristotle or even Moses. The greatest thinkers that mankind has ever known have never used their brain or their intellect to within a remote fraction of its potential. I think every single one of us knows and understands this, every person realizes that his brain or any brain is capable of much, much more

605

than he has ever done with it.

For example, I do a little bit of thinking myself, probably more than most men and yet I realize that I seldom allow myself to think constructively of different things. I allow my brain to be burdened and over-loaded with trivialities or thinking of the same thing over and over and over again. Now it has dawned upon me that I should be using my brain for bigger, better and more divergent things. The human brain should be trained to think of new things, of new horizons, of new schemes and new enterprises . . . to use even a small fragment of its capabilities.

So now I realize the great error of mankind . . . suggesting and requesting the diminishing use of our mental powers as we grow older. We are exhorted to lighten our load, relinquish responsibility, pass on the burdens to other younger people. Now don't you see the answer, don't you see what I'm driving at? Instead we should be increasing our mental work load as we grow older. We've only scratched the surface of the abilities of our intellect and we should be expanding it and increasing it so as to make greater use of its potential.

In my own life, as a youth I worked the least I could. I never ran if I could jog, I never jogged if I could walk, I never walked if I could stand, I never stood if I could sit and I never sat if I could lie down and I never just lay down if I could sleep and that was the story of my youth. It's as simple as this . . . I repeat, that I never did a stroke or a tap of work that I could avoid doing, in spite of the fact that I was exhorted or even pushed into work by my father.

I was in my mid 20's when suddenly I found out that I liked work, be it physical or mental and from that day onward I've consistently increased my work load. Now, past 66 I work harder and longer hours than I ever worked before in my life and I keep feeling younger and better with each succeeding day. I eat better, I feel better, I think better and my friends tell me I look better.

Now suddenly it has dawned upon me that age is just a state

of mind, it's something we have permitted ourselves to accept or become involved in and our brain or mental activity is the key to the whole problem. An active brain usually means an active body. It is more important to keep your brain active than your body because if your brain degenerates there will be no compulsion or desire for physical activity.

At last I have discovered why my mother wanted to die at 86 and why so many other people whom I have known wanted to get out of this vale of tears. It was because they and their friends and loved ones permitted their intellect to slowly go into senescence and become senile . . . and a sick brain means a sick body.

I observe, I investigate, I inquire and this is absolutely true. So now you have the answer to health and long life . . . it is an active brain. Do not shed your mental work load but slowly but progressively increase it. Your brain is capable of it, in fact your brain needs it, it demands it and you cannot grow old as long as you keep increasing the work load of your brain. The sure, the positive way to health and long life is an active, progressive mentality.

CHAPTER

99

SOIL . . . YOUR HEALTH, YOUR LIFE

There can never be and there never will be a healthy body without healthy food. And you cannot have healthy food without having a healthy soil. And you cannot have healthy soil without having healthy soil organisms. One follows the other just as night follows day. They are indivisible. They are parts of a whole. And failure to see or understand this can only lead to trouble or disaster.

I am acquainted with some of the most knowledgable men in the world in the field of biology, but unfortunately many or most of these men are so scientifically involved that they cannot lucidly explain themselves so as to be understood by the average individual. At the moment I am thinking of one man in particular who ranks as a foremost man in his field in America. He probably knows better than any other man in America the relationship of soil health to human health.

609

I have read his articles for years and in order to find a point explaining the relationship you have to pore through paragraph after paragraph, page after page, of scientific mumbo-jumbo. I don't think he can understand it or explain it himself. He knows what he wants to say but he can never put it down on paper so that anyone else can ever understand it. I have heard him deliver speeches and the same holds true. You come away with the idea that he sure knows his stuff but he's the only man there who does and he can't impart it to you or anyone else.

Some of you will no doubt recognize the man to whom I am referring.

I started in the nursery business in 1932 and have had my own nursery for nigh on 40 years. About 20 years ago I began to become keenly interested in health and I found that my botanical or biological training and experience were tremendous assets. I have yet to find anyone in the entire health field who has had a practical biological background.

Most of the experts regarded me as a Johnny-come-lately and ignored or refused to accept my statements and findings. But as the years went by, the public — who is the judge and jury — recognized that I had an earthy flavor about my writing on health, which none of the others could claim. And the public accepted me while the experts passed me by.

I have always related the soil to the health of the people. One of America's foremost health authorities, whom I respect as one of the most knowledgable men in the entire field of health and nutrition, made the tragic error of disregarding the importance and the value of the soil and human health. He learned his lesson . . . but fifty years too late . . . and he is paying for it with the loss of his own health. And this is a tragedy because this man helped more people than any man I know and I often think what a man he would have been and what work he could have done if only he had had a biological background . . . especially a practical one.

610

There are few people in America today who can accept the fact that nature is still greater than the scientists. Millions are spent annually on propaganda that literally compels us to accept and believe that we cannot feed our population without chemical fertilizers and chemical sprays, dusts and other treatments.

The sale of fertilizers grows by tremendous leaps each and every year and thus they have more and more millions to spend on propaganda. I do not know of one single experimental station that recommends the organic way of farming. I do not know of one experimental station in America that conducts even a trial with organic gardening methods.

In fact, I know of only one organization (New Bell's Farms, Haughley, Newmarket, Suffolk, England) in the entire world that actually puts it to the acid test. They have for 30 years conducted experiments showing the results of (1) farming the chemical way, (2) farming the organic way, and (3) farming with half chemicals and half organics. This organization has carried on these experiments for almost 30 years and conducted them strictly scientifically with established details and records and under the supervision of a respected Ph.D. Any common sense individual who actually did some honest thinking would know and understand that nature's way would come out best. Furthermore, the organic way proved that it was more practical, more profitable and more healthful.

This group is known as the Soil Association and by becoming a member you can avail yourself of their literature and publications. It is supported by individuals, most in Great Britain, but also a few others in other parts of the world.

Therefore, there is irrefutable evidence, scientifically prepared and recorded, to demonstrate that nature's way is better than the scientific or the chemical way, whichever you want to call it.

Actually, I should not refer to it as the scientific way because true science will clearly demonstrate the superiority of the natural way . . . but where do you find true science, except this one single

611

experiment that I mentioned?

This experiment conclusively proved that by farming organically you will have healthy soil organisms, healthy soil, healthy plants, healthy animals and, of course, healthy people.

Never lose sight of the fact that chemical fertilizers and chemicals in general tend to destroy soil organisms and without them you cannot have a healthy soil.

You will hear contra-arguments by the proponents of the chemical way that soil fertility cannot be maintained without the use of chemical fertilizers. This argument has been proven wrong by simply looking towards China where for thousands of years they have kept and maintained the fertility of the soil without the use of chemical fertilizers.

There are about 700,000,000 Chinese and at least up until a few years ago they did not have the so-called benefits of chemical fertilizers. Today they are challenging the world in a bid for supremacy. They have now learned how to use chemical fertilizers and in my opinion this will prevent them from achieving this supremacy.

It is a positive fact that something must be done to maintain the fertility of the soil and the best and the most natural way to achieve soil fertility is by returning the waste to the soil from which it was taken. Good soil can be maintained fertile in perpetuity by the simple expedient of returning the waste back to the soil . . . yes, including human and animal excrement. I have for over a third of a century maintained that one of the most serious blunders of our civilization is the fact that we do not return the human excrement back to the land. By dumping it into our waterways we are polluting the waterways. To a degree we are enriching the lake and ocean bottoms, whereas we should be enriching our soil. No doubt this will all balance out in the long run — that is, over a period of thousands or hundreds of thousands of years — but in the interim it may cause serious disruption. Let me assure you that chemical fertilizers would not be the answer . . . in fact, they would speed up the time of destruction.

There is a rather strange phenomenon that I have noted in my lifetime and that is that the proponents of chemical fertilizers will never debate the issue with organic minded people at any public meeting or public forum. Nor will they even allow the issue to be presented in any magazine or newspaper. They have the money to buy the mass media in any form in America and they do buy it and control it . . . and they do not brook any interference by those who are organic minded. And they brush off conflicting evidence and argument like a horse's tail brushes off flies. But still we persist and of late we have been making our presence felt and we are causing them a great deal of concern and worry.

We know that time is on our side but unfortunately millions will be sick and die in the interim. Isn't it a pity that it has to happen this way? But I know I'm doing what I can about it and I can take solace in this manner. But I assure you it is meagre comfort.

I would like to leave one message with you . . .

Mother Nature begins with the soil and all elements are required by nature and form a part of the whole. Soil organisms are as important as the soil, soil is as important as the plant, the plant is as important as the animal, and the animal is at least as important as man . . . although we know that man is an animal.

Let me prove to you that all of these are more important than man. That's right, they are! Soil organisms can live without us, the soil will exist without us, the plant can exist without us, the animal can exist without us, but we cannot exist without them. Man needs them all but they do not need man.

So if you as an individual have any illusions of supremacy or greatness or grandeur, think this over very, very carefully and last but not least, remember this . . . the greatest culture is agriculture.

CHAPTER 100

IS BACK TO NATURE THE ANSWER?

You can see my head nodding in the affirmative so fast that you wonder it doesn't fall off as I say, "Sure, back to nature is the answer!"

Ah, but how do we get back to nature?

You may wonder why a chapter on back to nature appears in a book on health? My answer is direct . . . I know of no factors more important to a human being's health than living in the country, drinking pure water, breathing unpolluted air and eating home grown organic food. So why wouldn't a chapter on "Back to the land", belong in a book on health?

From the latest information I understand that there is still some homesteading land left in Canada . . . in fact, quite a bit. And there is still some mighty cheap land left in the United States. If you want to know about it, get yourself a copy of "Our Public Lands", the official publication of the Bureau of Land Management, U.S. Department of the Interior; for sale by Superintendent of Documents, U.S. Government Printing Office, Washington, D.C. 20402. Subscription price is $1.00 per year (4 issues).

Therefore, any man who has the guts and the courage to go back to the land and live as nature intended man to live can still do it, even without money, or perhaps I should say with very little money. And with the wages that a man can earn today, even for pushing a broom, there should be no problem getting enough money to get that homestead or little farm. From there on out you're on your own . . . and that should be good, but you probably think it's bad.

One of the first things that some wise guy might come up with when I start telling about going back to the land is, "What you are telling us to do, would probably get us sick and we'd die before our time. Statistics tell us that because of our civilized way of life and because of the advances made by the medical profession we have extended our life span more than 20 years in the past few decades."

I've always said in countering this kind of statement that figures don't lie but liars sure know how to figure. The true fact concerning that statement is that the life expectancy has not increased in the past 20 years . . . in fact, it has dropped. Secondly, with statistics telling that untrue story, one must remember that the big gain in the life expectancy figures came about when the infant mortality rate was cut from 250 per 1,000 to 27 per 1,000. So with the saving of approximately 220 lives out of every 1,000, that alone is more than enough to account for the tremendous increase in the life span. But in spite of that gain things have levelled off, which means, if you have any common sense, that we definitely are worse off now than we were before. Or doesn't that make sense to you?

If you had the common sense and the guts to go back to nature tomorrow with your family you would have a lot of wonderful things working for you and the chances are you would live a long healthy life. And the same would hold true for your wife and your children.

Of course, we must face the sober fact that man has so polluted his atmosphere and done so much harm to his environment that our lives are in danger. Still, on a little farm of your own you would be subjected to a great deal less danger than the others in your society. Therefore, going back to nature is still the safest and most sensible course to follow.

No, I am not suggesting that you get yourself an axe and a knife or perhaps a rifle and maybe a canoe and go out into the country and seek to live in that way. But I would suggest that you get a piece of land and try to build yourself a habitable and comfortable house and grow crops that will feed your family and perhaps allow some extra to realize a satisfactory or livable income. In this way you would be your own boss and you would work whenever you liked and not work whenever you didn't like. Although you'd probably find out that you would work many more hours than you would work for an employer . . . and work a lot harder and a lot better. You see, you have to pay for the privilege of being your own boss and being independent.

It isn't necessary that you go off a million miles from nowhere, although that's probably where the free or cheap land is. But even if you bought more expensive land, remember, it will always be worth as much or more when you go to sell it again.

I have lived on a farm or owned a farm for about 35 years and that's probably the only good thing I've done in my entire life. On many occasions, on walking around or through or across my property, I felt pretty good to think that I owned this valuable 30 or so acres. I owned 12 acres originally in the Niagara Peninsula and then I bought 6 more and later 14 more, all pieces adjoining each other. Now I have a 127 acre farm on Vancouver Island.

On your own bit of land you will eat better than you ever ate before. You will know that your food isn't poisoned and you will actually be earning your living by the sweat of your brow. A few acres can make you independent but no one can stop you from working at your trade or other form of employment at certain periods if you want to supplement your income. I know many people who do this. They have the benefit of a farm and the good food that they raise and they also earn money in the business world or in industry.

Getting back to nature is not as difficult as some people would make it appear to be. I doubt very much if you would be able to afford a Cadillac from the working of a few acres of land but I do know a goodly number of people who make a clean honest living from only a few acres . . . and who are very happy doing so, and whose children are happier and healthier than those raised in the urban areas.

No, you don't need any experience. It's just like breathing and eating. You learn instantly. You can learn how to till your fields. You can learn how to milk a cow. You probably know how to drive a tractor. So I can't see any reason why any normal individual can't make a success of a small holding.

The size that you would require for making a living would vary according to the area in which you lived and also to the extent that you wanted to become involved in a back to nature movement on the land. But if you were going to make a living from a piece of land and you wanted to be completely independent and not work elsewhere, then you would need anywhere up to 15 acres, depending again on the type of crops you wanted to raise. If you were considering market gardening, well, you could do very well on five or ten acres and concentrate on such crops as can be harvested in a few weeks or months. I know a man who makes a very good living on 15 acres of fruit. I'm sure you could make a good living from 10 or 15 acres in berries, whether it be strawberries, raspberries or some other form of berry. You can grow a lot of berries on 10 or 15 acres and your gross can easily be $10,000 or $20,000.

I have a 14 acre orchard and vineyard from which my gross runs about $10,500. I do not work it myself — I have a neighbor do it — and my expenses in this manner run between $4,000 and $5,000. But if I depended on it for a living, I would do most of the work myself or all of it and in this way I would also increase my gross to probably $12,500 and would no doubt show a clear profit of at least $5,000 or $6,000 after all expenses were paid ... and my living expenses taken off as well.

So there you have a concrete example. Whether it suits you or not I do not know. Maybe you wouldn't be content with a gross of $10,000. Well, you could get more land and increase your income in that manner.

There is no reason why you can't have as little as two acres and then work to supplement your income. On the two acres you could have your own fruits and vegetables and even a goat or a cow, and of course chickens and ducks if you wanted them. You could attend to your farm evenings and weekends and of course you would have the help of your wife and your family. Then your food would cost you practically nothing.

There is a further advantage. You can buy a little farm or a little bit of land and a house in the country cheaper than you can buy a house in the city.

Yes, you can go back to nature and live as nature intended a man to live ... to your benefit, healthwise and dollarwise.

619

INDEX